Patient teaching made Incredibly Easy!™

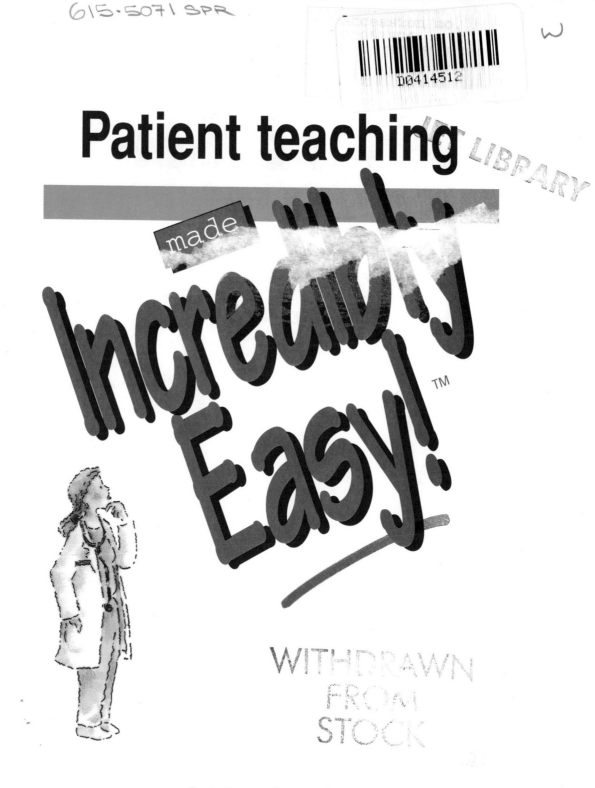

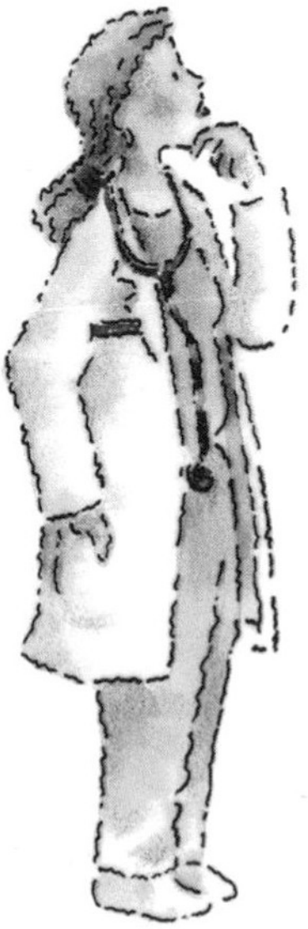

Springhouse Corporation
Springhouse, Pennsylvania

Staff

Vice President
Matthew Cahill

Clinical Director
Judith A. Schilling McCann, RN, MSN

Art Director
John Hubbard

Managing Editor
Michael Shaw

Clinical Editors
Carla M. Roy, RN, BSN, CCRN (project manager); Joanne M. Bartelmo, RN, MSN, CCRN; Clare M. Brabson, RN, BSN, CCRN; Jill M. Curry, RN, BSN, CCRN; Beverly Tscheschlog, RN; Tracy L. Yeomans, RN, BSN, BA, CCRN;

Editors
Kevin Haworth, H. Nancy Holmes, Anthony Prete, Patricia Wittig, Doris Weinstock

Copy Editors
Cynthia C. Breuninger (manager), Mary T. Durkin, Stacey A. Follin, Brenna H. Mayer, Pamela Wingrod

Designers
Arlene Putterman (associate art director), Mary Ludwicki (book designer), Joseph Clark

Illustrator
Bot Roda

Typography
Diane Paluba (manager), Joyce Rossi Biletz, Valerie Molettiere

Manufacturing
Deborah Meiris (director), Patricia K. Dorshaw (manager), Otto Mezei (book production manager)

Editorial Assistants
Beverly Lane, Liz Schaeffer

Indexer
Barbara Hodgson

The clinical treatments described and recommended in this publication are based on research and consultation with nursing, medical, and legal authorities. To the best of our knowledge, these procedures reflect currently accepted practice. Nevertheless, they can't be considered absolute and universal recommendations. For individual applications, all recommendations must be considered in light of the patient's clinical condition and, before administration of new or infrequently used drugs, in light of the latest package-insert information. The authors and the publisher disclaim any responsibility for any adverse effects resulting from the suggested procedures, from any undetected errors, or from the reader's misunderstanding of the text.

Printed in the United States of America.

IEPT-011098

A member of the Reed Elsevier plc group

Library of Congress Cataloging-in Publication Data

Patient teaching made incredibly easy.
p. cm.
Includes index.
1. Patient education—Study and teaching.
2. Nurse and patient. 3. Health education.
I. Springhouse Corporation.
[DNLM: 1.Patient education—methods nurses' instruction. W 85P29887 1998]
RT86.3.P38 1998
615.5'071—dc21
DNLM/DLC 98-36727
ISBN 0-87434-959-1 (alk. paper) CIP

Contents

Contributors and consultants *iv*
Foreword *v*

1 Cardiovascular disorders 1

2 Respiratory disorders 39

3 Neurologic disorders 79

4 Gastrointestinal disorders 115

5 Immune and hematologic disorders 151

6 Musculoskeletal disorders 187

7 Renal and urologic disorders 219

8 Endocrine disorders 249

9 Reproductive disorders 281

10 Cancer 307

Appendix and index 331

Patient teaching for additional disorders 332
Index 339

Contributors and consultants

Karen T. Bruchak, RN, MSN, MBA
Assistant Administrator, Cancer Clinical Programs
University of Pennsylvania Cancer Center
Philadelphia

Nancy Cirone, RN,C, MSN
Director of Education
Allegheny University Hospitals
Warminster, Pa.

Jacqueline Crocetti, RN,C, MSN, CRNP
Nursing Professor
Northampton Community College
Bethlehem, Pa.

Deborah Fischer O'Reilly, RN, BSN, CCRN
RN Surgical/Trauma Intensive Care Unit
Abington (Pa.) Memorial Hospital

Athena A. Foreman, RN, MSN
Nursing Coordinator
Stanley Community College
Albemarle, N.C.

Ellen J. Mangin, RN, MSN, CRNP, CS
Director of Resident Services
Rydal (Pa.) Park

Andrea Marino, RN, BSN, CCRN
Staff Nurse CCU
Allegheny University Hospitals
Elkins Park, Pa.

Linda M. Ourach, BSN, CED, MBA, CNS
Clinical Nurse Specialist, Diabetes
Abington (Pa.) Memorial Hospital

Robert Rauch
Medical Economics Manager
Amgen, Inc.
Maple Glen, Pa.

Charee Y. Reckner, RN, BSN, MBA
Home Care RN
Grandview Home Care
Sellersville, Pa.

Maryann Summers, RN, BS, MS
Certified School Nurse
Philadelphia School District

Deborah Watkins Bruner, RN, MSN, PhDc
Director, Prostate Cancer Risk Assessment Program
Fox Chase Cancer Center
Philadelphia

Bonnie Zauderer, RN, MS, CNS
Assistant Professor of Clinical Nursing
University of Texas-Houston School of Nursing

Foreword

Patient teaching is a paradox. It's the most subtle nursing skill and the most powerful. During your interaction with patients, you may act as a teacher without being aware of it. Many times, the only equipment you use is your caring, knowledge, and imagination. The effect of your efforts is difficult to quantify. Nevertheless, your teaching may be the single most important factor in improving a patient's quality of life.

Good teaching provides patients with the knowledge they need to question health care providers and administrators, seek treatment options, make informed decisions, manage self-care, and take responsibility for their health. There is no better way to be a patient advocate than to empower your patients with clear, precise explanations of their condition and care.

But what is the secret of powerful patient teaching? The answer is effective communication — the ability to make information perfectly clear and relevant to a patient's life. Unfortunately, all too many patient-teaching references for nurses are dull, dry tomes, without any spark of enthusiasm.

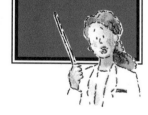

The paradox of patient teaching

- Subtle nursing skill (you may not even realize you're doing it)
- Powerful effect on the patient's quality of life

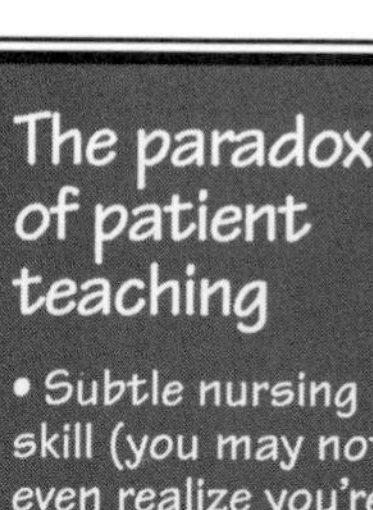

To help you motivate patients, a patient-teaching guide should be lively and exciting. That's why the clinical experts at Springhouse created *Patient Teaching Made Incredibly Easy.* This remarkable book infuses your patient teaching with a spirit of joy. In so doing, it helps you teach patients more effectively.

Each of the first nine chapters in *Patient Teaching Made Incredibly Easy* is devoted to a major body system. Together these chapters cover a broad variety of illnesses. You'll find teaching information for such disorders as coronary artery disease, hypertension, chronic obstructive pulmonary disease, Alzheimer's disease, cerebrovascular accident, Parkinson's disease, acquired immunodeficiency syndrome, sickle cell anemia, osteoporosis, chronic renal failure, diabetes mellitus, breast cancer, and dozens more.

You'll find clear, concise explanations to help patients and caregivers understand each disorder. You'll also find information to teach your patients about diagnostic tests, the goals of treatment, and all aspects of care — activity restrictions, drugs, diet, surgery, and more. Best of all, this information is presented in the unique *Incredibly Easy* style.

The tenth chapter is dedicated to teaching patients with cancer. In it, you'll learn about teaching at each stage of cancer. The chapter also features an easy-to-use chart to help you discuss your patient's specific type of cancer. In the book's appendix, you'll find another chart covering patient-teaching points for dozens of additional disorders.

Patient Teaching Made Incredibly Easy is filled with features that make the book refreshingly lively and entertaining. *Memory joggers* provide clever tricks for remembering key points. Checklists, in the style of a schoolroom blackboard, provide at-a-glance summaries of important points. Cartoon characters appear occasionally to spark laughter. A *Quick quiz* at the end of each chapter helps you assess your understanding. Special logos throughout alert you to essential information:

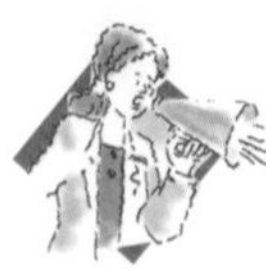

Listen up highlights crucial points for you to discuss with your patient.

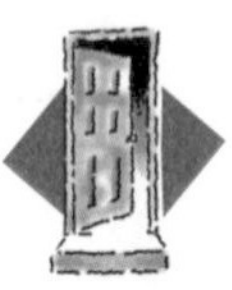

No place like home offers home care tips to help both patient and family cope with illness.

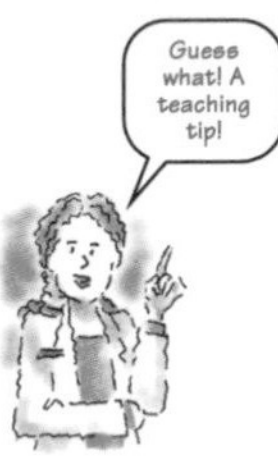

Teaching tip provides insight on how to teach patients confidently and effectively, covering such topics as motivation, learning styles, and goal setting.

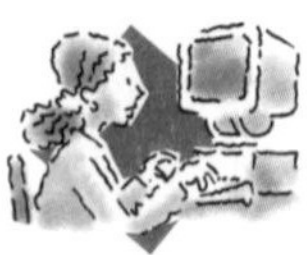

Getting connected provides names and addresses for sites on the Internet that provide valuable health-related information.

To remain effective, patient teaching can't be allowed to become rote or routine. That's why you need a patient-teaching reference that's packed with fun and surprises. To reinvigorate your teaching efforts, I heartily recommend *Patient Teaching Made Incredibly Easy.* It will help you resolve the paradox of patient teaching. Enjoy teaching — and learning.

Nancy Cirone, RN, MSN
Director of Education
Allegheny University Hospitals
Warminster, Pa.

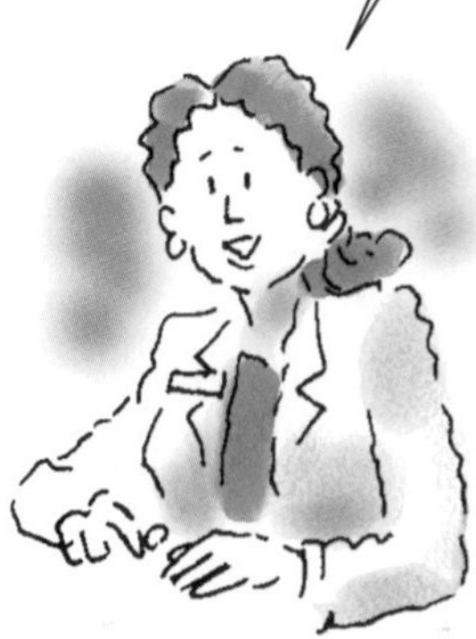
Don't forget to visit the Springhouse Web site: www.springnet.com

Cardiovascular disorders

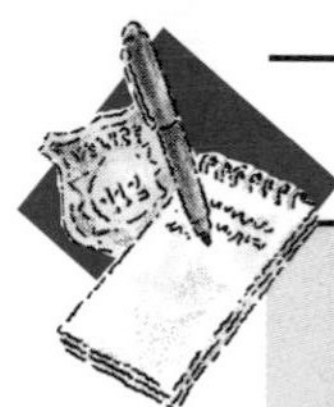

Just the facts

In this chapter, you'll learn how to teach patients with the following cardiovascular disorders:

- arrhythmias
- arterial occlusive disease
- coronary artery disease
- heart failure
- hypertension
- myocardial infarction.

Arrhythmias

Arrhythmias range from mild, asymptomatic disturbances, such as sinus arrhythmia, to life-threatening emergencies, such as ventricular fibrillation. The wide variety of arrhythmias requires you to be familiar with various degrees of illness. You may also find yourself teaching patients with diverse learning needs, ages, and health histories. Your goal is to tell each patient about his or her specific arrhythmia and its treatment.

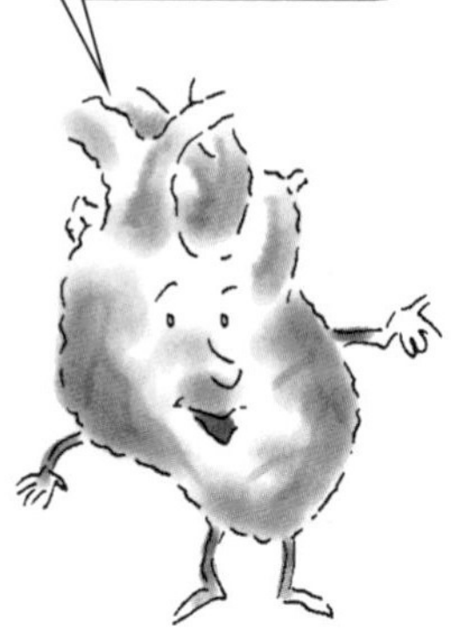
An arrhythmia is an abnormal change in my rate, rhythm, or both.

What is an arrhythmia?

Begin your teaching by telling the patient what an arrhythmia is — an abnormal change in heart rate, heart rhythm, or both. Explain that, normally, electrical impulses make the heart contract. Any disruption of the electrical impulse's pathway can produce arrhythmia.

Tell me more

Explain that arrhythmia alters the heart's output (the volume of blood pumped out of the heart to provide oxygen to tissues). This can lead to a wide range of complications. (See *Complications of arrhythmia*.)

Complications of arrhythmia

- Dizziness
- Fainting
- Blood clots
- Cardiac arrest

Why?

In your teaching, make sure you describe the possible causes of arrhythmia, including:

- congenital abnormalities
- inadequate blood flow to the heart
- myocardial infarction (MI)
- heart disease
- drug toxicity.

Teaching about tests

There are several ways to diagnose arrhythmia and discover its possible cause.

Blood tests

Tell the patient that the doctor may order blood tests to measure levels of serum electrolytes, such as potassium, or certain drugs, such as quinidine and digoxin.

Drug tests

If the doctor suspects an illicit or street drug as the underlying cause of the arrhythmia, he may also order tests for such drugs as heroin, amphetamines, and cocaine.

More tests

Other tests commonly used to identify the specific arrhythmia and to monitor antiarrhythmic therapy include electrocardiogram (ECG), Holter monitoring, stress testing, and electrophysiologic studies. (See *Teaching patients about cardiovascular tests*, pages 3 to 6.)

Teaching about activity and lifestyle

Treatment of an arrhythmia depends on the severity of the symptoms. Emphasize that the patient shouldn't restrict his normal activities. In fact, a medically supervised exercise routine can improve his cardiovascular fitness.

(Text continues on page 6.)

Teaching patients about cardiovascular tests

Test and purpose	What to teach the patient
Abdominal ultrasonography • To detect an abdominal aortic aneurysm	• He will lie on an examining table while a technician applies conductive jelly to his abdomen. The technician then moves a transducer slowly over the abdominal area to scan the blood vessels. • Sound waves bouncing off anatomic structures are translated into graphic images, which are then displayed on a monitor or printed as a sonogram.
Holter monitoring (ambulatory monitoring) • To detect arrhythmias and their relationship to activity • To evaluate arrhythmias in relationship to chest pain • To evaluate the effectiveness of antiarrhythmic therapy	• This test takes 24 hours and causes no discomfort. • The technician cleans, dries and, possibly, shaves different sites of the patient's body and applies electrodes at these sites. • The patient needs to log his usual activities (such as walking, sleeping, urinating), emotional upsets, physical symptoms (such as chest pain, palpitations, dizziness, or fatigue), and medication administration in a diary. • He shouldn't tamper with the monitor or disconnect leadwires or electrodes. He must avoid magnets, metal detectors, high-voltage areas, and electric blankets. The patient must learn how to check for improper function. Light flashes, for example, may indicate a loose electrode.
Angiography (arteriography) • To examine arteries or veins for suspected abnormalities, such as aneurysms, thrombi, and atherosclerotic obstructions • To detect vessel compression from an extravascular tumor • To evaluate the patency of arterial grafting and reconstruction	• This test may take 30 minutes to 4 hours, depending on the vessels examined. • An area of the patient's body is shaved and cleaned. After a local anesthetic is injected, a catheter is inserted into a vessel and advanced as necessary. • A contrast medium is injected into the vessels. Then a series of X-ray films follows the contrast medium's passage. Any flushing sensation, nausea, or unusual taste will pass quickly. • When the catheter is removed, pressure is applied to the insertion site for 15 to 30 minutes. After bandaging, additional pressure is applied by using sandbags or clamps on the affected limb. The patient must keep the arm or leg extended and immobile for approximately 6 hours.
Cardiac blood pool imaging • To assess left ventricular function • To detect motion and structural abnormalities of the ventricular wall	• This 30- to 45-minute test evaluates how well the main chamber of the patient's heart (left ventricle) pumps. • Electrodes are attached to various sites on the patient's body. • The patient lies on his back, and a mildly radioactive contrast medium is injected into a vein. A scintillation camera records the contrast medium's passage through his heart and is then synchronized with an electrocardiogram (ECG) to correlate subsequent images with ECG waveforms. The patient must remain still during scanning.
Cardiac catheterization • To assess valve and cardiac wall function • To diagnose various abnormalities, such as valvular insufficiency or stenosis, septal defects, and congenital anomalies	• This test usually takes 2 to 3 hours. He shouldn't eat or drink anything after midnight before the procedure. • The patient lies on a padded table, and his groin area is shaved and cleaned. The nurse starts a peripheral I.V. line and attaches electrodes to various sites. The patient receives a mild I.V. sedative to help him relax.

(continued)

Teaching patients about cardiovascular tests *(continued)*

Test and purpose	What to teach the patient
Cardiac catheterization *(continued)* • To evaluate coronary artery bypass graft patency • To detect pulmonary artery hypertension • To evaluate the effectiveness of drug therapy	• The doctor injects a local anesthetic into the patient's groin, inserts a catheter, and threads it through an artery to the left side of the heart or through a vein to the right side of the heart to the patient's lungs. Next, the doctor may inject a contrast medium through the catheter, which can cause flushing, nausea, or chest pain. These sensations should pass quickly. The patient should follow instructions to cough or breathe deeply to provide a better view of the heart. He may receive nitroglycerin during the test to expand coronary vessels and aid visualization. • The doctor slowly removes the catheter and bandages the site. The nurse closely monitors the patient during the procedure. The patient should keep the bandaged arm or leg straight and still for up to 6 hours. To help keep him from moving, the arm or leg may be splinted or weighed down with a sandbag or clamp. Once he's allowed to resume his diet, he should drink plenty of fluids to excrete the I.V. contrast medium.
Cardiac computed tomography scan • To perform rapid screening for aortic dissection • To detect and evaluate pericardial disease • To check bypass graft patency	• This noninvasive test produces X-ray images of the blood vessels. If a contrast medium is ordered, the patient must not eat or drink anything for 4 hours before the test. • The patient lies on a table in the appropriate position, and medical staff place a stabilizing strap across the body part being scanned. The scanner revolves around the patient, taking radiographs at preselected intervals. If the test calls for a contrast medium, it's infused I.V. The patient should report sensations of warmth, itching, or other discomfort immediately. • The patient will be able to communicate with the examiner during the procedure. • After the test, the patient can resume usual activities and diet. However, if he received a contrast medium, he needs to increase fluid intake for the rest of the day to help eliminate it.
Cardiac magnetic resonance imaging (MRI) • To identify anatomic effects of a myocardial infarction (MI) • To detect and evaluate cardiomyopathy • To detect and evaluate pericardial disease • To identify and evaluate masses within or near the heart • To detect congenital heart disease • To identify vascular disease, such as thoracic aneurysm and thoracic dissection • To assess the structure of pulmonary blood vessels	• This test takes up to 90 minutes. Although MRI is painless, the patient may feel uncomfortable because he must remain still inside a small space (in most facilities). If he suffers from claustrophobia, he may not be able to tolerate the procedure or may need sedation. • The patient must remove all jewelry and other metal objects. If he has shrapnel, a pacemaker, or any surgically implanted joints, pins, clips, valves, or pumps containing metal that could be attracted to the strong MRI magnet, he isn't able to have this test. • Medical staff check the patient at the scanner room door one last time for metal objects. He may receive a sedative. Then he lies in a supine position on a narrow bed, which slides into a large cylinder housing the MRI magnets. Radiofrequency energy is directed at the chest; resulting images are displayed on a monitor and recorded. • The scanner makes loud clicking, whirring, and thumping noises as it moves inside its housing to obtain different images, so the patient may receive earplugs or a headset for music. He'll be able to communicate with the technician at all times, and the procedure will be stopped if he feels claustrophobic. The patient must remain still during the procedure.

Teaching patients about cardiovascular tests *(continued)*

Test and purpose	What to teach the patient
Doppler ultrasonography • To aid diagnosis of chronic venous insufficiency, superficial and deep vein thromboses, peripheral artery disease, and arterial occlusion • To detect abnormalities of carotid artery blood flow associated with such conditions as aortic stenosis • To monitor patency of arterial grafting and reconstruction	• This test takes about 20 minutes. • The patient uncovers his leg, arm, or neck and loosens any restrictive clothing. • A transducer coated with conductive jelly is placed on the patient's skin and moved along the vessel to be examined. Blood pressure is checked at the calves, thighs, and arms. He may be asked to move his arms into different positions and perform breathing exercises to vary blood flow while measurements are taken.
Echocardiography • To diagnose and evaluate valvular abnormalities • To identify aneurysms • To aid diagnosis of cardiomyopathy • To detect atrial tumors • To evaluate cardiac function after MI • To detect pericardial effusion • To measure the size of the heart's chambers and effectiveness of contractility	• This test takes 15 to 30 minutes. • The technician applies conductive jelly to the patient's chest. • A transducer is angled over the patient's chest to observe different parts of the heart. He may be asked to breathe in and out slowly and to hold his breath. He must remain still during the test because movement may distort results.
Electrocardiography (ECG) • To help identify primary conduction abnormalities, arrhythmias, cardiac hypertrophy, pericarditis, electrolyte imbalance, myocardial ischemia, and the site and extent of MI • To evaluate the effectiveness of cardiac drugs • To monitor pacemaker performance	• This test takes 15 minutes. • The technician cleans, dries and, possibly, shaves different sites on the patient's body, such as his chest and arms, and applies electrodes at these sites. • The patient must lie still, relax, breathe normally, and remain quiet. Talking or limb movement distorts ECG recordings and requires additional testing time.
Electrophysiologic studies • To diagnose arrhythmias • To evaluate the effects of antiarrhythmic drugs	• These tests take 2 to 5 hours. The patient must avoid food, fluids, and nonprescription drugs for 6 hours before the tests. • A catheter insertion site at the groin is shaved and cleaned. • After injection of a local anesthetic, a catheter is inserted into the femoral vein and advanced into the right side of the heart. The patient receives an I.V. sedative to help him relax. The doctor may try to induce extra heartbeats with the catheter. • After the test, the catheter is removed and pressure and a heavy dressing are applied to the site to control bleeding. The patient may need to lie with his leg straight for a few hours after the test.

(continued)

Teaching patients about cardiovascular tests *(continued)*

Test and purpose	What to teach the patient
Exercise ECG (stress test, treadmill test, graded exercise test) • To help diagnose the cause of chest pain or other possible cardiac pain • To identify arrhythmias that occur during exercise • To evaluate the effectiveness of antiarrhythmic or antianginal therapy	• This test takes about 30 minutes, and a doctor or nurse will be present in the testing area at all times. The patient must not eat, smoke, or drink alcohol for 3 hours before the test. However, he should continue any drug regimen, as ordered. • He should wear comfortable shoes and loose, lightweight shorts or slacks. • A technician cleans, shaves (if necessary), and lightly rubs sites on the chest and, possibly, the back. Then the technician attaches electrodes at these sites. • If the patient is scheduled for a multistage treadmill test, the treadmill speed and incline increase at predetermined intervals and he'll be told of each adjustment. If he's scheduled for a bicycle ergometer test, resistance to pedaling increases gradually. • The patient may receive an injection of thallium. Then the doctor will evaluate coronary blood flow on a scanner. • The patient can stop the test if he experiences severe fatigue, chest pain, or leg pain. Typically, the patient will feel tired and be out of breath and sweaty. Nevertheless, he should report any sensations he feels during the test. Blood pressure and heart rate are checked periodically. • After the test, the patient's blood pressure and ECG are monitored for 10 to 15 minutes. He should wait at least 1 hour after the test before showering and should use warm water.
Technetium scan • To confirm the presence, size, and location of an acute MI	• This test takes 45 minutes. • The doctor injects an I.V. tracer isotope called technetium pyrophosphate into an arm vein about 3 hours before the test. • The patient lies on his back and a series of scans are taken at different angles. He should remain still.
Thallium scan (resting) • To assess myocardial perfusion • To locate and estimate the size of an acute or old MI • To evaluate the patency of a coronary artery bypass graft	• This test takes 45 to 90 minutes, although additional scans may be required. • Within the first few hours of MI symptoms, the patient lies on a table and receives an injection of radioactive thallium. After 3 to 5 minutes, scanning begins. The patient is placed in various positions to produce multiple images. • There is no known radiation danger from thallium.

Don't overdo it

Remind the patient to avoid overexertion and stop exercising immediately if he experiences dizziness, light-headedness, dyspnea, or chest pain. If his arrhythmia causes periodic dizziness or syncope, warn him not to drive a motor vehicle or operate heavy machinery. (See *Additional advice on arrhythmias.*)

Teaching about diet

Instruct the patient to follow any special diet the doctor prescribes.

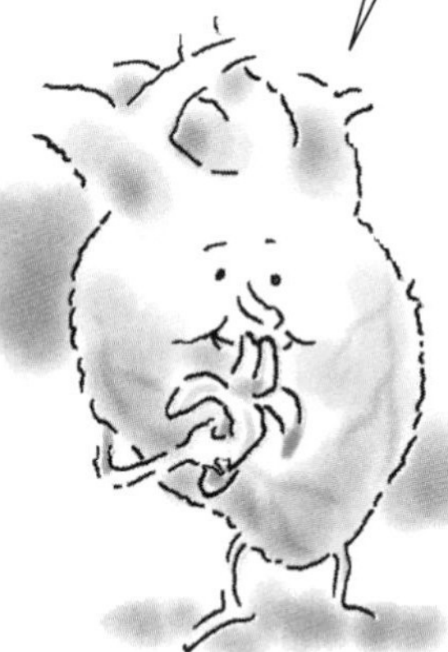
Encourage your patient to eat potassium-rich foods. Yum.

Have a banana

Because a low serum potassium level sometimes contributes to arrhythmia, encourage him to eat potassium-rich foods, such as:

- bananas
- prunes
- leafy green and cruciferous vegetables
- oranges.

Moderation in all things

Advise the patient not to overeat or consume too much alcohol or caffeine. If he smokes, urge him to stop. (See *Holiday heart syndrome,* page 8.)

Teaching about medication

Medications commonly used to treat arrhythmia include:

- antiarrhythmics such as digitalis glycosides
- beta blockers such as propranolol

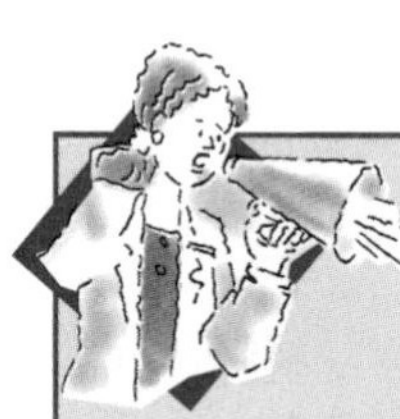

Listen up!

Additional advice on arrhythmias

Explain the following additional care measures to your patient who's treated for arrhythmia.

Keep a pulse on things

Teach the patient how to take his pulse. If the patient has a pacemaker, instruct him to keep an accurate record of daily pulse readings and to notify the doctor of any significant abnormalities, such as a rate that is 5 or more beats below the pacemaker's preset rate, a rate that exceeds 100 beats per minute, or any unusually irregular rhythm. Teach the patient with atrial fibrillation how to take a carotid pulse rather than a radial pulse.

A worthwhile effort

Suggest that at least one family member learn cardiopulmonary resuscitation. This training could make the difference between life and death if the patient develops sudden cardiac arrest or myocardial infarction.

Two more things

Discuss risk factors of cardiovascular disorders, such as stress, obesity, smoking, and sedentary lifestyle. Finally, tell the patient to contact the American Heart Association, Coronary Club, Heart Disease Research Foundation, or Heartlife for further information.

• calcium channel blockers such as diltiazem (Cardizem)
• angiotensin-converting enzyme (ACE) inhibitors such as captopril (Capoten).

Explain to your patient that drugs used to treat arrhythmia may be given in combination with other drugs to treat an underlying cardiovascular disorder.

Keep to the schedule

Point out that medications can only control, not cure, the arrhythmia. Emphasize that the patient must take antiarrhythmics and other prescribed drugs on schedule, even when he doesn't have symptoms. Warn him never to discontinue his medications without consulting the doctor.

Listen up!

Holiday heart syndrome

Warn the patient not to overindulge during the holidays. "Holiday heart syndrome" is a result of increased food and alcohol consumption, smoking, and emotional excitement associated with holiday get-togethers. Overdoing any of these can trigger or worsen arrhythmias.

Teaching about procedures

Depending on the patient's symptoms, there are several procedures that may be used to manage arrhythmia.

Valsalva's maneuver

In some arrhythmias, Valsalva's maneuver may enable the patient to restore normal heart rhythm. Tell the patient to follow these simple instructions:

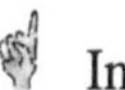 Inhale deeply.

Hold that breath and strain hard for at least 10 seconds before exhaling.

Explain that this maneuver increases chest pressure, which converts the arrhythmia to a normal rhythm. This procedure should be advised by a doctor because increasing chest pressure may be contraindicated in some patients.

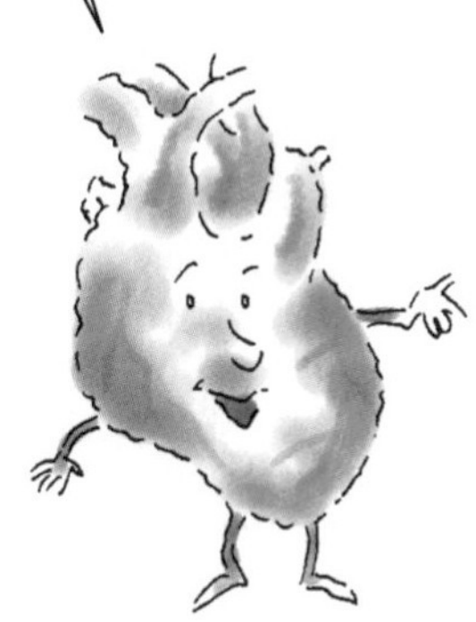
When my rate or rhythm is off, a pacemaker can help get me back on the beat.

Temporary pacemaker

If your patient is to receive a temporary pacemaker, explain that it's used to regulate the heart rate and rhythm. Then describe the basic procedure:

• The doctor first inserts a long, thin electrode leadwire into a vein.
• Guided by fluoroscopy, the doctor advances the leadwire through the vena cava to the right atrium and into the right ventricle.

• As soon as the electrode lead is in place, the doctor attaches its other end to a battery-powered pacemaker pulse generator.

Burn, sting, or flutter

Make sure you tell your patient what to expect during the procedure. He may feel:
• burning or stinging from the anesthetic used to numb the skin
• transient pressure at the insertion site as the catheter is placed
• his heart flutter as the pacemaker is activated or adjusted.

Tell your patient that, aside from the sensations described above, he should not experience any discomfort.

What next?

Tell the patient that the temporary pacemaker remains in use for several days — until the arrhythmia is controlled or until he undergoes other measures, such as permanent pacemaker insertion or cardiac surgery.

Remind him that, until these other measures are taken, activities must be limited and bed rest may be required.

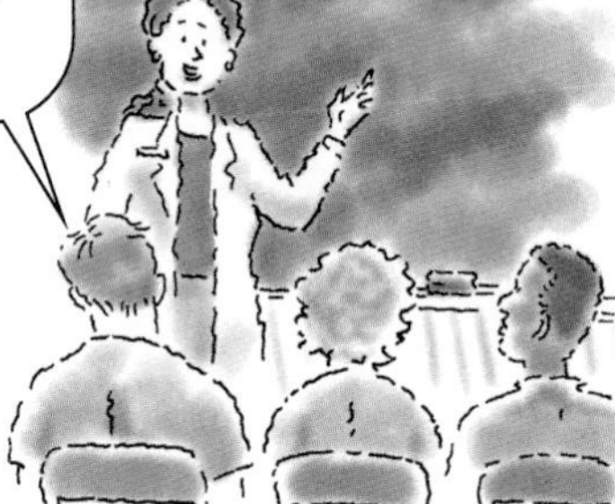
How long will I need my temporary pacemaker?
For several days — until the arrhythmia is controlled or new treatment is initiated.

Electrocardioversion

Electrocardioversion is used to convert unstable arrhythmias. Tell the patient that, in cardioversion, an electric current is used to restore a normal heart rate and relieve symptoms.

You'll get a charge outta this

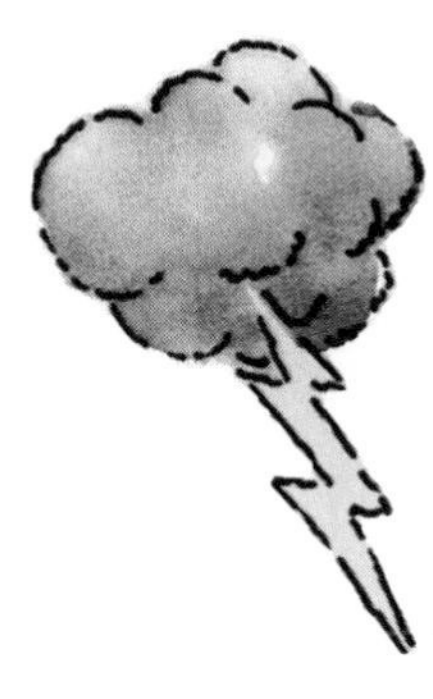

Before electrocardioversion is performed, pass on the following information:
• Explain that just before the procedure, he'll receive an I.V. sedative.
• Tell the patient that, while he's sedated, an electric current is delivered to the heart through paddles placed on the chest.
• Tell the patient that the procedure may be uncomfortable and that, on waking, he may feel some discomfort on the chest wall surface due to the electric current. The chest sites where the paddles were applied may also itch and be slightly reddened for a day or two.

• Tell the patient that he may eat and move about once the sedative wears off.

Teaching about surgery

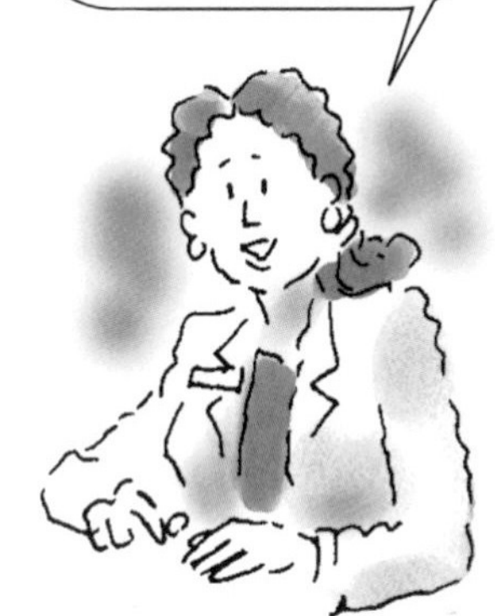
If an arrhythmia can't be controlled by medications or other conservative measures, surgery may be necessary.

If arrhythmias can't be controlled by medication or other conservative measures, the doctor may suggest surgery. The type of arrhythmia and any underlying cardiovascular problems determine the type of surgery performed. These types include:

- surgery to correct structural defects
- permanent pacemaker implantation
- in recurrent life-threatening arrhythmia, automatic implantable cardioverter defibrillator (AICD) insertion or ablation therapy (the elimination of the accessory conducting pathway that is causing the arrhythmia).

Permanent pacemaker implantation

During surgery to implant a permanent pacemaker, the pacemaker pulse generator is implanted under the skin in an unobtrusive area, and electrodes are threaded through a vein into the heart's right chamber. If your patient is to receive a permanent pacemaker, explain the function of a pacemaker and the implantation procedure. Also give preoperative and postoperative instructions.

AICD implantation

If the patient is scheduled to receive an AICD, explain that the device delivers an electric shock to the heart to correct an abnormal heart rhythm. Tell him that the implant is slightly larger than a deck of cards and weighs about ½ lb (0.23 kg).

Tell the patient that battery life is about 3 to 5 years, or 3,000 shocks. Hospitalization is required to replace the AICD battery. Instruct the patient to always carry an AICD information card and to wear a medical identification bracelet. Also instruct the patient to note on a calendar when he receives a shock. This information will be helpful to his doctor.

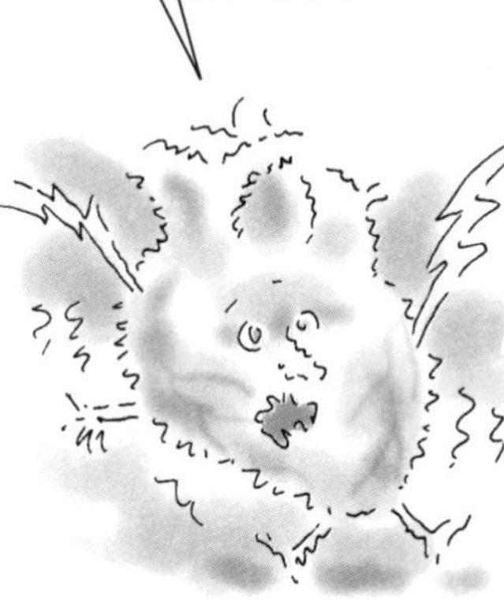
An AICD delivers an electric shock to the heart to correct an abnormal heart rhythm.

Ablation therapy

Explain to the patient that in this procedure a catheter is inserted, and the arrhythmia-producing pathway is identified and eliminated. This may be accomplished using a laser beam or radiofrequency waves.

Arterial occlusive disease

In arterial occlusive disease, arteries are narrowed, disrupting blood flow. Arterial occlusive disease often goes undetected until symptoms of arterial insufficiency force the patient to seek treatment. By the time symptoms appear, arterial damage is often extensive, limiting the effectiveness of treatment. Nevertheless, your teaching can help the patient cope with the demands of this chronic disorder.

In teaching about arterial occlusive disease, make sure you provide information about how the disease progresses. (See *How arterial occlusive disease progresses,* page 12.)

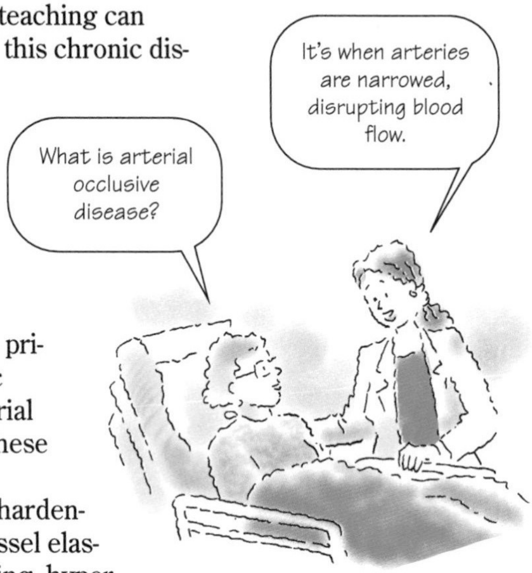

What is arterial occlusive disease?
It's when arteries are narrowed, disrupting blood flow.

What's happening to my blood vessels?

Point out that changes in blood vessels — primarily arteriosclerotic and atherosclerotic changes — cause varying degrees of arterial occlusion. Also, inform your patient that these changes may appear in combination.

In arteriosclerosis (commonly called hardening of the arteries), progressive loss of vessel elasticity is associated with such factors as aging, hypertension, and diabetes.

In atherosclerosis, gradual buildup of fatty, fibrous plaques on the inner arterial walls results from lipoprotein abnormalities, arterial wall injury, and platelet dysfunction.

What are the risks?

Explain that in arterial occlusive disease, the aorta and its major branches become narrowed. This interrupts blood flow, usually to the legs and feet, and prevents oxygen and nutrients from reaching the tissues. Such occlusion, or blockage, can cause severe ischemia, skin ulceration, and gangrene.

What causes these painful cramps?

Explain how arterial changes lead to intermittent claudication: Insufficient blood flow through occluded arteries causes an oxygen deficiency in the leg muscles — usually in the calves — resulting in a painful cramp.

The patient usually feels no symptoms while resting, but pain and weakness develop in the calf muscles after he walks a certain distance without resting. When he does rest, his symptoms disappear as blood supply to the calf muscles is restored.

How arterial occlusive disease progresses

- Arteries become narrow.
- Blood flow is disrupted.
- Tissues don't receive oxygen or nutrients.
- Oxygen-deprived muscles lead to painful cramps.

Teaching about tests

Help your patient understand how arterial occlusive disease is diagnosed. Tell him that:

- Blood clotting studies are done to check for blood clotting abnormalities or to evaluate the effectiveness of anticoagulant therapy.
- The doctor also may order measurement of blood cholesterol, triglyceride, and fat levels to assess for atherosclerosis.
- He must abstain from alcohol for 24 hours and from exercise for 12 hours before these tests.

Teach the patient about other diagnostic tests he may undergo to evaluate the extent of arterial occlusive disease and collateral circulation. These may include arteriography, Doppler ultrasonography, blood chemistry studies, and serum lipid and lipoprotein measurements. (See *Teaching patients about cardiovascular tests,* pages 3 to 6.)

Teaching about activity and lifestyle

Treatment of arterial occlusive disease may be medical, surgical, or a combination of these. (See *Treatment for arterial occlusive disease.*) Emphasize the importance of getting regular exercise to help prevent further arterial blockages. Point out that exercise also promotes development of collateral circulation, which reduces intermittent claudication and helps prevent leg ulcers. Depending on the patient's age and capabilities, the doctor may recommend daily walking, swimming, or bicycle riding.

Exercise, rest, resume

Tell the patient that daily progressive exercise may gradually reduce the severity of claudication. Emphasize that, in progressive exercise, the patient exercises until pain forces a halt, then rests, and then resumes the exercise. Instruct him to balance exercise and rest periods. (See *Additional advice on arterial occlusive disease,* page 14, and *Keep cool,* page 15.)

Treatment for arterial occlusive disease

- Risk reduction, including the importance of quitting smoking
- Exercise
- Dietary changes
- Foot and leg care
- Medication
- Angioplasty
- Bypass graft surgery
- Sympathectomy
- Endarterectomy

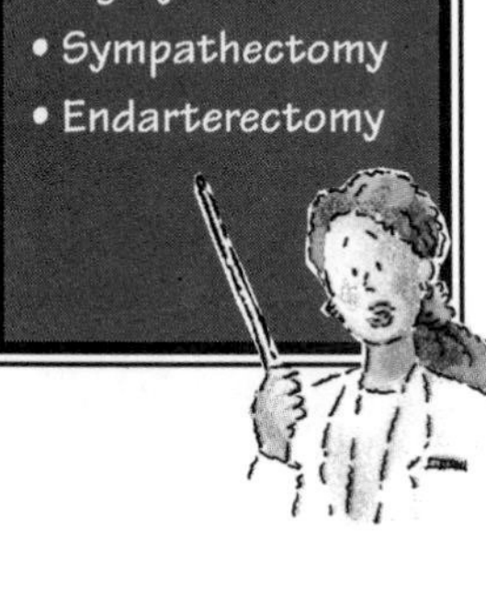

Teaching about diet

A person's diet can have a powerful effect on arterial health. Depending on what ailment lies behind your patient's arterial occlusive disease, the doctor may restrict his dietary intake of cholesterol, saturated fats, or salt.

To help maintain skin integrity and reduce the chance of infection and ulcers, advise your patient to consume adequate amounts of protein, vitamin B_{12}, and vitamin C.

Teaching about medication

The patient may receive such drugs as:
- anticoagulants
- vasodilators
- pentoxifylline (Trental).

For all prescribed drugs, make sure the patient is familiar with its purpose and adverse effects and any special instructions.

Anticoagulant advice

The purpose of drugs such as aspirin and dipyridamole (Persantine) is to reduce clot formation by interfering with platelet aggregation. If the doctor prescribes anticoagulants, tell the patient that he must take precautions to prevent bleeding. The patient must also stay alert for adverse effects, such as susceptibility to bleeding, while on anticoagulant therapy.

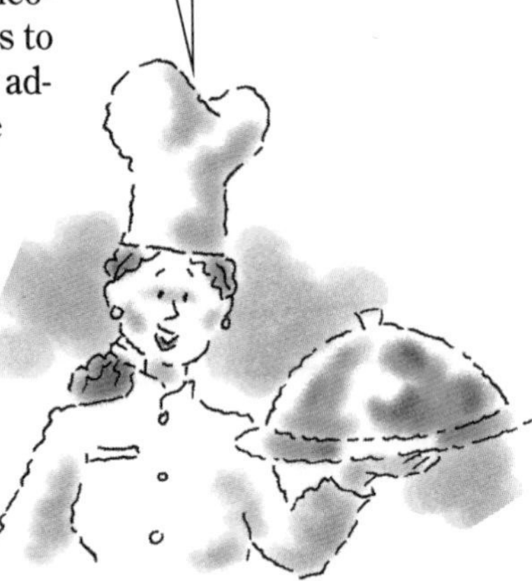
Enjoy today's special: protein, vitamin B_{12}, and vitamin C soufflé.

Expanding the arteries

If the patient is taking a vasodilator, such as isoxsuprine (Vasodilan), tell him that the drug eases symptoms by expanding the arteries. Warn him that it may cause symptoms of low blood pressure, such as dizziness, flushing, and headache — especially when he gets up from a sitting or lying position. To help prevent dizziness, advise him to rise slowly.

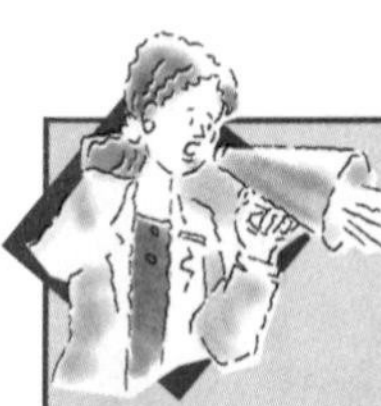

Listen up!

Additional advice on arterial occlusive disease

Long-term management of arterial occlusive disease typically involves reducing cardiovascular risk factors and taking steps to prevent infection and skin ulcers.

Why risk it?
Advise the patient to reduce cardiovascular risk factors by limiting his dietary salt and cholesterol intake, stopping smoking, losing weight, if necessary, and keeping hypertension or diabetes under control.

Move about and keep warm
If the patient's job involves standing for prolonged periods or working outdoors in cold weather, suggest changing position frequently and protecting the body by dressing warmly.

Protecting skin and feet
To help prevent infection and avoid skin ulcers, stress the importance of practicing meticulous skin care and avoiding any activity that could cause skin injury or irritation or that could apply pressure or heat to the skin.

To help safeguard the feet from injury and subsequent infection, instruct the patient to wash his feet daily with mild soap and warm water and to dry them carefully — especially between the toes.

Why comply?
If the patient has leg ulcers, explain that the prescribed dressing will help clean the ulcers and promote healing. Tell him to take prescribed pain medication about 30 minutes before changing dressings.

If the doctor prescribes an Unna's boot, tell the patient that this boot is a bandage that protects and medicates leg ulcers while preventing swelling.

Recognize and report
Teach the patient to recognize and immediately report early warning signs and symptoms of an embolism or aneurysm:
- sudden onset of excruciating pain
- abnormally pale skin or skin mottling (spotting with patches of color)
- difficulty breathing
- loss of pulse in the effected extremity
- paralysis in the affected extremity.

Want more info?
Refer the patient to the American Heart Association for more information and support.

Solving a sticky problem

If the patient is receiving Trental, explain that this drug aids blood flow through the blood vessels by making the blood less sticky. Tell him to report adverse effects to the doctor, especially dizziness, tremors, agitation, palpitations, and fainting spells.

Listen up!

Keep cool

Caution the patient not to exercise too vigorously because this generates a great deal of heat in leg muscles. Excessive exercise also places increased demands on already compromised leg circulation. These demands, in turn, worsen leg pain and increase the risk of infection. For the same reasons, the patient should avoid crossing his legs and raising the affected leg or applying heat to it.

Teaching about procedures

If medications don't prove sufficient, the doctor may employ a nonsurgical procedure as the next step.

Balloon angioplasty

Balloon angioplasty — also called percutaneous transluminal coronary angioplasty (PTCA) — allows the doctor to open a blocked or narrowed artery. Tell the patient that he will be awake but sedated and must lie flat during the 1- to 4-hour procedure.

Then describe the procedure to the patient. With X-ray guidance, the doctor threads the catheter through the blocked artery and confirms the presence of the blockage by angiography (X-ray examination of blood vessels after a contrast medium is injected). The doctor introduces a small, balloon-tipped catheter through the guide wire. After positioning the balloon tip in the blocked artery, the doctor inflates it. The inflated balloon compresses the cholesterol deposits against the arterial wall, widening the diameter of the artery.

Laser-assisted angioplasty

Explain that this alternative to standard angioplasty can be used to open vessels that are totally blocked or narrowed with dense plaque.

Describe the procedure to the patient. Include the following information:

- The doctor makes a small incision to expose the artery or inserts a needle into the artery.
- The doctor then inserts a small catheter into the artery and advances it to the blockage site.
- A contrast medium is injected to outline the blocked area. As soon as the blocked area is identified, the doctor opens the blood vessel with a laser catheter alone.

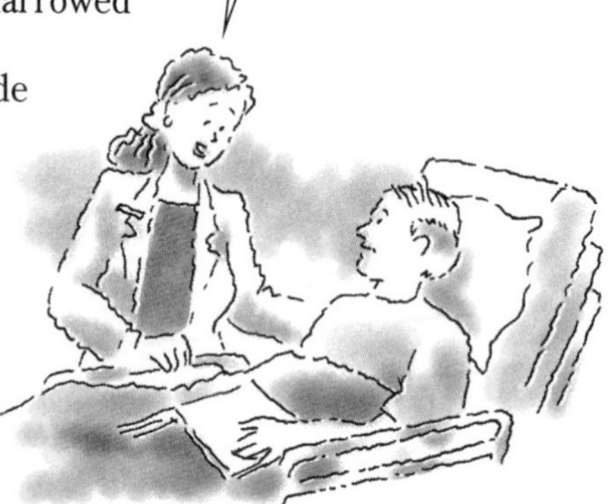
Balloon angioplasty is used to open a blocked or narrowed artery.

• If some blockage remains, the doctor may also use a balloon-tipped catheter.

Teaching about surgery

Some patients with arterial occlusive disease require surgery, typically for the following reasons:

- claudication interferes with walking
- a blocked carotid artery causes neurologic problems
- the procedure will improve blood supply to an ulcerated area.

Surgical procedures to treat arterial occlusive disease include bypass grafting, sympathectomy, and carotid endarterectomy.

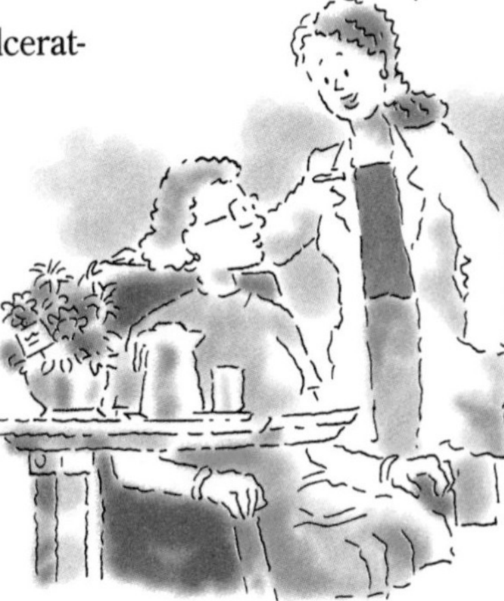
In bypass graft surgery, a graft is used to divert blood flow around the blockage.

Bypass graft surgery

If the doctor recommends this procedure, tell the patient that a graft is used to divert blood flow around the blockage. Tell him that bypass graft surgery is the most effective surgical treatment for his condition. Depending on the blockage site, surgery may involve an aortofemoral bypass, an axillofemoral bypass, or a femoropopliteal bypass graft.

Don't bypass this

If the patient is scheduled for an *aortofemoral* bypass, explain that he'll receive a general anesthetic and two or three incisions — one in the abdomen at the midline and one in the groin for each femoral graft done.

If he's scheduled for an *axillofemoral* bypass, tell the patient that he'll receive a general anesthetic and up to three incisions — one under the arm and one or two in the groin area. Explain that, after surgery, he won't be permitted to lie on the side of the graft. Advise him to avoid the following activities:

• heavy lifting
• carrying
• sudden or forceful use of the arm on the affected side
• reaching overhead.

Flex, extend, and wiggle

Explain that passive range-of-motion exercises can help your patient regain use of the affected limb. These exercises involve alternately flexing and extending the legs, wiggling the toes, and rotating and flexing the feet. As his condition allows, the patient will be allowed to begin active exercises. (See *After a bypass graft.*)

Tell the patient undergoing *femoropopliteal* bypass that this procedure can be done under general or spinal anesthesia. The surgeon may make several incisions from the ankle to the groin, depending on the specific procedure.

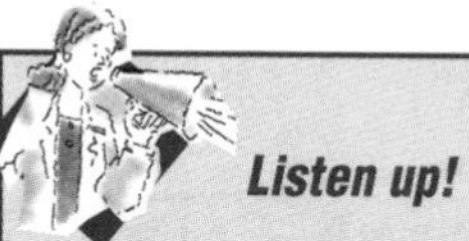

Listen up!

After a bypass graft

To prevent graft occlusion, caution the patient against sitting, crossing his legs, or standing for prolonged periods. Also caution the patient against wearing tight or constrictive garments (belts, girdles, or suspenders) over the graft.

Sympathectomy

Explain that a sympathectomy, which requires general anesthesia, is usually done in conjunction with other revascularization procedures.

Increasing blood flow

Sympathectomy involves the surgical removal of selected sympathetic nerve fibers. If successful, this surgery expands the arteries and increases blood flow to the limbs.

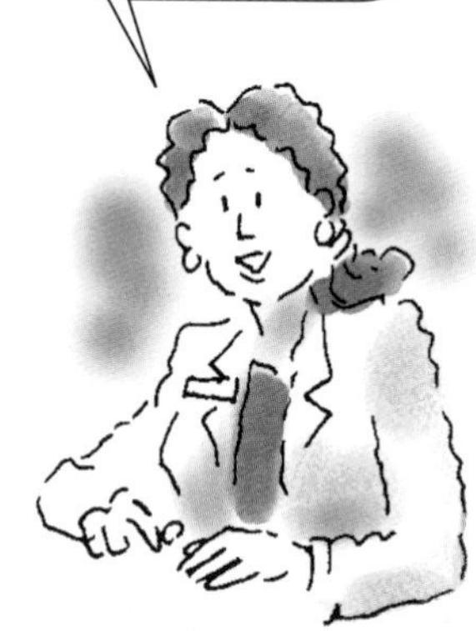
If successful, sympathectomy expands the arteries and increases blood flow to the limbs.

Carotid endarterectomy

Tell the patient scheduled for this procedure that it improves circulation in the brain by removing atherosclerotic plaque in the carotid artery that blocks blood flow. Mention that, after the procedure, he'll stay in the intensive care unit for at least 24 hours.

Instruct him to immediately report any changes in speech or level of consciousness, difficulty swallowing, hoarseness, paralysis or weakness in the arms or legs, or facial drooping. These symptoms could indicate neurologic damage.

Coronary artery disease

Coronary artery disease (CAD) claims more lives in the United States than any other disorder. Most patients lack symptoms until middle age or later, when the heart no longer receives an adequate blood supply for its needs.

Many patients with CAD first seek medical attention after experiencing chest pain.

What is CAD?

Tell the patient that CAD is characterized by narrowing or blockage of one or more of the coronary arteries, leading to diminished blood flow to the heart. This decrease deprives the heart of vital oxygen and nutrients, causing tissue damage.

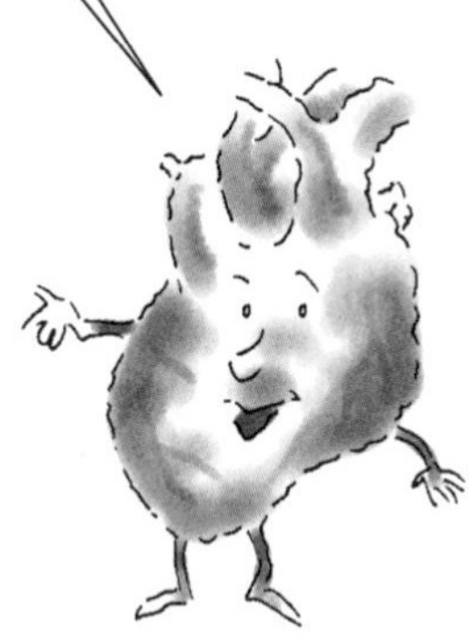
CAD deprives me of vital oxygen and nutrients, causing tissue damage.

Explain that atherosclerosis — a buildup of fatty, fibrous plaques on inner arterial walls — usually causes CAD. These plaques narrow the vessels and reduce the amount of blood that can be pumped through them. Review the risk factors linked to atherosclerosis. (See *Risk factors for CAD.*)

What can I do now?

Treatment for CAD typically includes:

 increased exercise

 diet change

 drug therapy.

Explain that, if these treatments don't improve or eliminate chest pain, the doctor may recommend cardiac catheterization to determine the size and location of blockages. Depending on these results, further interventions or surgery may be needed. Emphasize the importance of adhering to the treatment plan to reduce the risk of serious complications of CAD, such as:
- heart attack
- arrhythmia
- heart failure
- death.

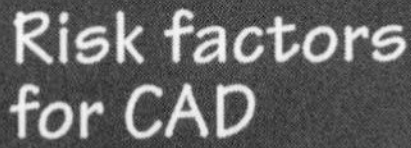

Risk factors for CAD

- Obesity
- Sedentary lifestyle
- Hypertension
- Smoking
- Over age 40
- Type A personality

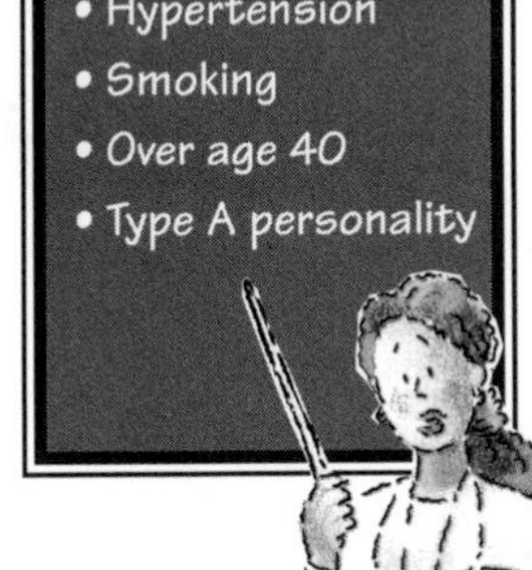

Teaching about tests

Help your patient understand the tests that are used to diagnose CAD. Tell the patient that:
- Blood tests are used to detect and classify the type of hyperlipidemia (high blood fat level) the patient has. These tests include total cholesterol level, triglyceride level, lipoprotein phenotyping, and lipoprotein-cholesterol

fractionation. Instruct the patient not to drink alcohol for 24 hours and not to eat for 12 to 24 hours before the tests.

• Periodic blood tests evaluate the effectiveness of drug and dietary therapy in reducing blood fat levels.

• Other ordered diagnostic tests may include additional blood tests, an echocardiogram, an electrocardiogram (ECG), or a stress test. (See *Teaching patients about cardiovascular tests*, pages 3 to 6.)

Benefits of exercise in CAD

- Increases serum HDL levels
- Promotes weight loss
- Lowers blood pressure
- Tones up entire cardiovascular system

Teaching about activity and lifestyle

Encourage your patient to follow recommended activity guidelines. Emphasize that a sedentary lifestyle contributes to CAD, encourages overeating, leads to obesity and hypertension, and unfavorably alters the ratio of high-density lipoprotein (HDL) to low-density lipoprotein (LDL). Suggest that the patient exercise regularly. (See *Benefits of exercise in CAD.*)

Drop the barbell

Advise against isometric exercise, such as weight lifting, because it increases blood pressure and taxes the heart and coronary arteries. Warn that occasional strenuous exercise may be more dangerous than no exercise.

Avoiding angina

Tell the patient to take prescribed nitrate medications before engaging in any activity that normally provokes angina, including exercise and sex. (See *More CAD teaching tips,* page 20, and *In case of angina,* page 21.)

Teaching about diet

Explain how diet adjustments can help modify three important CAD risk factors:

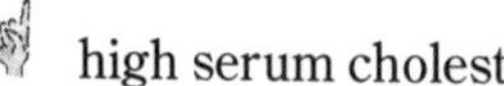

- high serum cholesterol
- high blood pressure
- obesity.

No more than 30%

Advise the patient to limit fat intake to no more than 30% of total daily calories, with saturated fats making up less than 10% of total calories. Also advise him to limit foods high in cholesterol.

Forgoing fat

Tell the patient to control fat intake by limiting consumption of:
- red meat
- processed meat
- lard
- whole milk products
- saturated tropical oils (coconut, palm, and palm kernel) found mostly in processed foods.

More steps

Here are some additional steps the patient can take to improve his diet:
- Trim visible fat from red meat.
- Remove the skin from poultry before cooking.
- Substitute fish and margarine for meat and butter.
- Broil, microwave, grill, or roast meat on a rack and avoid deep-frying.
- In restaurants, order foods cooked in unsaturated vegetable oils.

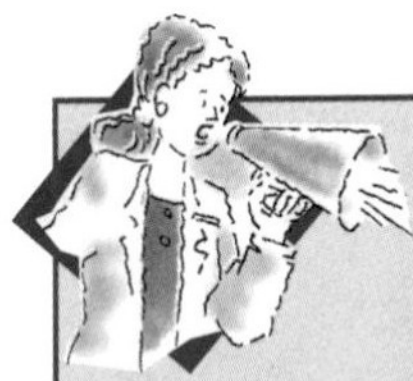

Listen up!

More CAD teaching tips

Here are some additional teaching points to help your patient manage coronary artery disease (CAD) long-term.

Establishing a program
Review the patient's prescribed exercise program. Stress the need to increase activity gradually and to establish realistic goals. Advise him to alternate light and heavy tasks and to rest between tasks.

On schedule
Make sure the patient understands the administration schedules for all prescribed medications and is familiar with possible adverse effects.

Two more risk factors
Emphasize that smoking and stress are also CAD risk factors. Urge the patient to stop smoking because smoking reduces the serum HDL level, constricts the arteries, and reduces the blood's oxygen-carrying capacity.

More info
To help your patient obtain further information, provide the address and phone number of the American Heart Association.

• Eat no more than three egg yolks in one week, including yolks in prepared foods.

There's more

To help the patient lower his blood pressure, advise him to eliminate caffeine and reduce sodium intake. If he's overweight, explain that obesity is closely linked to several other CAD risk factors. Explain that losing excess weight by itself affects CAD and also helps lower blood pressure. Tell him that the two best ways to lose weight are to limit caloric intake (especially of fats) and to exercise.

Listen up!

In case of angina

Tell the patient to follow these steps if he experiences angina:
- Stop activity immediately.
- Sit or lie down with head elevated.
- Breathe deeply and slowly to relax.
- Take the prescribed nitrate.

Tell the patient to have someone take him to the hospital emergency department if the angina persists longer than 10 minutes after he takes three spaced doses of the nitrate medication.

Teaching about medication

Explain all prescribed medications to the patient, including:
- antilipemics (to reduce the levels of certain proteins and fat combinations in the blood)
- antiplatelet drugs such as aspirin (to hinder clot formation)
- beta blockers (to lower blood pressure)
- calcium channel blockers (to reduce the frequency and severity of chest pain and to lower blood pressure)
- nitrates (to alleviate chest pain).

Teach the patient to check sodium levels and caffeine and aspirin content in nonprescription medications to avoid drug interactions.

Teaching about procedures

If drug therapy is unsuccessful in relieving chest pain, or the patient develops unstable angina, the doctor may plan a balloon angioplasty. Describe the procedure so that your patient knows what to expect. (See "Balloon angioplasty," page 15.)

Teaching about surgery

If the patient consents to the procedure, the doctor may schedule a coronary artery bypass graft (CABG) to relieve chest pain (and, possibly, to prevent MI). Describe the surgery, including preoperative and postoperative care measures.

A way around it

In your teaching, tell the patient that CABG restores normal blood flow to the heart. Explain that the doctor removes a portion of a healthy vessel from another part of the body (usually a portion of the saphenous vein or a mammary artery). He then grafts it above and below the blocked portion of the coronary artery. Circulation is then diverted through the graft.

What to expect before

Tell the patient that he'll be asked to shower with a special antiseptic soap and will be shaved from neck to toes. Tell him that he may be given a sedative the morning of surgery to help him relax.

If indicated, explain that the patient may undergo preoperative pulmonary artery catheterization. Tell him that the catheter remains in place after the surgery but that the catheter, arterial lines, special monitoring lines, and epicardial pacing wires cause minimal discomfort.

What to expect after

Explain the complex and often frightening equipment that supports the patient's vital functions after surgery. For example, prepare him for intubation and mechanical ventilation. Also, include the following topics in your patient teaching:

• Explain that an intra-aortic balloon pump may be inserted to provide circulatory support for several hours after surgery. A nasogastric (NG) tube, a mediastinal chest tube, and an indwelling urinary catheter will be in place for the first day or two, and the patient will be connected to a cardiac monitor.

• Teach the patient about short-term postoperative care measures. Start with the expected course of the hospital stay: how many days he'll spend in the critical care area, the step-down unit, and a regular room before discharge.

• Emphasize that his priority is to relax and rest; stress and anxiety only hinder recovery. Encourage him to request pain medication to avoid discomfort. When the endotracheal and NG tubes are removed, tell him that he will gradually be able to swallow liquids. Tell him that solid food will gradually be reintroduced to his diet.

• To enhance circulation and reduce swelling in a leg from which a saphenous vein was taken, the patient may

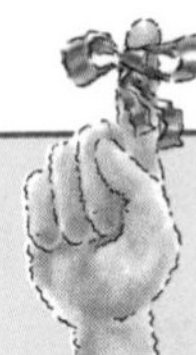

Memory jogger

A patient who has had the saphenous vein removed for a bypass graft can take steps to reduce the risk of lower leg swelling. Teach the patient to use the mnemonic *SWELL* to help him remember precautions:

Signs and symptoms to report are redness, tenderness, or drainage.

Wear support stockings.

Elevate your legs when sitting.

Loose clothes are better than tight ones.

Let your legs dangle; don't cross them.

also need to wear support stockings, elevate the leg frequently, and avoid crossing his legs.

A flight of stairs

Address the patient's concerns about sex after surgery. Tell him that once the doctor has given approval, sex is no more dangerous to the heart than walking up a flight of stairs.

Point out that a satisfying sex life can help speed recovery. However, advise your patient to reduce strain on the heart by avoiding sex right after a meal, after drinking alcohol, when fatigued or emotionally upset, or when in an unfamiliar and stressful situation (in a strange environment or with a new partner, for example). Also, suggest that he use positions that don't restrict breathing and avoid positions in which he must support his partner with his arms. Reassure him that impotence is fairly common but that it's almost always temporary.

Reducing reocclusion risk

Following surgery, emphasize that a diet low in cholesterol and saturated fats can reduce the risk of arterial reocclusion. Instruct the patient to report warning signs and symptoms of reocclusion or other serious complications. (See *Signs of reocclusion.*)

Signs of reocclusion

- Angina
- Persistent fever
- Swelling or drainage at the incision site
- Dizziness
- Shortness of breath at rest
- Rapid or irregular pulse
- Prolonged recovery time from exercise or sex

Two per day

With the doctor's permission, the patient may have up to two alcoholic drinks per day, beginning 2 to 3 weeks after surgery.

Usually temporary

Tell the patient that it's not uncommon after surgery to have postoperative depression. Tell him that such depression is usually temporary.

Sex is no more dangerous for me than walking up a flight of stairs!

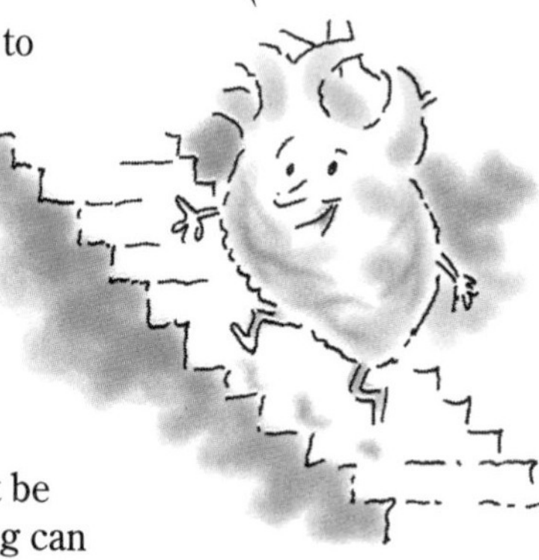

Heart failure

Over four million Americans experience heart failure and hundreds of thousands more are diagnosed each year. Although this disorder usually can't be cured, early intervention and comprehensive teaching can lessen its severity and improve the patient's outcome.

> **Heart failure**
>
> **Causes**
> - Myocardial infarction
> - Angina
> - Diabetes
> - Uncontrolled hypertension
>
> **Risk factors**
> - Cardiomyopathy
> - High cholesterol levels
> - Smoking
> - Chronic or excessive alcohol use
> - Family history of the disease

What's happening?

Tell the patient that heart failure occurs when the heart can't pump enough blood to meet the body's metabolic needs. Low cardiac output triggers a series of compensatory mechanisms, which may lead to pulmonary edema if they fail.

When does it happen?

Heart failure can occur at any age, although its incidence increases with advancing age.

How does it happen?

Help your patient understand the possible cause of his heart failure. Also, tell the patient about risk factors for this condition. (See *Heart failure.*)

What do you call it?

You or your patient may be more familiar with the term congestive heart failure. However, "congestive" is not really an accurate description because pulmonary and systemic congestion is only one aspect of the syndrome.

What is left-sided vs. right-sided heart failure?

Explain to your patient that the most common way to describe heart failure is as either left-sided or right-sided.

Left-sided heart failure causes mostly pulmonary symptoms, such as:

1. shortness of breath
2. dyspnea on exertion
3. moist cough.

Right-sided heart failure causes systemic symptoms, such as:

1. edema and swelling
2. jugular vein distention
3. hepatomegaly.

How is it treated?

The goals of treatment are to identify or prevent conditions that can bring on or worsen heart failure, reduce the heart's workload, improve pump performance, and control sodium intake and fluid retention. Specific measures may vary depending on the severity and cause of heart failure. (See *Heart failure treatment goals.*)

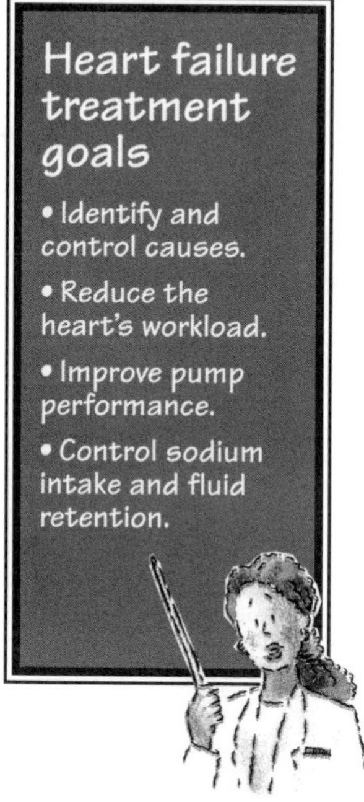
Heart failure treatment goals
• Identify and control causes.
• Reduce the heart's workload.
• Improve pump performance.
• Control sodium intake and fluid retention.

Teaching about tests

Explain that no single test confirms this diagnosis. Rather, blood tests and others are used in combination to help diagnose the condition.

Blood tests

Tell the patient that blood will be drawn so that the following measurements can be made:
- complete blood count
- serum albumin level
- liver function tests
- arterial blood gas analysis.

More tests

If the patient is over age 65 or has atrial fibrillation or evidence of thyroid disease, a thyroid-stimulating hormone test is conducted. Mention that a urine specimen will be collected for urinalysis.

A chest X-ray may be taken to determine the heart's size, evaluate the cardiac silhouette, and compare the sizes of major vessels. This test also reveals the extent of any pulmonary congestion. In addition, the doctor may order such tests as an ECG, an echocardiogram, cardiac catheterization, an angiogram, and a radionuclide ventriculogram (cardiac blood pool imaging). (See *Teaching patients about cardiovascular tests*, pages 3 to 6.)

Teaching about activity and lifestyle

In the past, patients with heart failure were advised to limit physical activity. However, recent research indicates that patients should stay as active as possible.

Urge your patient to pace himself to avoid fatigue, and stress the importance of following his doctor's recommendations on activity and exercise. Tell him to notify the doctor if activities seem to bring on or worsen shortness of breath, palpitations, or severe fatigue. (See *More about heart failure,* page 26.)

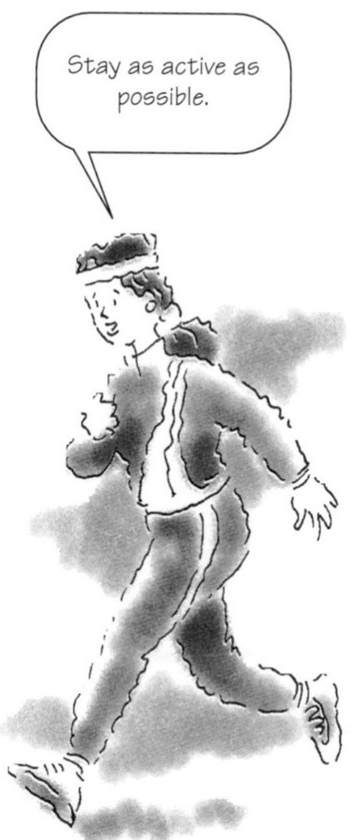
Stay as active as possible.

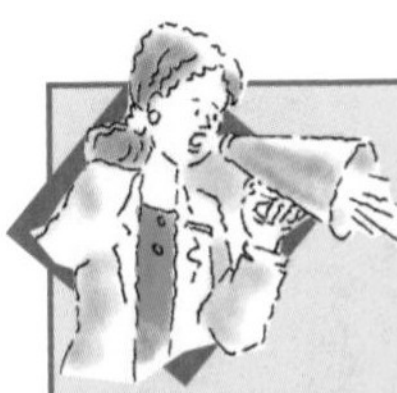

Listen up!

More about heart failure

Here are additional items to discuss with the patient who has heart failure.

Why risk it?
Heart failure puts the patient at risk for pneumonia and other respiratory infections. Advise the patient to limit exposure to crowds and to people with infections, when possible. Urge him to get annual pneumonia and influenza vaccinations.

Easy does it
Encourage the patient to learn ways to reduce his anxiety level. Remind him that anxiety may drive up blood pressure and speed his heart rate. The effects of anxiety can therefore affect cardiac output.

Early signs
Stress the importance of calling the doctor if he notices early signs of pulmonary edema, such as:
- difficulty breathing
- fatigue
- restlessness
- anxiety
- increased pulse rate
- weight gain
- anorexia
- dyspnea on exertion
- persistent cough
- frequent urination at night
- swelling of the ankles, feet, or abdomen.

More help
To help the patient cope with his condition, refer him to the American Heart Association.

Teaching about diet

Teach the patient to adhere to his prescribed diet to diminish fluid retention and thus decrease the heart's workload.

Pass (up) the salt

Point out that a low-sodium diet (2 to 3 g/day) promotes diuresis (urine excretion) and inhibits further fluid accumulation. Advise the patient to follow the doctor's instructions on how much sodium he may consume daily.

Follow up on fluid intake

Tell the patient that, although he should avoid excessive fluid intake, he need not restrict his fluid intake unless instructed by a doctor. To help monitor his fluid status, urge him to weigh himself daily, logging each measurement in a diary, and to report a weight gain of 3 lb (1.4 kg) or more in 1 week.

Because alcohol decreases the heart's ability to contract, caution the patient to restrict his alcohol intake according to the doctor's guidelines.

Potassium pointers

Depending on prescribed medication, the doctor may order a high- or low-potassium diet. As appropriate, help the patient identify foods high or low in potassium or refer him to a dietitian. (See *Shopping for potassium*.)

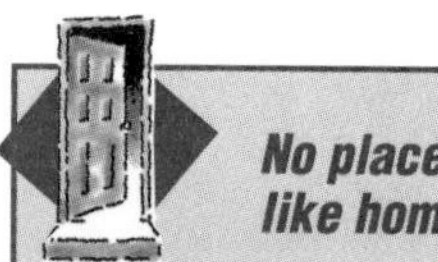

No place like home

Shopping for potassium

If the patient must follow a high-potassium diet, provide a copy of the following list.

Foods high in potassium
- Bananas
- Dates
- Salmon
- Carrots
- Potatoes
- Green leafy vegetables
- Cantaloupe
- Avocado

Teaching about medication

In acute heart failure, drug therapy may include a rapid-acting I.V. diuretic such as furosemide. In chronic heart failure, long-term drug therapy is likely to include:
- diuretics
- digitalis glycosides
- ACE inhibitors.

Relaxing blood vessels

Tell the patient that an ACE inhibitor, such as captopril (Capoten), relaxes the blood vessels, making it easier for the heart to pump. Instruct him to report adverse effects, such as a cough, dizziness, or a rash.

Removing excess fluid

Tell the patient that a diuretic eases fluid overload by removing excess fluid and salt from the body. These effects reduce stress on the heart. Also, provide the following pointers:
- Encourage the patient taking a loop diuretic (bumetanide, ethacrynic acid, or furosemide) to eat more high-potassium foods.
- If the patient takes a diuretic twice daily, advise him to take the second dose late in the afternoon rather than at night, to prevent nighttime urination.
- To minimize postural hypotension, recommend rising slowly from a sitting or lying position.

Strengthening cardiac contraction

If the patient doesn't improve with ACE inhibitors or diuretics, the doctor may prescribe a digitalis glycoside such as digoxin (Lanoxin). Explain that digitalis glycosides strengthen cardiac contraction and regulate the heart rate by slowing the pulse. Instruct the patient to measure his pulse rate daily and to notify the doctor if it falls below 60 beats per minute.

Tell the patient taking a digitalis glycoside to report the following adverse effects immediately:
- abdominal pain, dizziness, or drowsiness
- fatigue, headache, or loss of appetite
- malaise, nausea, visual disturbance, or vomiting.

Hypertension

Hypertension is an insidious disorder affecting as many as 60 million Americans. Because many patients are asymptomatic, the disease may go undetected until it's revealed during a routine checkup. Also, because of the "silent" nature of hypertension, the patient may need to be persuaded that he has a serious disorder.

What is it?

Explain that hypertension is abnormally high blood pressure. Blood exerts pressure against arterial walls as the heart pumps it through the body. In hypertension, this pressure is greater than it should be.

Making an adjustment

Tell the patient that a complex system involving the kidneys, brain, and nerves regulates blood pressure. The body makes adjustments through hormone release into the bloodstream when pressure is too high or too low. Other factors governing blood pressure include the following:
- the heart's strength and pumping ability
- circulating blood volume
- arterial condition.

Up or down

Emphasize that blood pressure normally fluctuates with age, activity, and emotional stress and rises and falls many times daily. Point out that sustained hypertension eventually damages blood vessels and reduces blood flow to tissues.

Primary or secondary

Tell the patient that hypertension can be:

- primary, also called essential hypertension
- secondary, resulting from another condition, such as kidney disease or an endocrine disorder.

In a blood pressure reading, the top number is the pressure that's exerted when the heart is at work.

At work and rest

Tell the patient that blood pressure is measured in millimeters of mercury (mm Hg) and that two values constitute a blood pressure reading. The first, or systolic, value measures maximum pressure, or that exerted when the heart is at work (contracting or beating). The second, or diastolic, value measures minimum pressure, or that exerted when the heart is at rest (relaxing between beats).

The bottom number is the pressure that's exerted when the heart is at rest.

Teaching about tests

Explain that blood pressure is measured with a device called a sphygmomanometer. Abnormally high pressure readings taken on at least three different days are necessary to confirm a diagnosis (unless a single reading is extremely high). Hypertension is diagnosed if the blood pressure exceeds 140/90 mm Hg.

Discuss, if appropriate, which diagnostic studies the doctor has ordered to rule out secondary causes of hypertension. These tests may include a chest X-ray, an angiogram, an ECG, an echocardiogram, and cardiac catheterization. (See *Teaching patients about cardiovascular tests*, pages 3 to 6.)

Teaching about activity and lifestyle

If the patient has newly diagnosed mild hypertension, the doctor will try to manage the condition by prescribing:

 a low-salt diet

 weight loss, if appropriate

 a regular exercise program.

If these measures fail, he will prescribe medications to lower blood pressure.

Make it a habit

Encourage your patient to get regular exercise to help lower blood pressure. Explain that the doctor recommends an exercise program based on the following factors:
- the patient's medical history
- the patient's age
- the patient's medication regimen.

Put down the barbell

Isometric exercises — such as weight lifting — aren't included in an exercise regimen to control hypertension because this type of exercise increases blood pressure.

An appropriate exercise program emphasizes aerobic exercise to accomplish the following:

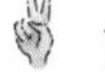 tone the cardiovascular system

lower blood pressure.

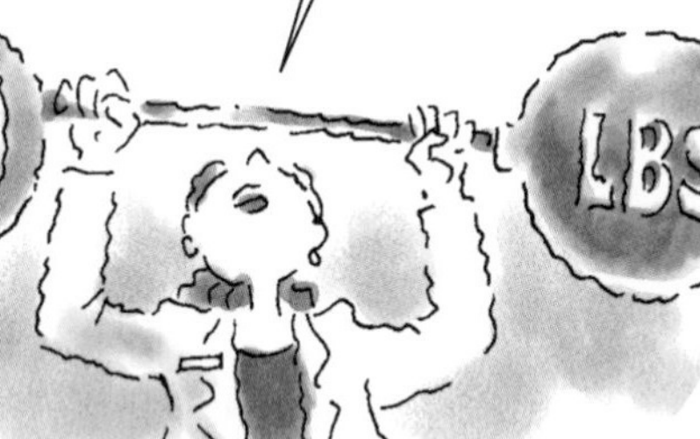
Because it increases blood pressure, weight lifting isn't included in the exercise regimen for hypertension.
500
LBS

But don't overdo it

Caution the patient not to overdo exercise, because occasional bursts of extreme activity can be worse than no exercise at all. Remind him to exercise only to the extent specified by his doctor. Also emphasize that he must stop exercising well before the point of exhaustion. Instruct him to stop exercising at once and call the doctor right away if he becomes dizzy. (See *More about hypertension.*)

Teaching about diet

Perhaps the most talked-about nutrient in a discussion about hypertension is sodium. Explain that excessive sodium intake contributes to hypertension. Recommend that the patient reduce the sodium in his diet by avoiding or limiting salty foods, such as:
- most processed foods

- luncheon meats
- canned soups and vegetables
- most snack foods and condiments.

Spice advice

Advise him to use alternatives to table salt, such as:
- herbs
- spices
- sodium-free salt substitutes.

Think before you drink

Also urge him to limit the amount of caffeine and alcohol he consumes. Explain that most alcoholic beverages are high in calories, and beer contains considerable sodium.

Pass the potassium

If the patient is taking a potassium-depleting diuretic, suggest that he eat a potassium-rich diet. Mention that many foods naturally high in potassium are low in sodium. Also, tell the patient about foods that are high in potassium, such as bananas, dates, salmon, carrots, and potatoes.

Don't overwork your heart

Overweight people are three times more likely to have hypertension than are people who maintain normal weight. Under the doctor's supervision, encourage the patient to

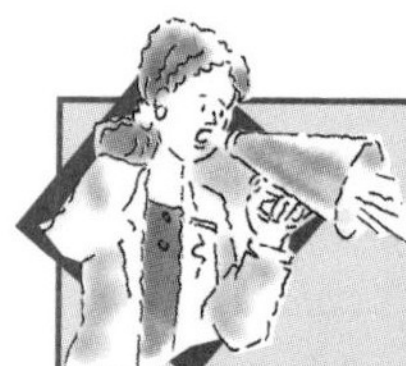

Listen up!

More about hypertension

Here are additional teaching points to share with your patient.

Easy does it

Because stress and hypertension often go hand in hand, encourage the patient to use stress-reducing techniques, such as relaxation exercises or meditation. Advise him to practice these techniques twice a day for 10 to 20 minutes.

Time to quit

If the patient smokes, give him information to encourage him to quit. Explain how nicotine constricts blood vessels, further increasing blood pressure. As appropriate, refer him to community programs, agencies, or support groups that can help him stop smoking and provide follow-up services after he stops.

More info

For more information about hypertension, direct your patient to the American Heart Association.

begin a weight-reduction program that emphasizes a balanced diet, regular exercise, and gradual weight loss. (See *Diet do's and don'ts.*)

Teaching about medication

If dietary restrictions and exercise fail to lower blood pressure sufficiently, drug therapy may be necessary. Initial therapy usually includes one or more of the following:

- a diuretic
- a beta blocker
- an ACE inhibitor
- a calcium channel blocker.

If the patient's blood pressure is still not under control after initial therapy, a combination of these drugs or other antihypertensive agents may be prescribed.

Cooperation = control

Help your patient understand the need to comply with the prescribed drug regimen. Stress that drugs can only control, not cure, hypertension. Tell the patient that he may need to take antihypertensive drugs for the rest of his life.

Even if feeling well

Emphasize the importance of taking prescribed medication even if the patient is feeling well. Warn him that reducing or discontinuing medications without medical guidance may lead to severe rebound hypertension, possibly triggering a life-threatening hypertensive crisis.

Over-the-counter caution

Make sure the patient understands that many over-the-counter medications contain ingredients that can make antihypertensives less effective. Also remind him that other over-the-counter drugs are high in sodium. These include:

- antacids
- laxatives
- diet pills
- cold remedies
- allergy medications.

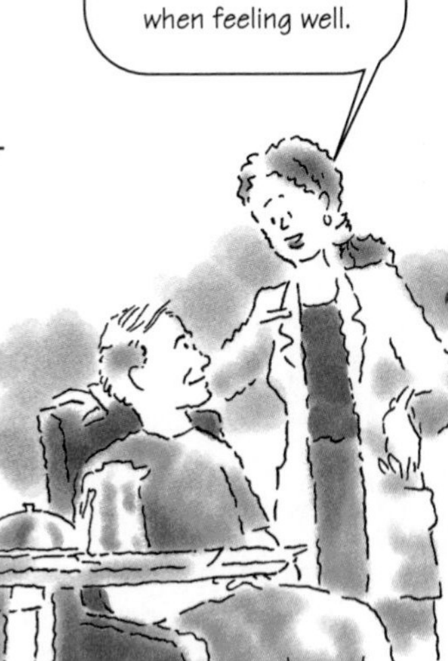
To control hypertension, you need to take medication even when feeling well.

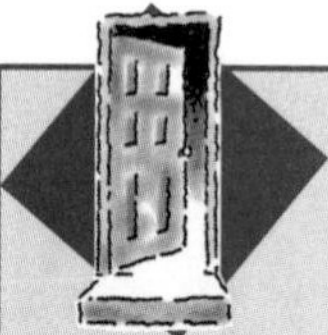

No place like home

Diet do's and don'ts

When teaching about diet, invite the patient's family to join the class, especially if the patient doesn't usually shop for groceries or cook for the household.

Putting a halt on salt
Tell the patient to reduce the sodium in the diet by avoiding or limiting salty foods, such as most processed foods, luncheon meats, canned soups and vegetables, and most snack foods and condiments.

Think before you drink
Advise the patient to limit intake of caffeine and alcohol.

Have a banana
If the patient is taking a potassium-depleting diuretic, suggest that he ask his doctor about following a diet high in potassium, including such potassium-rich foods as bananas, dates, salmon, carrots, and potatoes.

Ease your heart's workload
Point out that obesity raises blood pressure by increasing blood volume, thus adding to the heart's workload. Encourage the patient to begin a weight-reduction program that emphasizes a balanced diet, regular exercise, and gradual weight loss.

Myocardial infarction

Few disorders arouse as much anxiety in a patient as myocardial infarction (MI). The patient who has had an MI worries not just about his immediate survival, but also about the quality of life after recovery. When severe, anxiety can impair the patient's ability to learn and cooperate. It can also increase his risk of complications. Fortunately, thorough patient teaching can reduce anxiety.

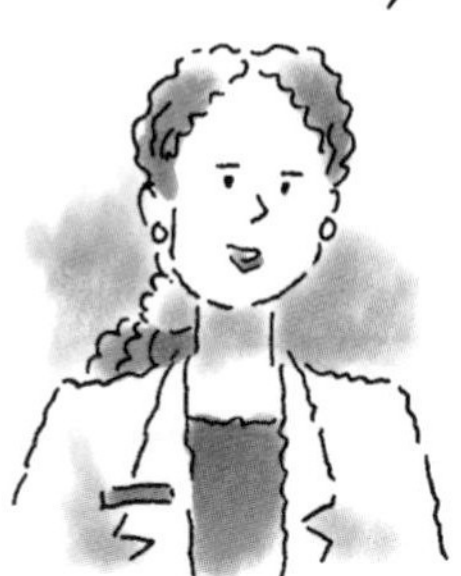
Make a difference. Educating patients can reduce anxiety, one of the major complications of MI.

What's the story?

Explain that MI results from reduced blood flow through one or more of the coronary arteries. The reduced flow, in turn, decreases blood supply to a portion of the heart, leading to ischemia, injury, and necrosis. (See *MI story,* page 34.)

What causes the pain?

Tell the patient that the chest pain of MI results from reduced oxygen supply to the heart, called myocardial ischemia. The pain may range from mild discomfort to a burning or crushing sensation that may radiate to the arm, jaw, neck, or shoulder blades.

What are the risks?

Point out that if blood flow isn't restored, tissue in the affected area of the heart is injured, becoming necrotic. Later, scar tissue forms but isn't able to contract. This further reduces the heart's ability to pump blood, placing the patient at risk for heart failure and another MI.

Why did this happen?

By far, the most common cause is atherosclerosis in one or more coronary arteries. Tell the patient that atherosclerosis is characterized by buildup of fatty, fibrous plaques that narrow or occlude the artery. Thrombosis, or clot formation, commonly occurs in atherosclerotic arteries and is a contributing factor in many MIs.

Tell the patient that some MIs result, not from atherosclerosis or thrombosis, but from a sudden spasm, or smooth-muscle contraction, in a coronary artery. The spasm blocks blood flow to part of the heart. Such spasms can occur in both normal and atherosclerotic arteries.

MI story

- Blood flow through a coronary artery decreases.
- Blood supply to a portion of the heart decreases.
- Oxygen supply to the heart is reduced.
- Heart tissue is destroyed.
- Scar tissue forms.
- Scar tissue can't contract.
- The heart's ability to pump blood decreases.

Teaching about tests

Help your patient understand the tests that are used to diagnose MI. Tell the patient with an acute MI that the condition is confirmed based on the following:

- the patient's symptoms
- serial blood studies
- ECG
- thallium and technetium scans.

Blood samples are collected regularly to detect fluctuations in cardiac enzyme levels, reflecting evidence of MI.

After the patient's condition stabilizes, tell the patient that the doctor may order additional studies, such as an exercise ECG (possibly with a thallium scan), an ambulatory ECG, or electrophysiologic studies. (See *Teaching patients about cardiovascular tests*, pages 3 to 6.)

Teaching about activity and lifestyle

Encourage the patient with an uncomplicated MI to perform activities as tolerated. The patient may be asked to sit in a chair or use a bedside commode if his condition is stable.

A bit more complicated

The patient who has a complicated MI or continues to have angina or hypotension remains on bed rest for the first 24 to 48 hours after an MI. This serves two purposes:

 reduces the demands on the heart

 improves the patient's chance of recovery.

Pass on the following pointers to your patient who's recovering from a complicated MI:

- Encourage the patient on bed rest to wiggle his toes regularly while in bed to reduce the risk of blood clots.
- Caution the patient not to perform any activity that strains the heart, such as pressing the feet against the footboard and raising the legs off the bed.
- Review the patient's prescribed activity program. Emphasize the need to resume activities gradually. Help him plan activities so that he alternates light and heavy tasks, takes frequent rest breaks, and shares the workload with a friend or family member. (See *Before you say goodbye*; *Birds do it, bees do it*, page 36; and *Safe sex after MI*, page 37.)

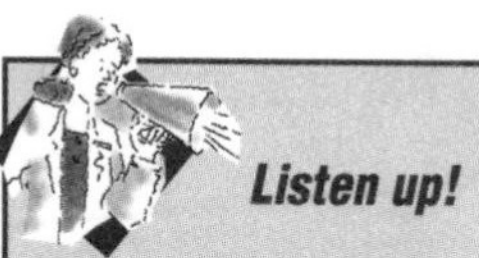

Before you say goodbye

Here are a few last-minute items to discuss with a patient recovering from MI.

Why risk it?
Educate the patient about the importance of correcting or reducing risk factors for MI, such as obesity, excessive stress, and smoking.

Follow up
Mention that to aid the patient's recuperation, the doctor may recommend a cardiac rehabilitation program and prescribe medications. Urge him to follow the treatment regimen closely. Also refer him to such sources of information as the American Heart Association.

Teaching about diet

For the first 24 hours after an MI, the patient receives only clear fluids. Depending on the patient's tolerance of the fluids, the diet is advanced to a cardiac diet, which has few calories from fat. Tell the patient to avoid caffeine, which stimulates the heart.

Teaching about medication

If the doctor discovers a coronary artery thrombus, explain the purpose of thrombolytic drugs.

Too late

If it's too late to administer thrombolytic therapy (it should be given in the first few hours after an MI) or if such therapy is contraindicated, emergency interventions such as surgery may be required.

O_2 for a day or two

Supplemental oxygen is given through a nasal cannula for the first 24 to 48 hours and as needed after that. Tell the patient that this therapy keeps the heart and other tissues well oxygenated.

More drugs

If the doctor orders nitroglycerin or morphine, explain that these drugs relieve chest pain by increasing oxygen supply to the heart. Also, describe the purpose of other prescribed medications, such as, nitroprusside (which lowers blood pressure, thereby reducing demands on the heart), lidocaine (which controls arrhythmia), dopamine or dobutamine (which strengthens cardiac contractions).

Still more drugs

Discuss other prescribed drugs. For instance, the doctor may order a stool softener to prevent straining during defecation, a sedative to decrease anxiety, and a sedative to promote rest.

Yet more drugs

As treatment progresses, the doctor may prescribe drugs to help regulate cardiovascular function and prevent complications, such as antiarrhythmics, diuretics, antilipemics, antihypertensives, and anticoagulants.

Birds do it, bees do it

Inform the patient that most patients can resume having sex 3 to 4 weeks after a heart attack. Explain that sex is a moderate form of exercise — no more stressful than a brisk walk. However, sex can place a strain on the heart if it's accompanied by emotional stress.

Your place or mine
Advise the patient to choose a quiet, familiar setting with a comfortable room temperature.

Breakfast in bed
Recommend having sex when rested and relaxed. A good time is in the morning, after he has had a good night's sleep.

Not tonight
Caution the patient not to have sex when he's tired or upset or after drinking a lot of alcohol. Also tell him to wait a few hours after a big meal.

Experiment
Advise the patient to choose positions that are relaxing, permit unrestricted breathing, and don't require him to use his arms to support himself or his partner.

Teaching about procedures

If treatment through medication is not successful, the doctor may order balloon angioplasty, pulmonary artery catheterization, or an intra-aortic balloon pump.

Balloon angioplasty

The patient may undergo a balloon angioplasty, or PTCA. Provide clear, simple explanations of patient preparation, how the procedure is done, and postprocedure care. Even if the patient or family members don't absorb all the details, your concern and reassurance can improve the patient's prospects for recovery.

Review information about the type of PTCA procedure the patient will have so that he knows what to expect. (See "Balloon angioplasty," page 15, and "Laser-assisted angioplasty," page 15.)

Pulmonary artery catheterization

The doctor may insert this catheter if the patient develops heart failure, hypotension, hypertension, or oliguria. He may also use it to assess cardiac function or monitor the effects of drug therapy.

Intra-aortic balloon pump

The doctor may insert an intra-aortic balloon pump (IABP) to increase the supply of oxygen-rich blood to the heart and decrease the heart's oxygen demand. Tell the patient that the IABP displaces blood within the aorta by means of a balloon attached to an external pump console. Explain that the balloon catheter will temporarily reduce the heart's workload to promote rapid healing of the ventricular muscle. Assure him that it will be removed after his heart can resume an adequate workload.

Tell the patient that crucial pressures will be measured while the IABP is in use, and that he will gradually be weaned from the intra-aortic balloon — usually about 24 hours after balloon insertion. For 24 hours or so after balloon removal, the patient is restricted to bed rest and is monitored closely.

Teaching about surgery

If the patient will undergo CABG to treat acute MI or complications associated with cardiac catheterization or PTCA, explain that CABG will restore normal blood flow to his heart.

Mention that, before surgery, the patient will shower with a special antiseptic soap and may be shaved from neck to toes. Tell him he won't be allowed to eat or drink anything after midnight before the day of surgery, although he can request a sleeping pill. Tell him that he may receive a sedative the morning of surgery to help him relax.

Discuss what will happen during surgery: The doctor will excise a portion of a healthy vessel from another part of the body and graft it above and below the blocked coronary artery. Tell the patient that his circulation will then be diverted through the graft.

Safe sex after MI

Instruct the patient to ask the doctor if he should take nitroglycerin before having sex. This medication can prevent angina attacks during or after sex. Point out that it's normal for pulse and breathing rates to increase during sex, but that they should return to normal within 15 minutes.

Call me

Instruct the patient to call at once if he has any of these symptoms after sex:

- sweating or palpitations for 15 minutes or longer
- breathlessness or increased heart rate for 15 minutes or longer
- chest pain that's not relieved by two or three nitroglycerin tablets (taken 5 minutes apart), a rest period, or both
- sleeplessness after sex or extreme fatigue the next day.

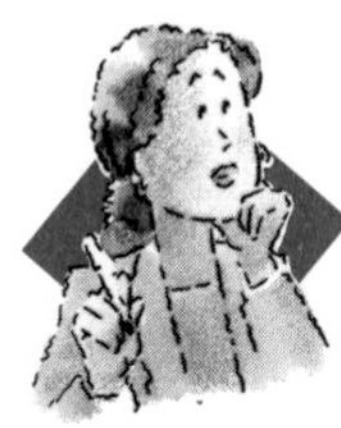

Quick quiz

1. The most important reason to encourage an arrhythmia patient to eat bananas is that they:

A. reduce oxygen demand.
B. are high in potassium.
C. are a natural alternative to antiarrhythmic drug therapy.

Answer: B. Because a low serum potassium level sometimes contributes to arrhythmia, patients should be encouraged to eat potassium-rich foods like bananas.

2. An appropriate explanation to give to a patient regarding how anticoagulant drugs achieve their effect is that they:

A. ease symptoms by expanding the arteries.
B. aid blood flow through vessels by making blood less sticky.
C. reduce clot formation by interfering with platelet function.

Answer: C. Anticoagulants achieve their effect by interfering with platelet function. Vasodilators ease symptoms by expanding the arteries. The drug Trental aids blood flow through vessels by making blood less sticky.

3. The advice you would not give to a patient with CAD regarding exercise would be to:

A. exercise regularly.
B. take a prescribed nitrate before participating in exercise that might provoke angina.
C. develop a weight-lifting routine.

Answer: C. Advise against weight-lifting and other isometric exercises when teaching a patient with CAD. Such exercise increases blood pressure and taxes the heart and coronary arteries.

Help for the heart

For more information about cardiovascular disorders, direct the patient to the following Web sites:

- American Heart Association (www.americanheart.org)
- National Heart, Lung, and Blood Institute (www.nhlbi.nih.gov/nhlbi/nhlbi.htm)
- Texas Heart Institute (www.tmc.edu/thi/his.html#Heart Information Service).

Scoring

☆☆☆ If you answered two or three questions correctly, good job. For all practical purposes, you've gotten to the heart of the matter.

☆☆ If you answered fewer than two questions correctly, take heart. Nine more quick quizzes to go!

Respiratory disorders

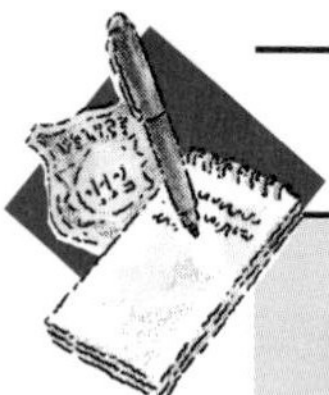

Just the facts

In this chapter, you'll learn how to teach patients with the following respiratory disorders:

- ♦ chronic obstructive pulmonary disease
- ♦ pleural disorders
- ♦ pneumonia
- ♦ pulmonary embolism
- ♦ tuberculosis.

COPD

Chronic obstructive pulmonary disease (COPD) is the second leading cause of disability in the United States. Although COPD can't be cured, thorough teaching can make a tremendous difference in a patient's quality of life.

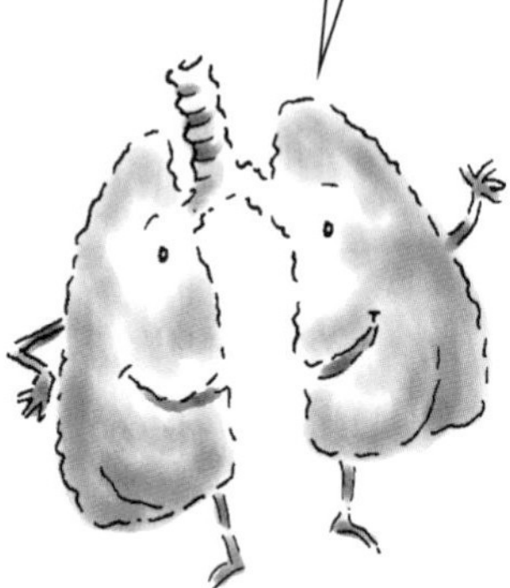

Good teaching will help your patients breathe easy.

What is it?

Begin your teaching by telling the patient that COPD is the name given to a group of respiratory conditions characterized by airflow resistance. This resistance may be caused by:

- mucus obstruction, as in asthma and chronic bronchitis
- lack of elastic recoil in the lungs, as in emphysema.

Tell your patient that COPD is a progressive condition. The chronic inability to breathe easily leads to exhaustion.

Review with the patient his particular type of COPD, such as:

- chronic bronchitis

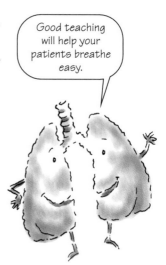

- emphysema
- asthma.

What is chronic bronchitis?

If the patient has chronic bronchitis, explain that repeated exposure to irritants such as dust or pet dander inflames the airways, causing them to swell and clog with mucus. This leads to airflow obstruction.

What is emphysema?

Tell the patient with emphysema that this condition is marked by airway inflammation. The inflammation eventually destroys air sacs (alveoli) in the lungs and small airways (bronchioles).

Explain to the patient that he may experience ruptured blebs and bullae (rupture of small vesicles on the lung surface) leading to spontaneous pneumothorax (in which the lung collapses for no known reason) or pneumonia.

Make sure your patient with emphysema understands the importance of calling the doctor immediately if he experiences signs of spontaneous pneumothorax. (See *Spotting spontaneous pneumothorax.*)

Listen up!

Spotting spontaneous pneumothorax

The chief sign of spontaneous pneumothorax is a sudden, sharp chest pain. The condition is worsened by chest movement, breathing, and coughing. If the patient experiences these symptoms, he should call the doctor immediately.

What is asthma?

Explain to the patient the characteristics that distinguish asthma: smooth airway muscle spasm that can constrict the airway, mucosal edema, and thickening mucus. Tell the patient that two types of factors can cause this condition:

1. intrinsic factors (internal, nonallergic)
2. extrinsic factors (external, allergic).

Teach your patient how to identify and avoid factors that might trigger his asthma. (See *Avoiding asthma.*) In addition, teach your patient how to deal with an acute asthma attack if it does occur. (See *How to control an asthma attack,* page 42.)

Tell the patient that although there are other predisposing factors that can cause asthma (as well as chronic bronchitis and emphysema), smoking is the most important. Encourage your patient to quit smoking.

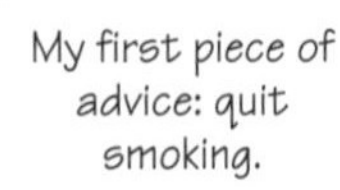
My first piece of advice: quit smoking.

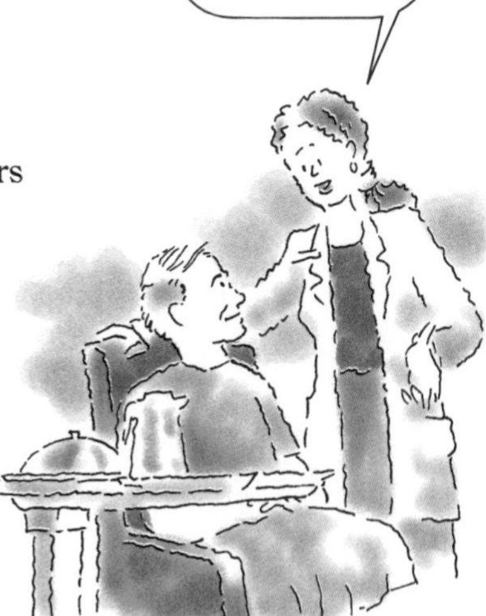

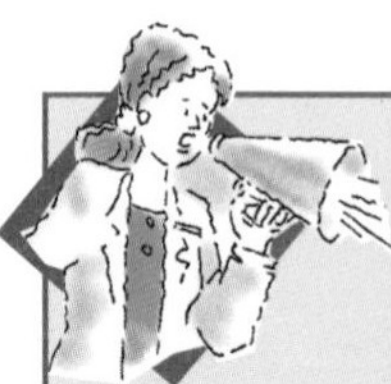

Listen up!

Avoiding asthma

To make it easier for your patient to live with asthma, teach him to avoid common asthma triggers and monitor his activity, diet, and drug use.

Asthma triggers

The patient must watch for asthma triggers at home, in the workplace, and outdoors.

At home

- Foods, such as nuts, chocolate, eggs, shellfish, and peanut butter
- Beverages, such as orange juice, wine, beer, and milk
- Mold spores; pollen from flowers, trees, grasses, hay, and ragweed (If pollen is the offender, advise the patient to install a bedroom air conditioner with a filter and avoid long walks when pollen counts are high.)
- Dander from rabbits, cats, dogs, hamsters, gerbils, and chickens (Suggest that the patient consider finding a new home for the family pet, if necessary.)
- Feather or hair-stuffed pillows, down comforters, wool clothing, and stuffed toys (Advise the patient to use smooth [not fuzzy], washable blankets on his bed.)
- Insect parts such as those from dead cockroaches
- Medicines such as aspirin
- Vapors from cleaning solvents, paint, paint thinners, and liquid chlorine bleach
- Fluorocarbon spray products, such as furniture polish, starch, cleaners, and room deodorizers
- Scents from spray deodorants, perfumes, hair sprays, talcum powder, and cosmetics
- Cloth-upholstered furniture, carpets, and draperies that collect dust (Tell the patient to hang lightweight, washable cotton or synthetic-fiber curtains and to use washable, cotton throw rugs on bare floors.)
- Brooms and dusters that raise dust (Instead, advise the patient to clean his bedroom daily by damp dusting and damp mopping. Also instruct him to keep the door closed.)
- Dirty filters on hot-air furnaces and air conditioners that blow dust into the air
- Dust from vacuum cleaner exhaust

In the workplace

- Dust, vapors, or fumes from wood products (western red cedar, some pine and birch woods, mahogany); flour, cereals, and other grains; coffee, tea, or papain; metals (platinum, chromium, nickel sulfate, soldering fumes); and cotton, flax, and hemp
- Mold from decaying hay

Outdoors

- Cold air, hot air, or sudden temperature changes (when going in and out of air-conditioned stores in the summer)
- Excessive humidity or dryness
- Changes in seasons
- Smog
- Automobile exhaust

Anywhere

- Overexertion, which may cause wheezing
- Common cold, flu, and other viruses
- Fear, anger, frustration, laughing too hard, crying, or any emotionally upsetting situation
- Smoke from cigarettes, cigars, and pipes (Advise the patient not to smoke and not to stay in a room where people are smoking.)

Diet, drugs, activity

Instruct the patient to:

- drink six to eight 8-oz (237-ml) glasses of fluid daily
- take all prescribed medications exactly as directed
- tell his doctor about any and all medications he takes — even nonprescription ones
- avoid sleeping pills or sedatives to promote sleep during a mild asthma attack (Explain that these medications may slow down his breathing and make it more difficult. Instead, suggest that he try propping himself up on extra pillows while waiting for antianxiety medication to work.)
- schedule only as much activity as he can tolerate and to take frequent rests on busy days.

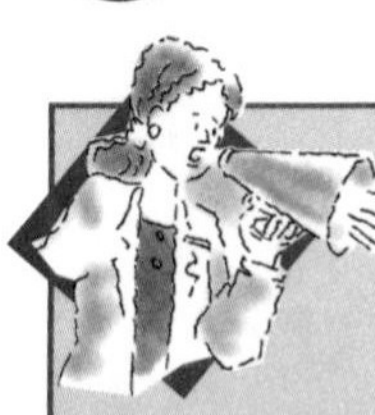

Listen up!

How to control an asthma attack

Tell your patient that an asthma attack is usually preceded by warning signs that say it's time to take action. Tell him to watch for:

- chest tightness
- coughing
- awareness of breathing
- wheezing.

Don't ignore it

After having a few asthma attacks, the patient should have no trouble recognizing these early warning signs. Emphasize that he *must not ignore them.* Instead, tell him to follow the steps discussed below.

No worse

Instruct the patient to take prescribed medicine with an oral inhaler, if directed, to prevent the attack from getting worse.

Relax

Encourage the patient to try to relax as the medicine goes to work. Although he may understandably be nervous or afraid, these feelings only worsen shortness of breath.

To help him relax, give your patient the following instructions: Tell him to sit upright in a chair, close his eyes, and breathe slowly and evenly. Then he should begin consciously tightening and relaxing the muscles in his body. Tell him to first tighten the muscles in his face, counting to himself: "one-1,000; two-1,000." Tell him not to hold his breath. Then he should relax these muscles and repeat with the muscles in his arms and hands and then legs and feet. Finally, he should let his body go limp.

Regaining control

Instruct the patient to perform the pursed-lip breathing exercises he's been taught to regain control of his breathing. Tell him not to gasp for air. He should continue pursed-lip breathing until he no longer feels breathless.

Cough it up

If the attack triggers a coughing spell, help the patient control his cough so that it effectively brings up mucus and helps clear the airways. Tell him to lean forward slightly, keeping his feet on the floor, then breathe in deeply and hold that breath for a second or two. Tell him to cough twice, first to loosen mucus and then to bring it up, and to be sure to cough into a tissue.

Finally

Instruct the patient to call the doctor right away if the attack gets worse after he has followed these steps.

What's at risk?

No matter which form of COPD the patient has, be sure to explain that an untreated respiratory infection can lead to life-threatening respiratory failure. Also mention that COPD increases the risk of lung collapse from mucus plugs that block the bronchi.

What else?

If COPD involves the pulmonary blood vessels, tell the patient that pressure in these vessels may rise too high and the right side of the heart may fail. This failure may lead to:

- increased difficulty breathing
- swollen ankles, lower back, and scrotum

• bluish or mottled skin
• productive cough with frothy, pink-tinged expectorated sputum.

Teaching about tests

Tell the patient that the doctor typically relies on pulmonary function tests and chest X-rays to assess respiratory impairment or detect complications. However, he also may order the following tests:
• computed tomography (CT) scan or magnetic resonance imaging (MRI) of the chest
• exercise electrocardiogram (ECG)
• arterial blood gases.

If the doctor suspects a coexisting respiratory infection, tell the patient that he'll undergo a complete blood count and sputum analysis, or possibly other respiratory diagnostic tests. (See *Teaching patients about respiratory tests*, pages 44 to 48.)

Treatment for COPD

• Daily exercise
• Limits on activity
• Dietary changes
• Drug and oxygen therapy
• Chest physiotherapy
• Self-care measures

Teaching about activity and lifestyle

Although treatment for COPD involves a number of factors, exercise is likely to play an important role. (See *Treatment for COPD*.) After evaluating the results of the patient's exercise ECG, the doctor may prescribe an exercise program to boost endurance and strength without causing severe breathing difficulty.

Do it!

Encourage regular participation in exercises, such as riding a stationary bicycle and walking.

Warm up, cool down

Advise the patient to perform several minutes of warm-up exercises (slow walking, bending, stretching) and to finish with cool-down exercises.

Start slow

Instruct the patient to start slowly and gradually increase the pace and duration of activity. The doctor reevaluates the patient's exercise tolerance from time to time and modifies the program as necessary.

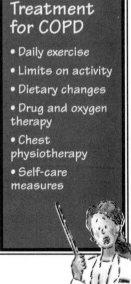

(Text continues on page 49.)

Teaching patients about respiratory tests

Test and purpose	What to teach the patient
Arterial blood gas analysis • To evaluate the efficiency of gas exchange in the lungs • To assess the integrity of the ventilatory control system • To determine the acid-base level of the blood • To monitor respiratory therapy	• The patient must breathe normally while an arterial puncture is performed to collect a blood sample. He may experience a brief cramping or throbbing pain at the puncture site.
Bronchoscopy • To help identify the cause of dyspnea and other respiratory symptoms • To visually examine a possible tumor, secretions, or another obstruction demonstrated on X-ray • To help diagnose bronchogenic carcinoma, tuberculosis, interstitial pulmonary disease, or fungal or parasitic pulmonary infection by obtaining a tissue or mucus specimen for examination • To locate a bleeding site in the tracheobronchial tree • To remove foreign bodies, mucus plugs, or excessive secretions from the airways	• This test takes 45 to 60 minutes. • The patient must not eat or drink for 6 hours before the test. However, he should continue taking prescribed drugs unless the doctor orders otherwise. • If the test will be done with a local anesthetic, the patient may receive a sedative to help him relax. He should be prepared for the unpleasant taste and coolness of the anesthetic throat spray used to suppress the gag reflex and ease passage of the bronchoscope. • The patient is usually placed in a supine position on a table or bed, although he may be asked to sit upright in a chair. He must remain relaxed, with his arms at his sides, and breathe through his nose during the test. The doctor inserts the bronchoscope tube through the patient's nose or mouth into the airway. Then he flushes small amounts of anesthetic through the tube to suppress coughing and wheezing. Although the patient may experience dyspnea during the test, he won't suffocate. Also, oxygen will be given through the bronchoscope. • The patient's blood pressure, heart rate, and breathing are monitored for about 15 minutes. He should lie on his side or sit with his head elevated at least 30 degrees until his gag reflex returns. Food, fluid, and oral drugs are withheld for about 2 hours or until his gag reflex returns. Hoarseness or a sore throat is temporary. He can have throat lozenges or liquid gargle when his gag reflex returns. • The patient should report bloody mucus, dyspnea, wheezing, or chest pain immediately.
Chest X-ray (chest radiography) • To detect respiratory disorders, such as pneumonia, atelectasis, pneumothorax, pulmonary bullae, and tumors • To detect mediastinal abnormalities (such as tumors) and cardiac disease • To evaluate the effectiveness of therapy	• This test takes only minutes, but the technician or doctor will need additional time to check the quality of the films. • The patient should remove all jewelry from his neck and chest. • The patient stands or sits in front of the X-ray machine. He must take a deep breath and hold it for a few seconds while the X-ray is taken and must remain still for those few seconds. • He'll be exposed to only slight amounts of radiation.

Teaching patients about respiratory tests *(continued)*

Test and purpose	What to teach the patient
Computed tomography scan (CT scan, thoracic computed tomography) • To locate or monitor lesions in the lungs, mediastinum, thoracic lymph nodes, blood vessels, or other tissues	• This test takes 30 to 60 minutes and causes little discomfort. • If a contrast medium will be used, the patient must fast for 4 hours before the test. He should remove all jewelry. • The patient lies in a supine position on an X-ray table. To restrict movement, a strap is placed across the body part to be scanned. The table then slides into the large, tunnel-shaped machine. When the contrast medium is injected, the patient may experience transient nausea, flushing, warmth, and a salty taste. He must not move during the test, but should relax and breathe normally. • He can resume his usual activities and diet immediately after the test.
Electrocardiography (ECG) • To help identify changes in heart activity that may suggest pulmonary embolism	• This test takes 15 minutes. • The technician cleans, dries and, possibly, shaves different sites on the patient's body, such as the chest and arms, and applies electrodes at these sites. • The patient is asked to lie still, relax and breathe normally, and remain quiet. Talk or limb movement will distort ECG recordings and require additional testing time.
Exercise ECG (stress test, treadmill test, graded exercise test) • To help diagnose the cause of breathing problems • To help evaluate the effectiveness of bronchodilator therapy • To assess the degree of pulmonary dysfunction • To help plan or evaluate an exercise program	• This test takes about 30 minutes. A doctor or nurse will be present in the testing area at all times. The patient must not eat, smoke, or drink alcohol for 3 hours before the test. However, he should continue his prescribed drug regimen. • The patient should wear comfortable shoes and loose, lightweight shorts or slacks. • A technician cleans, shaves (if necessary), and lightly rubs sites on the chest and, possibly, the back. Then he attaches electrodes at these sites. • If the patient is scheduled for a multistage treadmill test, the treadmill speed and incline increase at predetermined intervals and he'll be told of each adjustment. If he's scheduled for a bicycle ergometer test, resistance to pedaling increases gradually as he tries to maintain a specific speed. He'll be asked to breathe in and out of a mouthpiece during the test and may need to wear a noseclip. • The patient can stop the test if he experiences severe fatigue or dyspnea. Typically, he'll feel tired, out of breath, and sweaty. Nevertheless, he should report any sensations he feels during the test. He may receive low-flow nasal oxygen during the test to determine if this therapy improves his cardiopulmonary function. • The patient's blood pressure and ECG are monitored for 10 to 15 minutes after the test.
Lung perfusion scan • To detect and assess a pulmonary vascular obstruction such as a pulmonary embolism	• This test takes about 30 minutes. • The patient lies in a supine position on a table as a radioactive protein substance is injected into an arm vein. This substance travels through the bloodstream to the lungs, where it's detected by a large scanning camera. Pictures are taken while the patient is supine, lying on one side, prone, and sitting. More contrast medium is injected when the patient is positioned on his stomach. • The radioactive substance exposes him to minimal radioactivity. However, he may experience some discomfort from the venipuncture and from lying on a cold, hard table.

(continued)

Teaching patients about respiratory tests *(continued)*

Test and purpose	What to teach the patient
Magnetic resonance imaging (MRI) • To help diagnose respiratory disorders by providing high-resolution, cross-sectional images of lung structures and by tracing blood flow	• This painless, noninvasive test relies on a powerful magnet, radiowaves, and a computer to produce clear cross-sectional images of the chest. The test doesn't expose the patient to radiation but does involve exposure to a strong magnetic field. • Although MRI is painless, the patient may feel uncomfortable because he must remain still inside a small space (in most facilities). If he suffers from claustrophobia, he may not be able to tolerate the procedure or may need sedation. • The patient must remove all jewelry and other metal objects. If he has shrapnel, a pacemaker, or any surgically implanted joints, pins, clips, valves, or pumps containing metal that could be attracted to the strong MRI magnet, he won't be able to have this test. • The patient is checked at the scanner room door one last time for metal objects. He may receive a sedative. Then he lies in a supine position on a narrow bed, which slides into a large cylinder housing the MRI magnets. Radiofrequency energy is directed at the chest; the resulting images are displayed on a monitor and recorded. The scanner will make clicking, whirring, and thumping noises as it moves inside its housing to obtain different images; the patient may receive earplugs. He'll be able to communicate with the technician at all times, and the procedure will be stopped if he feels claustrophobic.
Mediastinoscopy • To visualize and obtain a biopsy of the mediastinal area to confirm an occupational respiratory disorder • To detect bronchogenic carcinoma, lymphoma, or sarcoidosis • To determine staging of lung cancer	• The patient must not eat or drink for 8 hours before the test. He'll receive an I.V. sedative before the test and then a general anesthetic. • After inserting an endotracheal tube, the surgeon makes a small transverse suprasternal incision. Then he inserts a mediastinoscope through this incision to obtain tissue specimens for analysis. • The patient may remain intubated for several hours or overnight. He may experience pain or tenderness at the incision site, a sore throat, and hoarseness; however, these effects soon pass.
Pleural biopsy • To differentiate between nonmalignant and malignant disease • To diagnose viral, fungal, or parasitic disease, and collagen vascular disease of the pleura	• This test takes 30 to 45 minutes, although the needle remains in the pleura less than 1 minute. • Blood is drawn for various studies, and chest X-rays are taken. The biopsy site is cleaned and a local anesthetic is injected. • The patient may sit on the edge of the bed and lean forward on the overbed table with arms resting on a pillow and feet resting on a stool, he may straddle a chair, or he may sit in bed in semi-Fowler's position. The doctor will probably use an ultrasound device to guide a needle (an Abrams' or a Cope's needle) through the thorax wall to obtain a sample of pleural tissue. The patient may feel some pressure as the needle enters the chest cavity. He must not move, breathe deeply, or cough while the needle is in place. • The doctor applies pressure and a bandage to the catheter insertion site, and a chest X-ray is taken to check for complications. The patient should tell the doctor if he feels faint or has increased breathing difficulty, chest pain, or an urge to cough.

Teaching patients about respiratory tests *(continued)*

Test and purpose	What to teach the patient
Pulmonary angiography (pulmonary arteriography) • To confirm diagnosis of a pulmonary embolism	• This test a takes about 1 hour. • The patient must fast for 6 hours before the test, or as ordered. He may continue taking prescribed drugs unless the doctor orders otherwise. • The patient should remove his clothing, except for socks, and put on a gown that fastens in the front. He's asked to void just before the test. • The patient must remove the gown, but will be covered with sheets and sterile drapes. He lies in a supine position on a table and ECG electrodes are attached to his arms and legs to monitor his heart. A blood pressure cuff is wrapped around his arm and an I.V. line is started. After injecting a local anesthetic, the doctor makes a small incision or a percutaneous needle puncture in an antecubital, femoral, jugular, or subclavian vein. The patient may feel pressure. Next, the doctor inserts and advances a catheter through the vein to the right side of the heart and the pulmonary artery, where he measures pressures and withdraws blood samples. A radiopaque contrast medium is injected into the catheter. The patient may experience a flushed feeling, nausea, or a salty taste for a few minutes after contrast medium injection. X-ray films are taken as the contrast medium circulates through the pulmonary vessels. When the test is completed, the doctor withdraws the catheter and applies a pressure dressing to the insertion site. • The patient should tell the doctor if he experiences shortness of breath, palpitations, chest pain, persistent nausea, numbness or tingling, or wheezing during the test. • The patient's vital signs are monitored during the first 1 to 2 hours, and the catheter insertion site is checked. If a femoral or antecubital vein was used, the patient may need to restrict activity in the affected limb for 4 to 6 hours. He should report wheezing, palpitations, chest pain, itching, nausea, vomiting, irritability, or euphoria after the test as well as redness, swelling, or bleeding at the insertion site.
Pulmonary function tests • To determine the cause of breathing problems • To determine whether a functional abnormality is obstructive or restrictive • To estimate the degree of pulmonary dysfunction in obstructive and restrictive diseases • To evaluate the effectiveness of therapy, such as use of bronchodilators or steroids	• The patient should put on loose, comfortable clothing. If he wears dentures, he should keep them in to help form a tight seal around the mouthpiece. Just before the test, he must void. • The patient sits upright and wears a nose clip. Alternatively, he may sit in a small, airtight box called a *body plethysmograph* and won't need the nose clip. Inside the plethysmograph, he may experience claustrophobia. • He may be asked to breathe in a certain way for each test; for example, to inhale deeply and exhale completely or to inhale quickly. He may receive an aerosolized bronchodilator and may then repeat one or two tests to evaluate the drug's effectiveness. An arterial puncture may also be performed during the test for arterial blood gas analysis. • The test will proceed quickly if the patient follows directions, tries hard, and keeps a tight seal around the mouthpiece or tube to ensure accurate results. • The patient may experience dyspnea and fatigue during the test but will be allowed to rest periodically. He should tell the technician if he experiences dizziness, chest pain, palpitations, nausea, severe difficulty breathing, or wheezing.

(continued)

Teaching patients about respiratory tests *(continued)*

Test and purpose	What to teach the patient
Sputum analysis • To identify the cause of pulmonary infection, thus aiding diagnosis of respiratory diseases (most frequently bronchitis, tuberculosis, lung abscess, and pneumonia)	• The patient should drink plenty of fluids the night before and avoid brushing his teeth before collection. If the specimen will be collected by bronchoscopy, he should fast for 6 hours before the procedure. • If the specimen will be collected by expectoration, the patient should take several deep abdominal breaths. When he's ready to cough, he should take one more deep abdominal breath, bend forward, and cough into the provided sterile container. • If the specimen will be collected by tracheal suctioning, the patient receives oxygen before and after the procedure, if necessary. The doctor passes a suction catheter through the patient's nostril and advances it into the trachea. Then he applies suction briefly to obtain the specimen. The patient will experience some discomfort as the catheter passes into the trachea. • If the specimen will be collected by bronchoscopy, a local anesthetic is sprayed into the patient's throat or he gargles with a local anesthetic. Next, the bronchoscope is inserted into the bronchus. Secretions are then collected, and the bronchoscope is removed. • After tracheal suctioning, the patient is given a drink of water. After bronchoscopy, he's observed for possible complications. He can have liquids as soon as his gag reflex returns.
Thoracentesis (pleural fluid aspiration) • To obtain a specimen of pleural fluid for analysis • To relieve lung compression caused by pleural fluid, blood, or air • To obtain a lung tissue biopsy specimen	• The patient puts on a hospital gown, and the area around the needle insertion site is shaved. • The patient is comfortably positioned — either sitting with his arms on pillows or lying partially on his side in bed. The doctor cleans the needle insertion site with a cold antiseptic solution, then injects a local anesthetic. The patient may feel a burning sensation as the doctor injects the anesthetic. After the patient's skin is numb, the doctor inserts the needle, obtains the necessary sample, and withdraws the needle. The patient will feel pressure during needle insertion and withdrawal. He should remain still and avoid coughing, breathing deeply, or moving. He should inform the doctor right away if he experiences dyspnea, palpitations, wheezing, dizziness, weakness, or diaphoresis, which may indicate respiratory distress. After withdrawing the needle, the doctor applies slight pressure and then an adhesive bandage. • The patient's vital signs are monitored frequently for the first few hours. He should report any fluid or blood leakage from the needle insertion site and any signs of respiratory distress. A chest X-ray will be taken to detect any posttest complications.
Ventilation scan • To assess general and regional lung ventilation • To help diagnose respiratory disorders, such as pulmonary embolism and chronic obstructive pulmonary disease	• This test takes about 30 minutes. • The patient must not eat large meals, drink a large volume of fluid, or smoke for 3 hours before the test. He may continue to take his medications unless the doctor orders otherwise. Before the test, he must remove all jewelry and metal objects. • The patient sits down and breathes a radioactive gas through a mouthpiece or a tightly fitted face mask. A nuclear scanner monitors gas distribution in his lungs. The patient is instructed to breathe deeply, hold his breath, breathe out, and then breathe normally. He should remain still when he's asked to hold his breath. The amount of radioactive gas used is minimal and mixed with air. He should report any dyspnea or wheezing during the test.

Low flow

If the patient needs low-flow oxygen during exercise, instruct him and his family on how to use oxygen at home. Show the patient how to take an accurate radial pulse to monitor exercise effects.

Plan

Counsel the patient on how to plan daily activities that conserve energy and how to best cope with breathing difficulty. (See *Stop and notify.*) Advise him to alternate light and heavy tasks, rest frequently, practice pursed-lip breathing, minimize body movements, and use labor-saving devices as appropriate. (See *Overcoming shortness of breath,* page 50.)

Take care of yourself

Also discuss with the patient other self-care measures that can help manage his condition. (See *Self-care for COPD,* page 51.)

Stop and notify

Tell the patient to stop exercising and notify the doctor immediately if he experiences increased difficulty breathing, heart fluttering, extreme fatigue, nausea, dizziness, or muscle cramps or if his skin becomes pale, mottled, or clammy.

Teaching about diet

Point out that a well-balanced, nutritious diet helps compensate for the extra calories the patient expends in breathing. Because difficulty breathing and increased sputum production can discourage eating and lead to weight loss, help the patient maintain caloric intake. (See *How to improve appetite.*)

Eight glasses a day

Encourage the patient to drink plenty of water — at least eight 8-oz (237-ml) glasses daily — to thin secretions and make expectoration easier, unless the patient is on a fluid-restricted diet. Explain that adequate fluid intake also helps prevent constipation and avoid breathlessness caused by straining during defecation.

A loss is a gain

Obesity interferes with movement of the diaphragm and adds to the heart's workload. This, in turn, can increase the work of breathing. If the patient is overweight, urge him to follow a medically supervised weight-loss diet.

Listen up!

How to improve appetite

To stimulate the patient's appetite and enjoyment of food, advise him to:

- maintain good oral hygiene
- chew food slowly
- eat small and more frequent meals to reduce fatigue and air swallowing
- continue oxygen therapy while eating, as instructed by the doctor.

Beforehand

Also recommend that he perform breathing exercises 1 hour before meals so secretions won't interfere with eating. Tell the patient to rest before eating.

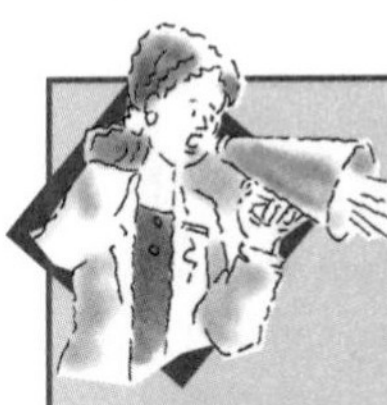

Listen up!

Overcoming shortness of breath

Breathing exercises may help a patient with chronic obstructive pulmonary disease feel better. Provide instructions on performing these exercises, and tell the patient to practice them twice a day for 5 to 10 minutes until her endurance increases.

Abdominal breathing

Instruct the patient to lie comfortably on her back and place a pillow beneath her head. Tell her to bend her knees to relax her stomach.

Next, tell her to press one hand on her stomach lightly but with enough force to create slight pressure. She should rest the other hand on her chest.

Then instruct her to breathe slowly through her nose, using the stomach muscles. The hand on her stomach should rise during inspiration and fall during expiration. The hand on her chest should remain almost still.

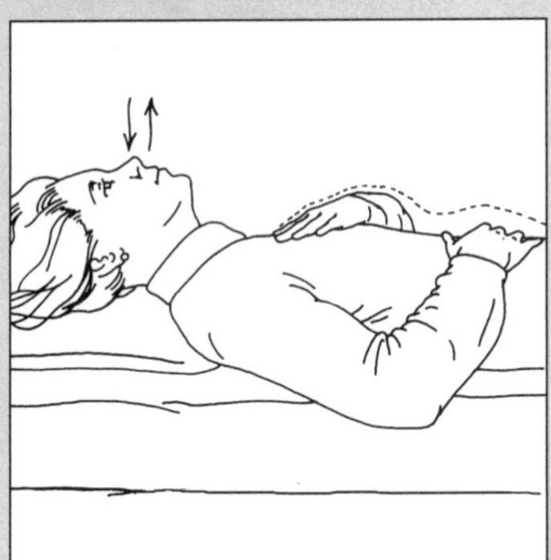

Pursed-lip breathing

Instruct the patient to breathe in slowly through her nose to avoid gulping air. Tell her to hold her breath as she counts to herself: "one-1,000; two-1,000; three-1,000."

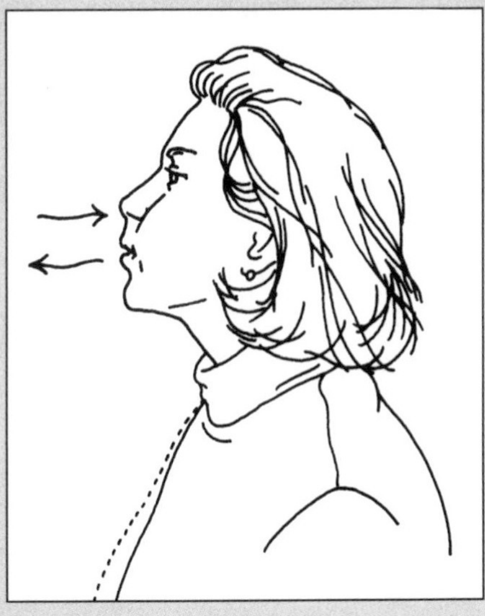

Next, tell her to purse her lips as if she's going to whistle. Then have her breathe out slowly through pursed lips as she counts to herself: "one-1,000; two-1,000; three-1,000; four-1,000; five-1,000; six-1,000."

Tell her that she should make a soft, whistling sound while she breathes out. Explain that exhaling through pursed lips slows her breathing and helps get rid of the stale air trapped in her lungs.

Describe how to perform pursed-lip breathing during activity: The patient inhales before exerting herself and then exhales while performing the activity.

If the recommended counting rhythm feels awkward to the patient, tell her to find one that feels more comfortable. Remind her to breathe out longer than she breathes in.

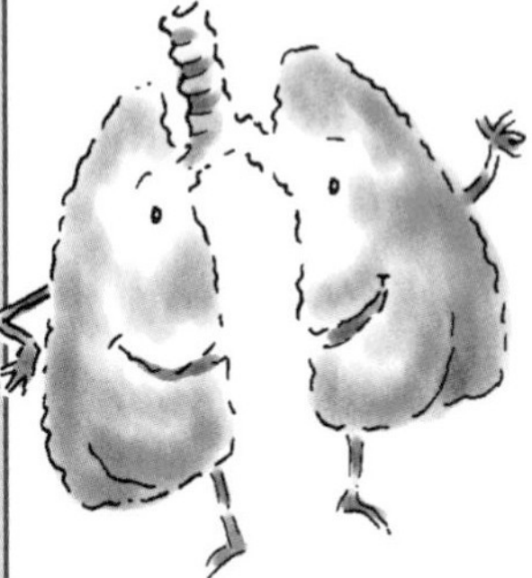
This sounds like good advice to me!

Teaching about medication

To treat COPD using medication, the doctor may choose from several options, including:
- inhalers
- oral bronchodilators
- corticosteroids
- antibiotics.

Inhalers

Inhaled bronchodilators, used in treating bronchospasms, are fast-acting, well tolerated, and highly effective. Make

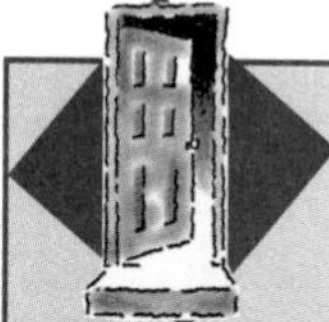

No place like home

Self-care for COPD

Self-care measures can improve the patient's quality of life and prevent a long, severe attack of chronic obstructive pulmonary disease (COPD). Explain to your patient that employing these measures may also eliminate the need for hospitalization.

Tell 'em

Urge the patient to report these early signs and symptoms of COPD complications:
- increased breathing difficulty
- wheezing
- fatigue
- change in cough or sputum production.

Why risk it?

The COPD patient's limited pulmonary reserve makes him susceptible to respiratory infection. To reduce his risk of infection, encourage the patient to do the following:

 Get prompt treatment for infection.

 Use proper hand-washing technique.

 Avoid people with infections.

Traffic, smog, cold, heat

Make sure the patient understands that pollutants and irritants can worsen his symptoms and that he should adhere to the following precautions:
- Whenever possible, he should try to avoid heavy traffic and smog. Also, counsel him to refrain from using aerosol sprays and to keep his home as dust-free as possible. Of course, smoking is extremely harmful.
- Tell the patient that exposure to blasts of cold or dry air can trigger bronchospasm, and that dry air can also thicken mucus. Whenever possible, he should avoid cold winds or cover his mouth with a scarf or mask when outdoors in cold weather.
- Point out that heat can also be dangerous. Urge him to stay indoors, keep the windows closed, and use an air conditioner on hot days when the air quality is poor. Instruct him to maintain environmental humidity at levels between 40% and 50% whenever possible.

Get comfy

Teach your patient how to position himself for comfort. If your patient is orthopneic (able to breath easily only when upright), teach him to prop himself up in bed with pillows, or teach him the tripod position (sitting down and leaning forward using arms for support), which promotes full lung expansion.

More info

To help the patient cope with his condition, give him the address and phone number of the American Lung Association. For help in quitting smoking, refer the patient to the American Cancer Society.

sure the patient understands the correct use of an inhaler, which requires a certain degree of mind-muscle coordination. (See *How to use an inhaler.*)

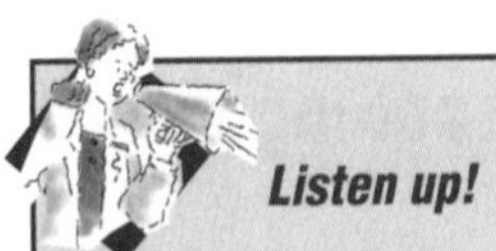

How to use an inhaler

When teaching your patient how to use an inhaler, tell him to:

- remove the cap and shake the inhaler to mix the contents (if a spacer is prescribed, attach it to the mouthpiece)
- breathe out to exhale as much air as he can
- tilt his head back
- put the inhaler mouthpiece in his mouth, keeping his tongue flat, or hold the inhaler upright $^3/_4$" to $1^1/_2$" (2 to 4 cm) from his mouth
- breathe in slowly and deeply and immediately depress the canister
- continue to breathe in slowly for 5 to 10 seconds
- hold his breath for 10 seconds or as long as is comfortable
- breathe out slowly
- wait one minute (if more than one puff is prescribed) and then repeat the procedure.

Enough of a puff?

Teach your patient to be aware of the number of "puffs," or actuations, that are in each medication vial. Advise the patient to keep a record of the number of puffs he takes to avoid using an empty vial or one that merely dispenses propellant when medication is needed.

Tell 'em

Tell the patient to notify the doctor if the inhaled drug seems to have lost its effectiveness or if he experiences tremors, nausea, vomiting, or rapid or irregular pulse.

Away from heat

Instruct the patient to store the medication away from heat. Tell him not to take nonprescription medications such as cold preparations because of potential interactions with the inhaler.

Oral bronchodilators

Oral bronchodilators such as theophylline (Theo-Dur) are sometimes used when inhalers alone don't effectively control bronchospasm. (See *How to take an oral bronchodilator.*)

Oral bronchodilators are slower acting than inhalers. They're rarely used as a primary treatment because of adverse effects, such as tremors, fast pulse, and palpitations.

Corticosteroids

Corticosteroids are anti-inflammatory drugs that are a mainstay in the treatment of asthma and other airway diseases. When administered by inhalation, the drug is delivered directly to the bronchial wall. Aerosol administration causes fewer overall adverse effects but may lead to thrush, a yeast infection in the mouth.

Stay alert

Warn the patient using an inhaled corticosteroid, such as beclomethasone dipropionate (Beclovent) or flunisolide (AeroBid), to stay alert for signs and symptoms of systemic absorption, including weight gain, increased thirst, and polyuria, and to notify the doctor if these occur.

More than one

If the patient uses more than one inhaler, provide the following advice:

• Tell the patient to inhale the bronchodilator 15 minutes before he inhales the corticosteroid.

• Advise the patient to rinse his mouth after using the inhaler to reduce the risk of oral fungal infections.

• Instruct the patient to call the doctor if he notices a decreased response to the drug, develops a fever, or develops local irritation.

Or else oral

Take an oral corticosteroid with food or milk.

In more severe cases, the doctor may prescribe an oral corticosteroid such as prednisone (Deltasone). Instruct the patient on long-term oral corticosteroid therapy to watch for adverse effects, such as weight gain, stomach ulcers, and fluid retention. To minimize these effects, the doctor may prescribe alternate-day therapy.

If the doctor prescribes an oral corticosteroid, provide the following pointers:

• Explain that this therapy suppresses the immune system.

• Suggest that he take the drug with food or milk to decrease the risk of stomach irritation.

• Warn the patient not to stop taking the drug abruptly because serious complications could result.

Antibiotics

If infection complicates COPD, the patient may need antibiotic therapy. Culture and sensitivity testing is used to identify the infecting organism.

Drugs to avoid

Warn your patient against using over-the-counter drugs that may interfere with prescription drugs. (See *Medications to avoid,* page 54.)

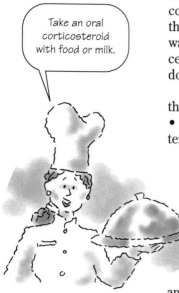

Listen up!

How to take an oral bronchodilator

If your patient is taking a xanthine-derivative bronchodilator (such as aminophylline [Aminophyllin] or theophylline), pass on this advice.

How
Take the bronchodilator with a full glass of water at mealtimes if GI upset occurs.

When
Take the medication at regularly scheduled intervals.

What not to do
Don't combine the drug with over-the-counter products, such as cold preparations, because of possible interactions. Avoid foods and beverages high in caffeine—such as coffee, tea, cola, and chocolate—because they may increase adverse effects of bronchodilators and cause tremors and palpitations.

Teaching about procedures

In addition to medication, the doctor may prescribe procedures to be performed by the patient or his family, such as chest physiotherapy and oxygen therapy.

Chest physiotherapy

Teach both the patient and a family member (or another caregiver) how to perform chest physiotherapy. Explain that this technique helps mobilize and remove mucus from the lungs. If the patient's caregiver has limited arm strength, recommend use of a mechanical percussor.

Oxygen therapy

The doctor may prescribe home oxygen therapy, specifying the type of system, flow rate, and hours of use. Give instructions for using the system to both the patient and caregivers. (See *How to use home oxygen equipment.*)

Acquaint and advise

Acquaint the patient and family with the types of oxygen delivery devices and advise them to investigate different oxygen suppliers before choosing one.

Exactly as prescribed

Make sure the patient understands that oxygen should be treated as a medication. Advise him to use it exactly as prescribed.

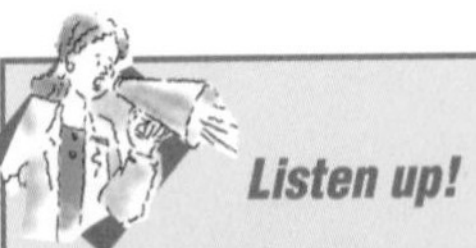

Listen up!

Medications to avoid

Tell your patient with chronic obstructive pulmonary disease to avoid the following over-the-counter drugs:
- cough suppressants
- sedatives
- sleep aids.

Why?
- These drugs can cause respiratory depression.
- Coughing is an important reflex that helps clear secretions from the airway.
- Suppressing a productive cough can worsen oxygen deficiency.

Pleural disorders

Begin by explaining to your patient that a pleural disorder affects the membranes that surround the lungs and line the chest cavity. Then describe how normal pleural function allows the lungs to operate smoothly and efficiently. Finally, review the patient's specific disorder. (See *Pleural disorders,* page 56.)

What's pleural effusion?

If the patient has pleural effusion, explain that his signs and symptoms are caused by excess fluid in the pleural space (the space between the membranes that surround the lungs and line the chest cavity).

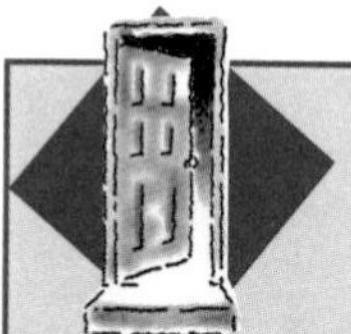

No place like home

How to use home oxygen equipment

When a home oxygen system is ordered, provide these instructions for using the equipment.

Setting up, checking, cleaning

When the patient receives his home oxygen system from a medical equipment supplier, he'll learn how to set it up, check for problems, and clean it.

The system will include a humidifier to warm and add moisture to the prescribed oxygen and a nasal cannula or a face mask through which he'll breathe the oxygen. Advise the patient to keep the supplier's phone number handy in case of problems. Also, recommend getting a backup system suitable for use in an emergency.

How to do O_2

When using an oxygen tank, an oxygen concentrator, or liquid oxygen, tell your patient to follow these important guidelines:

- Check the water level in the humidifier bottle often. If it's near or below the refill line, pour out any remaining water and refill the bottle with sterile or distilled water.
- If your nose dries, use a water-soluble lubricant such as K-Y Jelly.
- If the tubing irritates your skin, use cotton balls or moleskin to protect your skin from the tubing.
- If you need a new supply of oxygen, order it 2 or 3 days in advance or when the register reads one-quarter full.
- Maintain the oxygen flow at the prescribed rate. If you're not sure whether oxygen is flowing, check the tubing for kinks, blockages, or disconnection. Then make sure the system is on. If you're still unsure, invert the nasal cannula in a glass of water. If bubbles appear, oxygen is flowing through the system. Shake off extra water before reinserting the cannula.

Keeping it safe

- Oxygen is highly combustible. Don't use it near electrical equipment or while using an electric razor. Alert your local fire department that oxygen is in the house, and keep an all-purpose fire extinguisher on hand.
- If a fire does occur, turn off the oxygen immediately and leave the house.
- Don't smoke — and don't allow others to smoke — near the oxygen system. Keep the system away from direct sunlight, space heaters and other sources of heat, and open flames, as on a gas stove.
- Don't run oxygen tubing under clothing, bed covers, furniture, or carpets.
- Keep the oxygen system upright.
- Make sure the oxygen is turned off when it's not in use.
- Keep oxygen concentrators away from the wall to allow air to circulate.

Not enough

Tell the patient he may not be getting enough oxygen if he has these signs:

- difficult, irregular breathing
- restlessness
- anxiety
- fatigue or drowsiness
- blue fingernail beds or lips
- confusion or distractibility.

Too much

Tell the patient he may be getting too much oxygen if he has these signs:

- headaches
- slurred speech
- sleepiness or difficulty waking up
- shallow, slow breathing.

Call immediately

If any of these signs develops, the patient should call the doctor immediately. Finally, tell him never to change the oxygen flow rate without checking with the doctor first.

What's empyema?

If the patient has empyema, explain that pus or dead tissue is found in the pleural space.

What's pleurisy?

If the patient has pleurisy, explain that this disorder is marked by inflammation of the pleural linings.

What's chylothorax?

If the patient has chylothorax, explain that this rare disorder occurs when chyle, a milky fluid produced during digestion, accumulates in the pleural space.

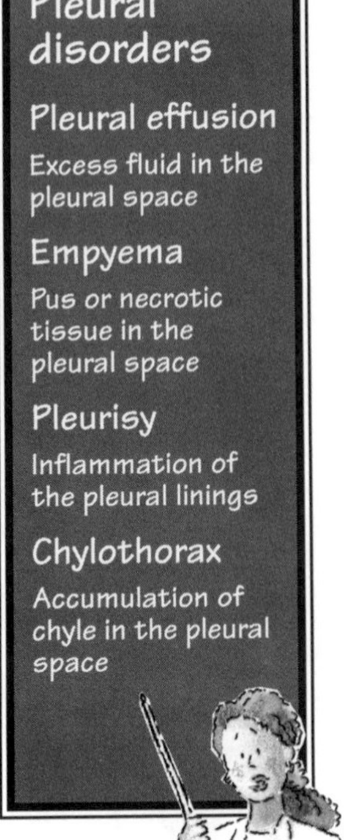

Pleural disorders
Pleural effusion
Excess fluid in the pleural space
Empyema
Pus or necrotic tissue in the pleural space
Pleurisy
Inflammation of the pleural linings
Chylothorax
Accumulation of chyle in the pleural space

Teaching about tests

Tell the patient with a suspected pleural disorder that the tests used in the diagnosis may include:
- chest X-rays
- CT scan
- pleural biopsy
- pleural fluid aspiration (thoracentesis) and analysis.

(See *Teaching patients about respiratory tests,* pages 44 to 48.)

Teaching about activity and lifestyle

Most patients with pleural disorders experience fatigue and breathlessness because the disorder deprives the body of adequate oxygen. The lower the patient's oxygen level, the greater his fatigue.

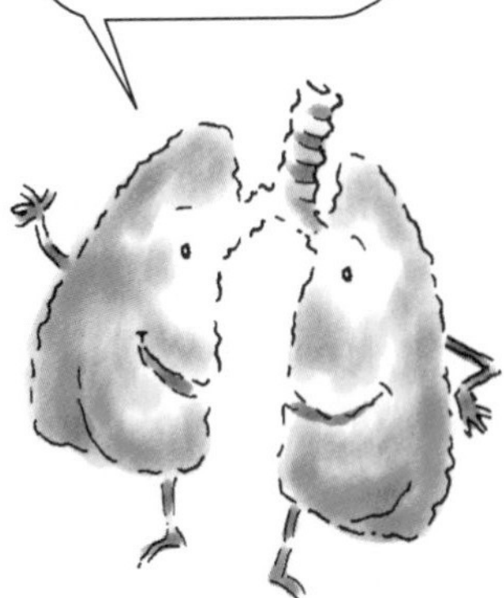

Less is more. The lower the oxygen level, the greater the fatigue.

Balancing act

Emphasize that the patient needs to find the right balance between rest (for healing) and activity (to prevent complications such as pneumonia). Suggest that he:
- take short naps (long ones may interfere with a good night's sleep)
- alternate exercise and rest periods
- schedule treatments and medications when they won't interrupt rest periods.

Pillow talk

If the patient has trouble breathing when lying down, recommend the orthopneic position: Instruct the patient to prop several pillows behind his back to keep him upright and to place several more on his lap (or on the overbed table). They'll help support and cushion the weight of his arms, shoulders, and head.

There's more

Also review additional teaching points for patients with pleural disorders. (See *Pleural disorders plus.*)

Teaching about diet

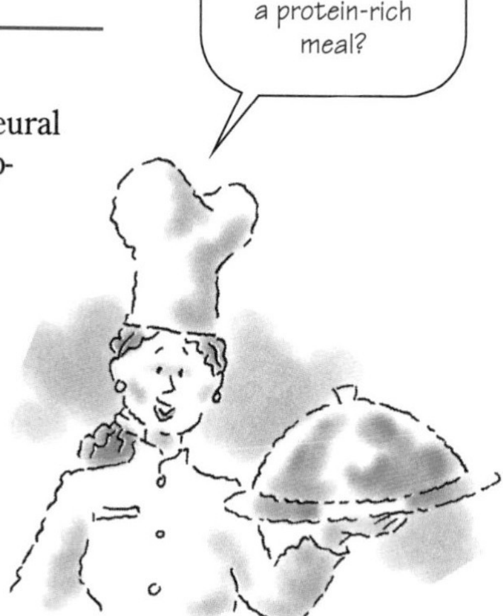
May I recommend a protein-rich meal?

Nutrition problems are common in patients with pleural disorders. The patient may complain of appetite-suppressing problems like the following:

- impaired taste and smell (from nasal congestion)
- coughing attacks that make eating difficult
- a bad taste in the mouth (from sputum and accompanying nausea).

Encourage the patient to do the following to boost the appetite:

- Brush and floss his teeth and rinse with mouthwash frequently, even if the mouthwash is half strength.

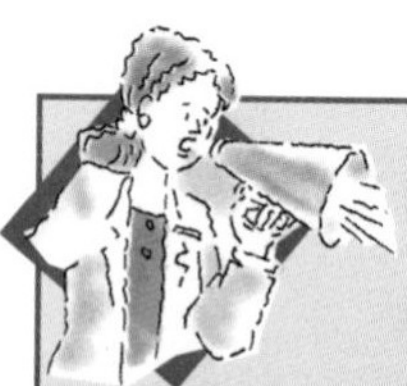

Listen up!

Pleural disorders plus

Here are a few more items to share with your patients with pleural disorders.

Chest support

If the doctor recommends chest support for a patient with pleurisy, show the patient how to tape the chest to provide support and firm pressure at the pain site. Even without chest binding, the patient can apply pressure to relieve discomfort, especially during coughing and deep breathing. Demonstrate how to use a folded blanket or pillow as a splinting device.

Other support

For information and support, refer the patient to an organization such as the American Lung Association.

- Eat small, protein-rich meals or snacks to conserve energy and ease digestion.
- Drink plenty of fluids, unless directed otherwise.

Teaching about medication

Tell the patient that medications are the primary treatment for pleural disorders. Discuss the drugs prescribed for the patient's particular disorder, explaining that they may be discontinued once the disorder is controlled.

Efforts to eliminate effusion

If the patient has pleural effusion, explain that he may receive a solution of tetracycline hydrochloride (Achromycin) or bleomycin sulfate (Blenoxane) through a chest tube to produce inflammation and adhesions. Explain that inflammations and adhesions in the pleural space may prevent repeated accumulation of pleural fluid.

Efforts against empyema

If the patient has empyema, tell him that high doses of antibiotic drugs may destroy the organism causing this infection. The drugs may be administered through a chest tube or I.V. or I.M.

Tell the patient that, before antibiotic therapy can begin, tests are used to find the cause of the infection.

Plans for pleurisy

Tell the patient with pleurisy that the goal of drug treatment is to relieve his symptoms. The doctor may recommend antitussive (anticough) therapy to control coughing. Teach the patient about possible adverse effects of cough suppressants. (See *Adverse effects of cough suppressants.*)

Extinguishing inflammation

If the doctor prescribes a nonsteroidal anti-inflammatory drug, such as ibuprofen, tell the patient that this drug reduces inflammation. Clarify the prescribed dosage. Caution him that, although they're usually mild with short-term therapy, the following adverse effects can be caused by this drug:
- dizziness
- GI upset
- insomnia.

Adverse effects of cough suppressants

- Insomnia
- Nervousness
- Irritability
- Unusual excitement
- Dizziness
- Drowsiness
- Stomach upset

For severe pain

If the patient needs a narcotic analgesic for severe pleuritic pain, the doctor may prescribe morphine (Duramorph), codeine, or meperidine (Demerol). Mention that some narcotic analgesics, such as codeine, have antitussive properties.

Yikes! Dry mouth, drowsiness

Point out the adverse effects of narcotic analgesics, such as constipation, dry mouth, and drowsiness. (See *A bad mix*.)

A bad mix

Drinking alcohol while taking a narcotic may:

- increase CNS depression
- worsen drowsiness and confusion
- lead to physical and psychological dependence (with prolonged use).

Teaching about procedures

Tell the patient that, in addition to medication, procedures used to control pleural disorders include oxygen therapy and thoracentesis.

Oxygen therapy

Tell the patient that oxygen therapy is usually necessary to treat pleural effusion or empyema. The flow rate, type of delivery system, and duration of therapy depend on the patient's disorder and the severity of his dyspnea.

Thoracentesis

Tell the patient with pleural effusion, empyema, or pleurisy with pleural effusion that thoracentesis may be performed. This procedure is used to drain the pleural space and relieve breathing difficulties.

Add that thoracentesis may be followed by insertion of a chest tube (to remove fluid or air) and closed drainage. Describe the chest tube insertion and drainage procedure.

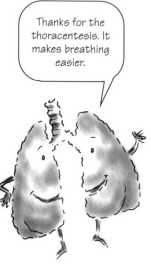

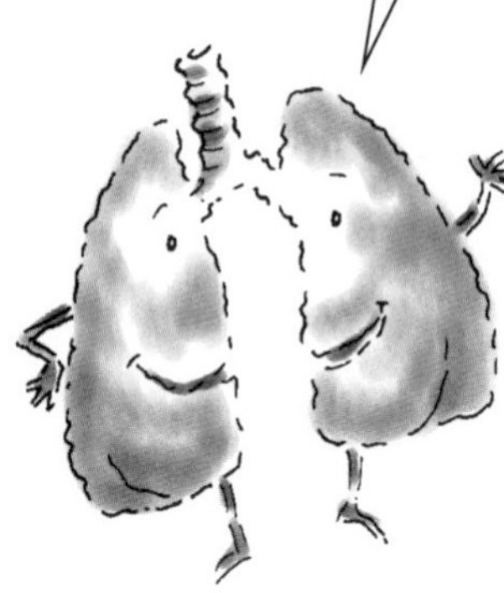

Thanks for the thoracentesis. It makes breathing easier.

Teaching about surgery

If the patient has severe empyema, explain that a surgical procedure called decortication may be performed. In this procedure, the membrane around the lung is removed. Rib resection may also be necessary to allow for drainage and lung expansion.

Pneumonia

Tell the patient that pneumonia is a lung infection that interferes with oxygen and carbon dioxide exchange.

How does it happen?

Explain that pneumonia develops when pathogens overwhelm the body's respiratory defenses. Normally, the upper and lower airways stop most pathogens from reaching the alveoli (air sacs in the lungs), where gas exchange takes place. The immune system provides backup by destroying any remaining pathogens. If all natural defenses fail, pneumonia can develop. (See *Signs of pneumonia.*)

Signs of pneumonia

- Fever
- Chest pain
- Shaking chills
- Difficulty breathing
- Rapid respiration
- Coughing

Why does it happen?

Pneumonia is usually a result of inhaling or aspirating a pathogen. The most common causative agents for primary pneumonia are:

- bacteria
- viruses
- fungi
- protozoa.

Pneumonia may also result from inhaling chemicals or toxins or the spread of bacteria to the lungs from elsewhere in the body. (See *Risk factors for pneumonia.*)

Where does it happen?

Pneumonia may be classified according to its location in the respiratory system:

- the distal airways and alveoli (bronchopneumonia)
- part of a lobe (lobular pneumonia)
- an entire lobe (lobar pneumonia).

What's the risk?

Emphasize that untreated or inadequately treated pneumonia can lead to life-threatening complications, such as septic shock, hypoxemia, and respiratory failure.

With inadequate treatment, the infection can spread within the lung, or it may spread by the bloodstream or by cross-contamination and infect other parts of the body, causing bacteremia, endocarditis, pericarditis, or meningitis.

Teaching about tests

Tell the patient about standard tests to detect and monitor the progression of pneumonia:
- sputum analysis
- blood studies
- chest X-ray. (See *Teaching patients about respiratory tests*, pages 44 to 48.)

If sputum analysis and blood culture results don't reveal the identification of the causative organism and the patient remains ill despite conventional therapy, the doctor may order more invasive studies, such as:
- bronchoscopy
- needle biopsy
- open-lung biopsy.

Risk factors for pneumonia

- Viral infection, such as a cold or influenza
- Age (under 1 year and over 65 years)
- Chronic illness and less efficient lung function
- Smoking and alcohol consumption
- Chronic lung diseases, such as emphysema and cystic fibrosis
- Depressed immune system
- Prolonged bed rest
- Use of narcotics and anesthesia
- Chest or abdominal surgery
- Neuromuscular disorders
- Exposure to contaminated air or water

Teaching about activity and lifestyle

Urge the patient to get adequate rest, which promotes a full recovery and helps prevent a relapse. (See *How long?* page 62.)

Home care

Also review with the patient important home-care measures for pneumonia. (See *Living with pneumonia*, page 63.)

Teaching about medication

Tell the patient that the doctor usually prescribes a broad-spectrum antibiotic, such as penicillin and erythromycin, based on results of the Gram stain of sputum. When pneumonia's cause is identified (through culture and sensitivity tests), the doctor may prescribe an antibiotic specific to the infecting organism.

Stick with it

Discuss the prescribed medication and reinforce instructions. Although the patient's condition may improve dramatically after only a few days of treatment, stress that he must take prescribed medication for the entire course of therapy (7 to 10 days) to prevent a relapse. Warn him that recurrent pneumonia can be far more serious than the initial illness.

Teaching about procedures

Other procedures to treat pneumonia may include breathing exercises, effective coughing, hydration therapy, chest physiotherapy, and oxygen therapy.

Breathing exercises

Show the patient how to perform deep breathing and pursed-lip breathing:
• Demonstrate the proper position for maximum effectiveness.
• Instruct the patient to sit upright, placing both feet on the floor.
• If he must remain in bed, tell the patient how to assume high Fowler's position.
• Demonstrate prolonged deep inspiration through the nose and slow exhalation through pursed lips.

Effective coughing

Tell the patient that effective coughing can help expel lung secretions. He should use the same position he uses for deep breathing. Show him how to flex his body at the waist if he's sitting or how to bend his knees if he's in a high Fowler's position. If he must lie flat, direct him to lie on one side and bend his knees. Then instruct him to breathe deeply through his nose, hold his breath for a few seconds, and cough twice to bring up any sputum. Finally, tell him to inhale by sniffing gently and then expectorate into a strong tissue. (Swallowed mucus can upset the stomach.)

Hydration therapy

Encourage the patient to drink 2 to 3 qt (2 to 3 L) of fluid per day to promote adequate hydration and keep mucus secretions thin for easier removal. Without adequate hydration, infected secretions become thick and tenacious. Fever and tachypnea also increase mucoid thickening, thereby providing an excellent medium for growth of the infecting organism.

How long?

Explain to your patient with pneumonia that convalescent time depends on:
• age
• health history
• severity of the infection.

Young vs. middle age
For example, a young, usually healthy patient can resume typical activities within a week of recovery, whereas a middle-aged or chronically ill patient may need several weeks before regaining his usual strength. Caution such a patient that he may tire easily, and encourage him to alternate activity with rest to conserve his energy.

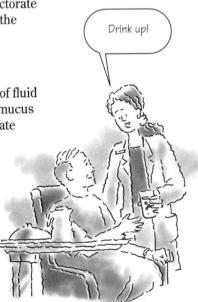

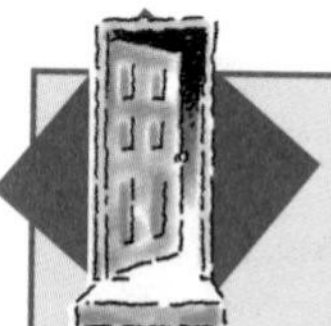

No place like home

Living with pneumonia

Here are more topics to discuss with your patient with pneumonia.

Nix the irritants
Urge the patient to avoid irritants that stimulate secretions, such as cigarette smoke, dust, and significant environmental pollution. Refer him to community programs that can help him stop smoking.

Protect others
To avoid spreading infection to others, remind the patient to sneeze and cough into tissues and to dispose of the tissues in a waxed or plastic bag. Advise him to wash his hands thoroughly after handling contaminated tissues.

Why risk it?
Because pneumonia caused by influenza usually carries a poor prognosis—even with treatment—encourage the patient to obtain yearly influenza immunization, unless he has a demonstrated allergy to eggs or to a previous influenza vaccine. Encourage the high-risk patient (over age 65, with chronic heart, renal, or lung disease, sickle cell anemia, or diabetes) to ask the doctor about pneumococcal pneumonia vaccination (Pneumovax 23).

More help and info
To promote a full recovery, advise the patient to contact the American Lung Association.

Chest physiotherapy

Include the patient's family when you discuss chest physiotherapy. Explain that postural drainage, percussion, and vibration help to mobilize and remove mucus from the lungs.

Show the patient how to position himself for gravity drainage of the affected lung segment or lobe. Ambulatory and upright positions naturally drain the upper lobes. The lower lobes (except for the superior segments) are best drained with the patient in Trendelenburg's position.

Oxygen therapy

If the patient will be receiving oxygen at home, teach him how to use the equipment. (See *How to use home oxygen equipment*, page 55.)

Pulmonary embolism

More than any other respiratory disorder, pulmonary embolism is likely to complicate the recovery of a hospitalized patient. As a result, many patients need to learn about the risk factors and warning signs of pulmonary embolism. Also, after an embolus resolves, some patients may not comply fully with prolonged anticoagulant therapy. In your teaching, encourage full compliance with treatment plans.

What happens?

Tell the patient that pulmonary embolism occurs when a mass, such as a dislodged thrombus or blood clot, lodges in an artery of the lung. (See *Why PE occurs.*)

What happens after that?

Tell the patient that the clot obstructs perfusion, or blood flow, to a portion of the lung; air in this part of the lung can't participate in gas exchange.

The patient must breathe faster and with more effort to avoid hypoxemia (oxygen depletion of the blood). The patient may also wheeze because of distal airway constriction. This is the body's attempt to shunt air from nonperfused to perfused areas of the lung.

Why PE occurs

Briefly discuss the most common cause of pulmonary embolism — a dislodged blood clot, or thrombus, usually originating in the deep leg veins, that results from one of the following:
- vascular wall damage
- venous stasis
- hypercoagulability of the blood.

A spontaneous journey
The thrombi may travel spontaneously during clot dissolution or become dislodged during trauma, sudden muscle action, or a change in peripheral blood flow.

Teaching about tests

Discuss the studies used to detect pulmonary embolism and to evaluate the patient's response to anticoagulant therapy, including the following:
- To help confirm pulmonary embolism, the doctor may order a lung perfusion scan, a ventilation scan, arterial blood gas measurements, pulmonary angiography, and an ECG.
- To detect peripheral venous thrombosis, the doctor may schedule Doppler ultrasonography or impedance plethysmography.
- To rule out other disorders, the doctor may order blood tests to determine the white blood cell (WBC) count, erythrocyte sedimentation rate, fibrin split products, and serum lactate dehydrogenase, aspartate aminotransferase, and bilirubin levels. He may also order a chest X-ray. (See *Teaching patients about respiratory tests,* pages 44 to 48.)

Clocking clot time

If the patient has acute pulmonary embolism, tell him that the doctor monitors the results of coagulation tests (clotting time, prothrombin time [PT], or activated partial thromboplastin time). Tell him that test results are used to evaluate his response to heparin therapy. The patient who's on heparin therapy needs daily coagulation studies.

Tell the patient that when he begins oral anticoagulants, the doctor will monitor PT until the desired anticoagulant level is reached.

Once a week

Remind the patient that when discharged and on anticoagulant therapy, he must return for periodic blood tests to monitor PT. Usually, blood is drawn once a week until PT stabilizes, then every 2 weeks and, eventually, once per month.

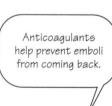

> **Preventing blood pooling**
>
> - Don't stand or sit with legs dangling or crossed.
> - Stop frequently for short walks during long car rides.
> - Periodically stroll up and down the aisle on airplane trips.

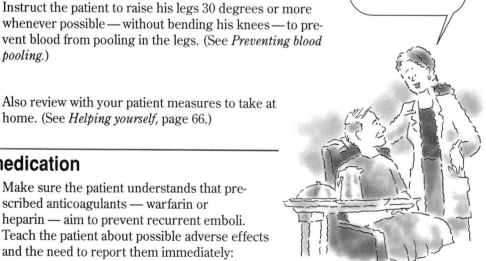

Teaching about activity and lifestyle

The good news is that most emboli resolve within 14 days. The goal of the treatment plan is to maintain adequate heart and lung function until the obstruction resolves and to prevent the embolism from recurring.

Rock, flex, extend

Tell the patient that prolonged standing, sitting, or inactivity can cause venous stasis, which sets the stage for blood clots in the legs. Encourage the patient to exercise his legs frequently to promote blood flow. Demonstrate exercises that can be done easily such as rocking on the heels or toes. If the patient is disabled or restricted to bed rest, instruct family members or other caregivers to perform passive leg exercises by flexing and extending his feet at the ankles.

30 degrees

Instruct the patient to raise his legs 30 degrees or more whenever possible — without bending his knees — to prevent blood from pooling in the legs. (See *Preventing blood pooling.*)

At home

Also review with your patient measures to take at home. (See *Helping yourself,* page 66.)

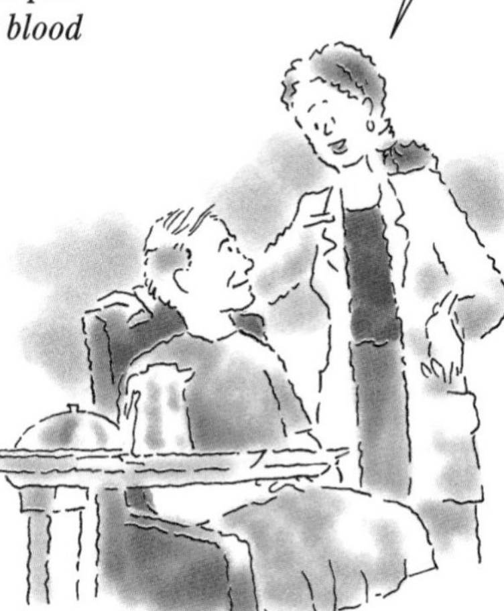
Anticoagulants help prevent emboli from coming back.

Teaching about medication

Make sure the patient understands that prescribed anticoagulants — warfarin or heparin — aim to prevent recurrent emboli. Teach the patient about possible adverse effects and the need to report them immediately:

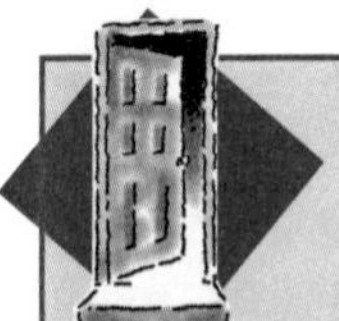

No place like home

Helping yourself

Here are some home care measures to discuss with your patient who has a pulmonary embolism.

Cough, breathe

Stress the importance of coughing and deep-breathing exercises to prevent atelectasis (lung collapse).

Take stock in stockings

Teach the patient how to apply antiembolism stockings or elastic bandage wraps, if ordered, to improve circulation in the legs. Emphasize that the stockings must fit properly and be applied smoothly. The patient should put the stockings on in the morning before getting out of bed and remove them at night once he's in bed.

Don't get thrown

To ensure safety, advise the patient to remove throw rugs and small objects from floors to help prevent falls. If the patient does fall, tell him to call the doctor, who may want to examine him to rule out internal bleeding.

Talk about it

Teach patients to recognize and immediately report the following signs and symptoms of complications:

- *thrombophlebitis* — calf pain (especially if pulling the toes backward toward the head makes the calf hurt more), swelling
- *postphlebitis syndrome* — lower leg swelling, ankle swelling, hyperpigmentation, ulceration
- *recurrent pulmonary embolism* — dyspnea, tachypnea, chest pain (especially when trying to take a deep breath), coughing up blood, apprehension or a feeling that "something isn't right," or a dry, annoying cough.

If the patient has underlying cardiopulmonary disease, instruct him to immediately report:

- fatigue
- swelling of the feet or ankles
- unexplained steady weight gain
- chest tightness.

Because pulmonary embolism can also trigger arrhythmias, such as atrial fibrillation or atrial flutter, tell the patient to report palpitations.

Info and support

If the patient is at high risk for recurrence of pulmonary embolism, refer him to the American Lung Association for information and support.

- bleeding gums
- nosebleeds
- bleeding hemorrhoids
- red or purple skin spots
- excessive menstrual flow.

War on clots

If the patient is taking warfarin, stress the importance of continuing this medication at home and returning for periodic blood tests. If the patient can't tolerate anticoagulants, the doctor may order aspirin or dipyridamole instead. Tell the patient to take these medications exactly as ordered.

Thwarting a thrombus

If the patient's embolism was caused by a thrombus, explain that treatment generally consists of anticoagulation with heparin as well as oxygen therapy as needed. He may also receive warfarin for 3 to 6 months, depending on his risk factors.

Within 14 hours

If the patient has a massive pulmonary embolism and shock, the doctor may prescribe fibrinolytic therapy with thrombolytic agents, such as streptokinase or urokinase. Explain that, when given early, thrombolytic agents dissolve clots within 14 hours. If the embolus causes hypotension, the patient may need a vasopressor such as dopamine.

A septic exception

Tell the patient who has a septic embolus that he will require antibiotic therapy specific to the causative agent, not anticoagulants, and that he will be evaluated for the infection source (most likely endocarditis).

Why risk it?

Emphasize that the patient can avoid or minimize atelectasis (lung tissue collapse) by strictly adhering to the treatment plan. Explain how atelectasis may worsen breathing distress. Note that the patient is at risk for atelectasis until the embolus resolves.

The "write" stuff

Have the patient read printed material to assess his ability to understand written information. If the patient has difficulty reading, use teaching tools other than reading materials. For example, make drawings of what you want the patient to do as you instruct him, or tape record step-by-step guidelines.

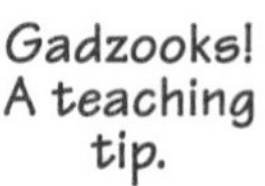
Gadzooks! A teaching tip.

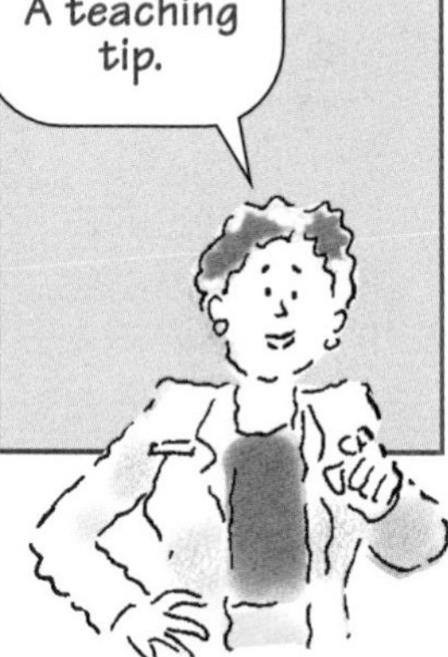

Teaching about surgery

A patient who can't take anticoagulants or who develops recurrent emboli during anticoagulant therapy may require surgery to insert a filter into the inferior vena cava. This umbrella-shaped device filters blood returning to the heart and lungs, trapping clots and avoiding emboli.

After surgery

Tell the patient that he may receive heparin or other medications to prevent blood clots after surgery. To prevent postoperative clotting problems (venous thromboembolism), pneumatic boots, sequential compression devices, or antiembolism stockings may be prescribed.

These devices may also be prescribed for patients who can't take anticoagulants.

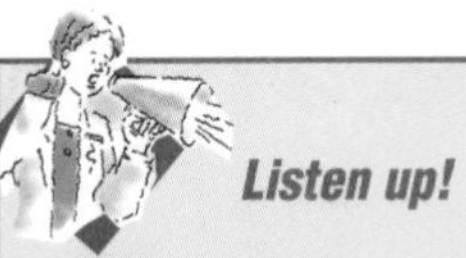

Listen up!

Two truths about tuberculosis

Your patient may know little about tuberculosis or may be misinformed. Clear up misconceptions by telling him the following:

- Chest X-rays and sputum cultures easily detect tuberculosis.
- New drugs and improved medical management can cure (not simply arrest) tuberculosis.

Tuberculosis

Despite better health care, improved drug therapy, and efficient screening programs, tuberculosis continues to infect many. Eight million new cases of tuberculosis are diagnosed in the world each year. As recently as 1996, 21,327 new cases were reported in the U.S. Factors contributing to the persistence of this disorder may include human immunodeficiency virus (HIV) infection, alcoholism, and drug abuse. (See *Two truths about tuberculosis.*)

What is it?

Tell the patient that this contagious disorder results from infection with an organism called *Mycobacterium tuberculosis*. It's transmitted through repeated inhalations of airborne bacteria from an infected person's sputum. The bacilli may disperse into the air when an infected person laughs, coughs, or sneezes.

What happens once you're infected?

Although many people may be infected with this organism, most fight off the infection and establish some immunity. Only a few people actually contract the disorder. The patient suspected of having tuberculosis is placed in respiratory isolation to prevent the spread of tuberculosis to others. Those exposed to the most bacilli are the most severely affected.

How does it happen?

Explain to your patient how a person commonly contracts tuberculosis. (See *How tuberculosis develops.*)

What is the infection like?

Signs and symptoms of the infection vary; after the incubation period, a patient with primary tuberculosis may be asymptomatic, or his symptoms may be vague, including:
- fatigue
- weakness
- anorexia
- weight loss

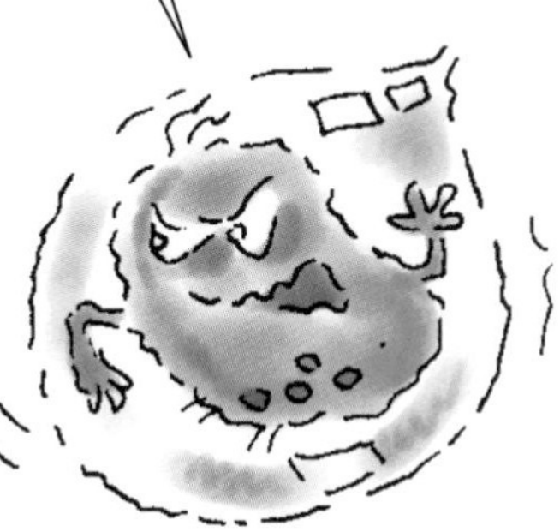
Tell your patient about the dangers of airborne bacteria in an infected person's sputum.

- night sweats
- low-grade fever.

If the patient becomes acutely ill, symptoms may include the following:

- intermittent or persistent fever
- cough
- dyspnea
- unexplained weight loss
- anorexia
- excessive sweating—especially at night.

Eventually, the patient may develop tubercular pneumonia, and exhibit these signs and symptoms:

- shortness of breath
- cough
- fever
- chest pain.

If tuberculosis spreads to the brain, heart, joints, or kidneys, the patient's signs and symptoms vary depending upon the body system affected.

What is secondary tuberculosis?

Point out that most patients with diagnosed tuberculosis have secondary tuberculosis; that is, they contracted the disorder months or years before diagnosis and treatment.

Some experts think that secondary tuberculosis erupts after a prolonged dormancy, when the patient's immune system encounters stress. Others argue that this disorder isn't reactivated tuberculosis but, instead, constitutes reinfection with new bacilli.

Regardless of the cause, the signs and symptoms resemble those of primary tuberculosis. Unfortunately, many patients endure signs and symptoms for a long time before seeking medical attention.

What's at risk?

Untreated tuberculosis can be fatal, with death usually resulting from pulmonary complications. Explain to your patient the dangers of neglecting treatment:

- Breathing difficulties increase as the disorder progresses.
- As cavities develop in the lungs, breakdowns occur in pulmonary blood flow and the areas for gas exchange.
- Thinning of the pulmonary artery walls heightens the danger of rupture.

Listen up!

How tuberculosis develops

When a person without immunity to tuberculosis inhales droplets of infected sputum, the bacilli lodge in the lungs. In most instances, the person's immune system contains them in nodules called tubercles.

The turning point

If the immune system can destroy the bacilli, the tubercles disappear or calcify. However, if the immune system only arrests the disorder, the live, encapsulated bacilli may lie dormant (possibly for years), reactivating and spreading later to cause active infection. Alternatively, if the bacilli overwhelm the immune system, active tuberculosis develops.

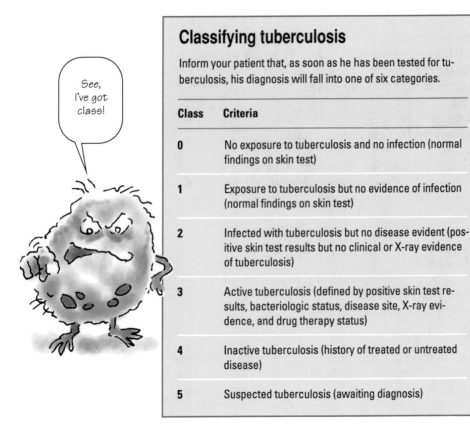

Classifying tuberculosis

Inform your patient that, as soon as he has been tested for tuberculosis, his diagnosis will fall into one of six categories.

Class	Criteria
0	No exposure to tuberculosis and no infection (normal findings on skin test)
1	Exposure to tuberculosis but no evidence of infection (normal findings on skin test)
2	Infected with tuberculosis but no disease evident (positive skin test results but no clinical or X-ray evidence of tuberculosis)
3	Active tuberculosis (defined by positive skin test results, bacteriologic status, disease site, X-ray evidence, and drug therapy status)
4	Inactive tuberculosis (history of treated or untreated disease)
5	Suspected tuberculosis (awaiting diagnosis)

- Lung tissue destruction can leave a hole between the bronchial tubes and the pleural space (bronchopleural fistula), which can lead to pneumothorax.
- Sepsis may develop from acute infection or from empyema associated with the contaminated thoracic cavity.
- Extensive lung tissue damage can lead to respiratory insufficiency and, eventually, respiratory failure.
- Occasionally, lung cancer develops in areas of tuberculosis granulation or scar tissue.

Teaching about tests

Diagnosis may involve the following tests:
- tuberculin skin test
- serial sputum analysis
- serial chest X-rays
- bronchoscopy (if the patient can't expectorate a satisfactory sputum sample).

The patient may also undergo CT scans or MRI to evaluate lung damage or to help confirm a difficult diagnosis. (See *Teaching patients about respiratory tests*, pages 44 to 48.)

Test findings are used to help classify the patient's tuberculosis and direct treatment. (See *Classifying tuberculosis*.) Some doctors simply classify the patient as having active or inactive tuberculosis, based on diagnostic test results.

Tuberculin skin test

Tell the patient that this simple test confirms exposure to the tuberculosis bacillus. Between 2 and 10 weeks after the initial infection, a skin test can detect an antibody response.

Using either a multipronged puncture device or an intradermal syringe and needle, the doctor or nurse injects a special solution into the patient's skin. Reassure the patient that he'll feel only a pinprick; the solution won't sting or burn.

Getting results

The patient may need to return in 48 to 72 hours for a skin evaluation. Tell the patient that a test not read within 72 hours must be repeated. If he's been exposed to tuberculosis, swelling and inflammation develop at the injection site.

Serial sputum analysis

Tell the patient that sputum analysis can isolate and identify the microorganism that causes tuberculosis.

First thing in the morning

Advise him to collect sputum samples first thing in the morning after secretions accumulate overnight. Instruct him to drink plenty of fluids the night before (to help thin mucus) and to wait until after the test to brush his teeth. Teach him how to prepare the specimen container. (See *Collecting a sputum sample*.)

Listen up!

Collecting a sputum sample

Instruct the patient on the following technique for collecting sputum. Make sure you show him how to avoid contaminating the container. Tell him to use this technique to collect sputum over several days, as specified by the doctor.

Here's how

- Open the sputum container, holding the lid in one hand and the container in the other.
- Avoid touching the inside of the container or the lid.
- Take several deep abdominal breaths.
- When ready to cough, take one more deep breath.
- Bend forward and make a soft, shortened cough into the container.
- Replace the lid and place the labels on the container.
- Place the sputum container in a sealable plastic bag.

Teaching about activity and lifestyle

Tell the patient that, when diagnosed, tuberculosis can be treated. (See *The tuberculosis treatment plan.*) Because fatigue is common, advise the patient to sleep 7 or 8 hours each night and to take at least one rest period during the day. Help him find ways to pace his daily routine to conserve energy. As he regains his strength, he can alter his schedule.

Don't let it happen

Also review with the patient ways to prevent the spread of tuberculosis. (See *Containing tuberculosis.*)

The tuberculosis treatment plan

- Medications to kill the bacilli
- Infection-control measures to prevent contagion
- Chest percussion and chest drainage to clear the lungs
- Rest and a high-calorie diet to promote healing and weight gain

Teaching about diet

Tell the patient that he'll need extra calories for breathing and healing damaged lung tissue. Also, because dyspnea and chronic infection can discourage eating and lead to weight loss, encourage him to follow a well-balanced, nutritious, high-calorie diet to replace calories and promote healing. As necessary, review nutritional guidelines or refer him to a dietitian.

Enhance appetite

Offer tips for enhancing the appetite, such as:

- Instruct the patient in regular oral hygiene (brushing his teeth after every meal, flossing daily, and rinsing with mouthwash). This may heighten the patient's desire to eat.
- If the patient has severe shortness of breath, suggest eating small, frequent meals to reduce fatigue.
- Advise the patient to chew food slowly and to eat nutritious snacks or drink liquid food supplements for additional nourishment between meals.

Drink up

Unless contraindicated, advise the patient to drink plenty of water to thin his mucus. Explain that adequate fluid intake also helps to prevent constipation and straining during bowel movements, which can cause breathlessness.

Have some more

Suggest eating raw fruits, vegetables, and bran to help prevent constipation. If your patient, like many tuberculosis patients, comes from a less affluent or immigrant population, help him to construct a nutritious and realistic meal plan that fits his budget and ethnic preferences.

Teaching about medication

Teach the patient about drug therapy for tuberculosis. As necessary, cover the following:
- first-line essential drugs
- first-line supplemental drugs
- second-line drugs
- preventive drug regimens.

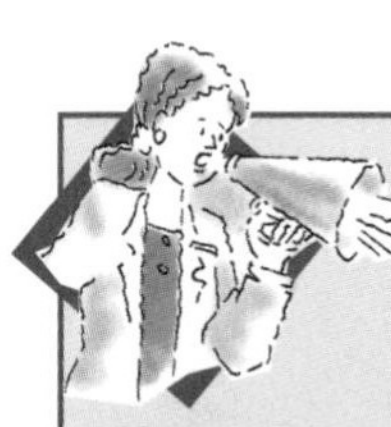

Listen up!

Containing tuberculosis

Here are some points to discuss with your patient and his family about preventing the spread of tuberculosis.

It's contagious

Be sure the patient, family, and any other caregivers understand that tuberculosis is contagious. Therefore, as long as mycobacteria live in the patient's sputum, he can spread the disorder to others.

Until tuberculosis becomes noninfective (a few weeks after drug therapy starts), caregivers must act to control infection, treating sputum as contaminated material.

Inside the hospital

Discuss infection control. Explain respiratory isolation and standard precautions. Tell him that he must have a private room to limit his exposure to others and that he should wear a mask when he's around people.

Who was that masked man?

People entering the patient's room also need to wear masks. If the patient leaves his room for treatments or tests, he and the people caring for him must wear masks.

Above all

Describe how to dispose of sputum. Direct the patient to cough and sneeze into tissues and to dispose of all secretions so that other people won't come into contact with them.

Above all, urge the patient to wash his hands thoroughly in hot, soapy water whenever he handles his own secretions.

Potential carriers

Stress the importance of identifying potential tuberculosis carriers, such as family members, friends, coworkers, or sexual partners, so they can be contacted, tested and, if necessary, treated.

When more help is needed

Refer the patient to appropriate sources of information and support such as the American Lung Association. If the patient can't care for himself, refer him and his family to the local visiting nurse agency or other appropriate caregivers. If he lives in crowded or unsanitary conditions, refer him to an agency to help find more suitable housing.

Be there!

Urge the patient to schedule and keep follow-up appointments.

First-line essential drugs

Explain to the patient that first-line essential drugs are antituberculars, and include isoniazid and rifampin (Rifadin). Tell the patient that these two drugs are essential components of any short-course therapeutic regimen. (See *Teaching about first-line drugs for tuberculosis.*)

First-line supplemental drugs

First-line supplemental drugs include pyrazinamide, ethambutol, and streptomycin. These drugs kill bacteria and are also used in short-course therapy.

Second-line drugs

Second-line antitubercular drugs are clinically effective in treating tuberculosis but frequently elicit severe reactions. They're used only against atypical mycobacterial infection or drug-resistant tuberculosis. Second-line drugs include para-aminosalicylic acid (PAS), ethionamide, cycloserine, kanamycin, amikacin, capreomycin, and thiacetazone.

Without category

Newer antitubercular drugs that haven't yet been placed in one of the three categories include rifabutin and the quinolones, especially ciprofloxacin, ofloxacin, and sparfloxacin. Tell the patient that he will usually take these drugs in combination to increase their effectiveness and decrease adverse effects.

Exactly as directed

Instruct the patient to take the medications exactly as directed for the specified duration to cure the disorder. Tell the patient that failure to comply with his drug regimen can lead to mutation of the tuberculosis strain and drug resistance. Discuss prescribed drug regimens in detail.

The end of isolation

Tell the patient that respiratory isolation will end after he has three negative sputum results.

If tuberculosis isn't active

If the patient is infected with tuberculosis bacilli but does not have active tuberculosis, explain that taking isoniazid daily for 6 to 12 months may prevent the disorder entirely. Adult patients with HIV infection usually receive treatment for 1 year after cultures are negative.

Teaching about first-line drugs for tuberculosis

Drug	Adverse reactions	What to teach the patient
First-line essential drugs		
isoniazid	Anorexia, arthritic symptoms, clumsiness or unsteadiness, dark urine, eye pain, jaundice, nausea or vomiting, unusual tiredness or weakness, visual changes, and burning, numbness, pain, tingling, or weakness in hands or feet as well as dizziness and GI upset	• Take this drug exactly as ordered, even if he feels better after a few weeks. • Treatment may last 1 year or more. • Don't take antacids containing aluminum because they interfere with this drug's absorption. • Take this drug with pyridoxine (vitamin B_6), as ordered, to avoid peripheral neuritis. • Avoid Swiss cheese and tuna fish while taking this drug because the combination can cause red or itchy skin, tachycardia, chills, sweating, headache, or light-headedness. Notify the doctor if these problems occur. • Don't drink alcohol while taking this drug because of potential liver problems. • Avoid activities that require mental alertness, such as driving a car or operating machinery, until it's known how his body responds to this drug.
rifampin (Rifadin, Rimactane)	Anorexia, bone and muscle pain, chills, dizziness, fever, headache, hematuria, nausea or vomiting, shortness of breath, sore throat, unusual bleeding or bruising, unusual drowsiness or weakness, and yellow eyes or skin as well as diarrhea, itchy or reddened skin, rash, reddish orange or reddish brown body fluids, sore mouth or tongue, and stomach cramps	• Take this drug exactly as ordered, even if he feels better after a few weeks. • Treatment may last 1 year or more. • Take a missed dose as soon as it's remembered, unless it's close to the time for the next dose (then skip the missed dose). Never double-dose. Take the drug on a regular schedule to avoid serious adverse effects. • Contact the doctor if symptoms worsen or don't improve after 2 to 3 weeks of therapy. • Take this drug on an empty stomach with 8 oz (237 ml) of water. However, if the drug upsets the stomach, take it with food. • Don't drink alcohol while taking this drug because of potential liver problems. • This drug will turn urine, stool, saliva, tears, and other body fluids reddish orange or reddish brown. If the patient wears soft contact lenses, they may become permanently discolored from this drug. However, the drug won't affect hard contact lenses. • This drug can decrease the effectiveness of many other drugs (for example, patients taking oral contraceptives may need to use

(continued)

Teaching about first-line drugs for tuberculosis *(continued)*

Drug	Adverse reactions	What to teach the patient
rifampin (Rifadin, Rimactane) *(continued)*		another method of birth control). Notify the doctor of other drugs being taken, so that dosage adjustments can be made. • Use toothbrushes, dental floss, and toothpicks carefully to prevent bleeding problems while taking this drug. • Avoid activities that require mental alertness, such as driving a car or operating machinery, until it's known how his body responds to this drug.
First-line supplemental drugs		
streptomycin	Clumsiness or unsteadiness, decreased urination, dizziness, hearing loss, hematuria, rash, vision loss, and burning, numbness, or tingling of the face or mouth as well as drowsiness and weakness	• It's important to keep appointments to receive I.M. injections of this drug, even if feeling better. • The doctor may recommend monitoring the patient's hearing while the patient is receiving this drug. • Drink at least eight 8-oz (237-ml) glasses of fluid per day to keep kidneys well hydrated. • This drug will be discontinued when serial sputum cultures are negative.
ethambutol (Myambutol)	Blurred vision or loss of vision, chills, eye pain, joint pain and swelling, and burning, numbness, pain, tingling, or weakness in hands or feet as well as dizziness, GI upset, itching, and rash	• Take this drug exactly as ordered, even if feeling better after a few weeks. • Treatment may last 1 year or more. • Contact the doctor if symptoms worsen or don't improve after 2 to 3 weeks of therapy. • Call the doctor immediately about eye problems, even though these problems usually subside when the therapeutic course is finished. • Avoid activities that require mental alertness, such as driving a car or operating machinery, until it's known how his body responds to this drug.
pyrazinamide (Tebrazid)	Anorexia, fever, jaundice, painful or swollen joints (especially in the big toe, ankle, or knee), and unusual drowsiness or weakness as well as dysuria, itching, nausea, photosensitivity, rash, and vomiting	• Take this drug exactly as ordered, even if feeling better after a few weeks. • Treatment may last 1 year or more. • Notify the doctor if symptoms worsen or don't improve after 2 to 3 weeks of therapy. • Limit time in the sun and don't use a sunlamp, especially if prone to sunburn. Notify the doctor of a severe sunburn.

Tell the patient on preventive treatment that he should be monitored with monthly blood tests to prevent toxicity. Make sure you instruct the patient on preventive therapy to report such signs and symptoms as abdominal swelling, jaundice, and nausea and vomiting.

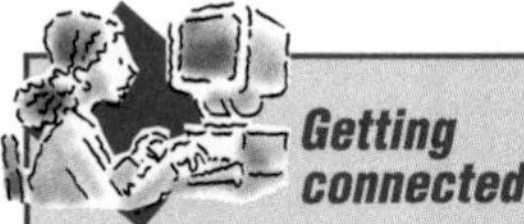

Logging on to lung info

For more information about respiratory disorders, direct the patient to the following Web sites:

- American Lung Association (www.lungusa.org)
- American Association for Respiratory Care (www.aarc.org/index.html)
- National Heart, Lung, and Blood Institute (www.nhlbi.nih.gov/nhlbi/nhlbi.htm).

Teaching about procedures

Tell the patient that chest percussion and chest drainage can loosen pulmonary secretions. Teach him or a caregiver how to perform these techniques, and then explain their purpose and the importance of performing them regularly.

Also, warn the patient to report any pain or dyspnea during chest percussion or in various chest drainage positions. If he can't tolerate certain positions, help him to adjust them so that he stays comfortable and the drainage remains effective. Help him to describe the expectorated sputum's amount, color, and type.

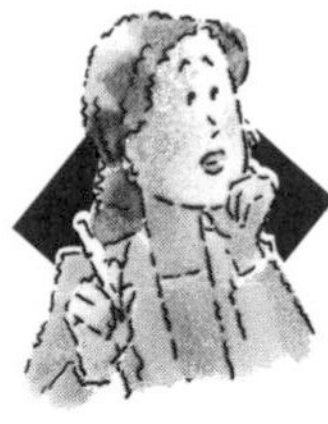

Quick quiz

1. COPD is characterized by:
A. airway resistance.
B. increased lung compliance.
C. an increase in airflow.

Answer: A. COPD — which includes chronic bronchitis, emphysema, and asthma — is characterized by airway resistance. Mucus obstructs air flow in asthma and chronic bronchitis, and lack of elastic recoil is the causative factor in emphysema.

2. It's important to keep track of the number of inhaler "puffs" that have been used in order to prevent:
A. overdosing.
B. addition.
C. running out of medication.

Answer: C. Each inhaler has a set number of puffs in each medication container. Knowing how many puffs have been used can prevent running out of medication. It can also prevent a trip to the emergency room if the patient administers propellant instead of medication.

3. Tell the patient with pleural effusion that he may undergo:

A. paracentesis.
B. thoracentesis.
C. cardiocentesis.

Answer: B. Thoracentesis is the removal of fluid from a pleural effusion to relieve breathing difficulties.

4. The patient on anticoagulants should report dangerous signs to his doctor immediately; these include all of the following except:

A. nosebleed and hematuria.
B. nervousness and back pain.
C. excessive bruising and menstrual flow.

Answer: B. These are not signs for the patient taking anticoagulants. The patients prescribed these medications are susceptible to bleeding easily.

5. All of the following are signs and symptoms of tuberculosis except:

A. increased WBC count, fever, night sweats, and fatigue.
B. headache, sore throat, and nausea.
C. weight loss, anorexia, and shortness of breath.

Answer: B. Headache, sore throat, and nausea aren't common signs and symptoms of tuberculosis.

Scoring

☆☆☆ If you answered all five questions correctly, congratulations. Your respiratory knowledge is free from obstructions.

☆☆ If you answered three or four questions correctly, good job. Your mastery of this chapter is clear and audible.

☆ If you answered fewer than three questions correctly, take a deep breath. Another review of this chapter should clear any blockages.

Neurologic disorders

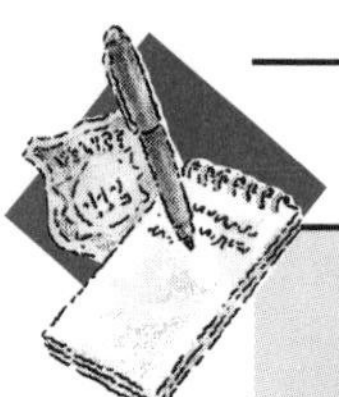

Just the facts

In this chapter you'll learn how to teach patients with the following neurologic disorders:

- Alzheimer's disease
- cerebrovascular accident
- Guillain-Barré syndrome
- multiple sclerosis
- myasthenia gravis
- Parkinson's disease
- seizures.

Alzheimer's disease

This degenerative brain condition affects approximately 3 million Americans. Your primary teaching goal is to prepare family members to meet the increasingly difficult demands of patient care.

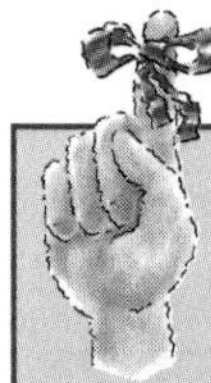

To help ensure that you provide family members with an accurate description of Alzheimer's disease progression, think FACT:

F is for Forgetfulness

A is for Activity decline

C is for Confusion

T is for Total deterioration.

What is it?

Explain that Alzheimer's disease causes progressive nerve atrophy in the brain. The cause of Alzheimer's disease is unknown, but several contributing factors are suspected, including:

- a deficiency in the brain's neurotransmitter substances
- viruses
- a genetic predisposition (First-degree relatives have four times the risk of developing the disease.)
- environmental toxins.

What are the signs?

Describe the subtle, early signs of Alzheimer's disease, such as forgetfulness. Later, the disorder produces progressive changes in the patient's intellect, personality, sensation, motor skills, and overall functioning. (See *Signs of Alzheimer's disease.*)

What happens?

Explain that the disease progresses in stages, but at an unpredictable rate. Eventually the patient suffers complete memory loss and total physical deterioration. (See *Stages of Alzheimer's disease.*)

Teaching about tests

When Alzheimer's disease is suspected, the diagnostic workup may be lengthy, requiring several trips to the hospital. Diagnosis includes a thorough patient and family history and several examinations and tests to rule out other diseases that cause dementia.

Who does what

Assessments typically include physical and neurologic examinations and a neuropsychological interview. Because several doctors may be involved in the diagnosis, discuss who performs each examination and where it's conducted.

Other tests include magnetic resonance imaging (MRI), EEG, cerebral blood flow studies, and cerebrospinal fluid (CSF) analysis. (See *Teaching patients about neurologic tests,* pages 83 to 86.)

Teaching about activity and lifestyle

Explain that exercise and activity help maintain the patient's mobility and prevent complications, such as pneumonia and other infections. Exercise also promotes a normal day and night routine. (See *Activities to ease anxiety,* page 82.)

Making life easier

Also, suggest measures family members can take at home to make life easier for the Alzheimer's patient and themselves. (See *Living with an Alzheimer's patient,* page 82.)

Signs of Alzheimer's disease

Intellectual

- Unaware of time, short attention span, distractable
- Unable to solve problems, make decisions, plan and complete activities
- Repetitive activity, poor motor skills and performance
- Perception of visual and auditory cues altered

Personality

- Inappropriate affect, uninhibited
- Self-involvement, won't participate
- Paranoia, hallucinations, delusions
- Hostility or helplessness

Stress tolerance

- Confusion
- Nighttime waking, pacing, wandering
- Fatigue
- Avoidance behavior
- Anxiety
- Violence

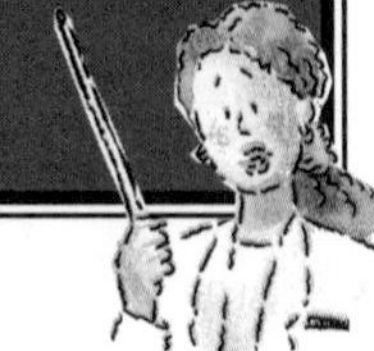

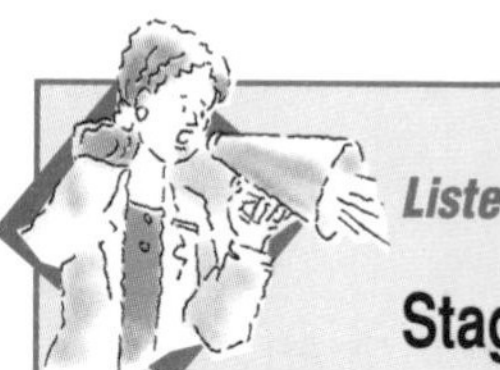

Listen up!

Stages of Alzheimer's disease

Counsel family members to expect progressive deterioration in the patient with Alzheimer's disease. Family members may have difficulty accepting the progress of the disease, so be sensitive to their concerns. If necessary, review the information again when they're more receptive.

Forgetfulness
Explain that in early stages of Alzheimer's disease, the patient becomes forgetful, especially of recent events. He frequently loses everyday objects such as keys. Aware of this loss of function, he may compensate by relinquishing tasks that might reveal his forgetfulness. Because his behavior isn't disruptive and may be attributed to stress, fatigue, or normal aging, he usually doesn't consult a doctor at this stage.

Activity decline
At this stage, the patient loses the ability to perform activities of daily living, such as eating or washing, without direct supervision. Weight loss may occur. The patient withdraws from the family and increasingly depends on the primary caregiver. Communication becomes difficult as the patient's understanding of written and spoken language declines.

Explain that agitation, wandering, pacing, and nighttime awakening are linked to an inability to cope with a multistimuli environment. The patient may mistake his mirror image for a real person (pseudohallucination). Inform caregivers that because they must be constantly vigilant, they may suffer physical and emotional exhaustion as well as a sense of loss and anger.

Confusion
Describe what happens as the disease progresses: The patient has increasing difficulty with activities that require planning, decision making, and judgment (such as managing personal finances, driving a car, or performing his job). However, he does retain everyday skills such as personal grooming.

Social withdrawal
Point out that social withdrawal occurs when the patient feels overwhelmed by a changing environment and his inability to cope with multiple stimuli. Travel is difficult and tiring. Forewarn the family that as the patient becomes aware of his progressive loss of function, he may become severely depressed.

Safety concerns
Safety becomes a concern when the patient forgets to turn off appliances or can't recognize unsafe situations such as boiling water. At this point, the family may need to consider day care or a supervised residential facility.

Deterioration
Point out that, in the final stage of Alzheimer's disease, the patient no longer recognizes himself, his body parts, or other family members. He becomes bedridden, and his activity consists of small, purposeless movements. Verbal communication stops, although he may scream spontaneously. Complications of immobility may include pressure sores, urinary tract infections, pneumonia, and contractures.

Risk of injury
Reinforce the need to take precautions as the disease progresses, to prevent the patient from injuring himself (by his own violent behavior, wandering, or unsupervised activity).

Immobility
In the final disease stage, patients typically are confined to bed and generally die of complications related to immobility.

Teaching about diet

Malnutrition and dehydration can occur if the patient forgets or refuses to eat. Stress the importance of a well-balanced diet with adequate fiber. If the patient is hyperac-

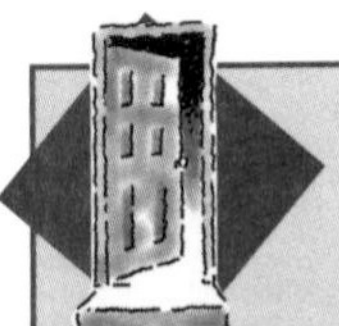

No place like home

Living with an Alzheimer's patient

Encourage the family to grant the patient as much independence as possible while ensuring his — and others' — safety. Stress that the patient can't control his behavior, although sometimes he may respond appropriately. And even if the patient no longer recognizes his family, urge them to keep including him in their activities. Suggest the following additional care measures for the patient at home.

Safety first
Teach home-safety measures, such as storing medication out of the patient's reach and removing throw rugs. If necessary, tell them to remove handles and buttons from appliances.

Ready for bed
Also, advise the family to avoid overstimulating the patient before bedtime and to limit fluids about 3 to 4 hours before bedtime so that the patient won't need to get up to urinate. Warn them that if he develops irregular sleep patterns and wanders at night, he may harm himself and others. If necessary, tell the family to lock doors and windows, barricade stairways, and use night-lights. If the patient is confused about his surroundings, tell the family to use pictures to guide him.

Combat confusion
To combat the patient's confusion, stress maintaining a routine in his activities. If the patient panics or becomes belligerent, advise the family to remain calm and to try distracting him.

Divide and guide
Recommend dividing the patient's daily tasks into short, simple steps and then guiding him through them. Tell the family to use activities that stimulate or calm him appropriately. Suggest repetitive tasks, such as sanding wood and listening to music.

Button up
If the patient has coordination problems suggest using Velcro straps instead of buttons and loafers or shoes with elastic shoelaces.

Seek support
Finally, emphasize to family members the importance of taking time for themselves. Refer them to a local Alzheimer's support group and to the Alzheimer's Association for further information and support.

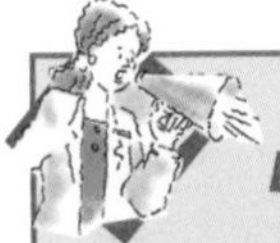

Listen up!

Activities to ease anxiety

Encourage family members to find physical activities that satisfy and occupy the patient. Activities might include repetitive chores, such as folding towels, scrubbing the floor, sweeping, or indoor stationary bicycle riding. Repetitive motions decrease the patient's stress level by eliminating the need for him to make decisions about what to do next.

tive, advise the family to increase his calorie intake with between-meal supplements. Also, tell them to avoid giving him stimulants, such as caffeine-containing coffee, tea, cola, and chocolate. (See *Making mealtime manageable*, page 87.)

Teaching about medication

Medications may be prescribed to help manage the patient's signs and symptoms. For example, antipsychotics

(Text continues on page 86.)

Teaching patients about neurologic tests

Test and purpose	Teaching points
Cerebral angiography (cerebral arteriography) • To detect disruption or displacement of the cerebral circulation by occlusion or hemorrhage	• This test, which takes about 2 hours, highlights the brain's blood vessels on an X-ray as a contrast medium circulates through them. It detects disruption or displacement of the cerebral circulation by occlusion or hemorrhage. • During the test, a technician shaves and cleans around the injection site — the carotid or femoral artery — and may immobilize the patient's head with tape or straps. If the carotid artery is used, the patient may have his face covered with a drape and his arms immobilized to maintain a sterile field. • He must lie still on an examining table and may feel discomfort from this prolonged stillness. The doctor injects a local anesthetic and inserts a catheter at the appropriate site for injection of the contrast medium. During the injection, the patient may sense pressure, warmth, a transient headache, nausea, or a salty taste. He should report any of these sensations. Immediately after the injection, he'll hear clacking sounds as the X-ray equipment takes pictures. Multiple injections of the contrast medium may be required to completely visualize the blood vessels. The patient should lie still to avoid blurring the films but should comply if the doctor tells him to move an arm or a leg. • After the test, the catheter is removed, and pressure is applied to the puncture site for about 15 minutes, followed by a pressure dressing and an ice pack. The patient must hold his head and neck (for the carotid approach) or leg (for the femoral approach) straight for 4 to 12 hours. He can resume his usual diet but should increase fluid intake for the rest of the day to help expel the contrast medium.
Cerebral blood flow studies • To measure cerebral blood flow • To detect abnormalities in cerebral perfusion • To evaluate the effectiveness of surgery, such as extracranial-intracranial bypass and cerebral aneurysm clipping	• Cerebral blood flow studies measure blood flow to the brain and help detect abnormalities. The test takes about 30 minutes, is painless, and exposes the patient to less radiation than a chest X-ray. • During the test, the patient lies still on a table with a frame placed around his head. He may inhale a radioactive gas, such as xenon, technetium, or krypton. Alternatively, he may receive an I.V. injection of the radioactive substance and breathe through a mask or dome while the isotope-sensitive detector probes measure the blood flow rate. He can resume his usual activities immediately after the test.
Cerebrospinal fluid (CSF) analysis • To help detect infection, multiple sclerosis, or cancer • To help detect obstruction of the subarachnoid space around the spinal cord • To inject medication or contrast medium into the central nervous system	• This test involves obtaining a sample of CSF for laboratory analysis during a procedure called a lumbar puncture. It takes about 15 minutes. The patient feels some pressure during the procedure as the needle is inserted, and he may become uncomfortable from the position assumed during the test.

(continued)

Teaching patients about neurologic tests *(continued)*

Test and purpose	Teaching points
Cerebrospinal fluid (CSF) analysis (continued)	*Lumbar puncture* • The patient sits with his head bent toward his knees or lies on the edge of a bed or table, with his knees drawn up to his abdomen and his chin resting on his chest. After cleaning the lumbar area, the doctor injects a local anesthetic. The patient should report any tingling or sharp pain. • The doctor inserts a hollow needle into the subarachnoid space surrounding the spinal cord. The patient should hold still to avoid dislodging the needle. He may be asked to breathe deeply or to straighten his legs. The doctor may apply pressure to the jugular veins. • The doctor removes the needle and applies an adhesive bandage. The patient lies flat for 4 to 24 hours to prevent headache. His head should be even with or below the level of his hips. Although he must not raise his head, he can turn from side to side. He should increase his fluid intake for the rest of the day to help replenish CSF and prevent a headache.
Computed tomography (CT) scan • To identify structural abnormalities, edema, and lesions, such as nonhemorrhagic infarction, hematomas, aneurysms, and tumors, in the brain and spinal cord	• A CT scan produces X-rays of the brain or spinal tissue. It takes about 30 to 60 minutes and causes no discomfort, although the patient may feel chilled because the equipment requires a cool environment. If the doctor will be using a contrast medium, the patient should restrict food and fluids for 4 hours before the test. • A technician will position the patient on an X-ray table and place a strap across the part of the body to be scanned to restrict movement. The table will then slide into the circular opening of the scanner. If a contrast medium is ordered, the patient will receive it through an I.V. site; the infusion takes about 5 minutes. He should tell the technician immediately if the infusion causes discomfort, a feeling of warmth, or itching. (The technician can see and hear him from an adjacent room.) He will hear noises from the scanner and may notice the machine revolving around him. • After the test, he can immediately resume his usual activities and diet. He should increase his fluid intake for the rest of the day to help expel the contrast medium.
Digital subtraction angiography • To evaluate the patency of cerebral vessels and to determine their position • To detect and evaluate lesions and vascular abnormalities	• Digital subtraction angiography visualizes the blood vessels in his head and neck. It takes about 30 to 45 minutes. The patient may experience a feeling of warmth or a metallic taste on injection of the contrast medium. He should restrict solid food for 4 hours before the test. • The patient lies on an X-ray table and an I.V. needle or catheter is inserted. He should lie still during the test. After the doctor injects a contrast medium, a series of X-ray images is taken. He should tell the doctor immediately if he feels any discomfort or shortness of breath.

Teaching patients about neurologic tests *(continued)*

Test and purpose	Teaching points
Digital subtraction angiography (continued)	• After the test, the doctor removes the needle or catheter. If the I.V. route was used, the patient can resume his normal activities. For the intra-arterial route, he'll need to restrict movement in his arm or leg for 4 to 12 hours. He should increase fluid intake for the rest of the day to help expel the contrast medium.
Electroencephalography (EEG) • To evaluate the brain's electrical activity in such disorders as seizures • To help identify the brain area in which the patient's seizures originate and determine the frequency with which they occur • To aid diagnosis of intracranial lesions, such as abscesses and tumors	• EEG records the electrical activity of the brain. The test is painless and the electrodes won't cause an electric shock. It takes about 45 minutes. • Pretest restrictions depend on the type of EEG. The patient should wash his hair 1 to 2 days before the test to remove hair spray, cream, or oil. • He is positioned comfortably in a reclining chair or on a bed. A technician will apply paste and attach electrodes to the patient's head and neck. The patient should remain still throughout the test. Depending on the type of EEG, he may be asked to perform activities, such as breathing deeply and rapidly for 3 minutes (hyperventilating) or sleeping. • After the test, the technician removes the electrodes. He also removes the paste, using acetone. (This may sting where the skin was scraped.) The patient should wash his hair to remove residual paste; then he can resume usual activities.
Electromyography (EMG) • To evaluate neuromuscular disorders such as myasthenia gravis	• EMG measures the electrical activity of specific muscles. It takes about 1 hour. • The patient lies down or sits up, depending on the muscle to be tested. A technician cleans the skin over the muscle. The patient may experience some discomfort as a needle attached to an electrode is inserted into the muscle. Then another electrode is placed on the patient's limb to deliver a mild electrical charge. This may cause discomfort as each muscle is stimulated to test its response at rest and during voluntary contraction. He should remain still during the test, except when asked to contract or relax a muscle. An amplifier may cause crackling noises whenever his muscle moves. • After the test, electrodes are removed and he can resume his usual activities.
Evoked potential studies (evoked responses) • To aid diagnosis of nervous system lesions and abnormalities • To assess neurologic function	• Evoked potential studies measure the nervous system's electrical response to a visual, auditory, or sensory stimulus. The test lasts about 1 hour and is painless. The patient should wash his hair 1 to 2 days before the test. • The patient lies on a bed or table or in a reclining chair. He must lie still during the test. A technician cleans his scalp and applies paste and electrodes to his head and neck. He may hear noises from the test equipment. He's asked to perform various activities, such as gazing at a checkerboard pattern or a strobe light and listening to a series of clicks. Alternatively, he may have electrodes placed on an arm and leg, and may be asked to respond to a tapping sensation. • After the test, the technician removes the electrodes. The patient can resume his normal activities. He should wash his hair to remove residual paste.

(continued)

Teaching patients about neurologic tests *(continued)*

Test and purpose	Teaching points
Magnetic resonance imaging (MRI) (nuclear magnetic resonance scan) • To aid diagnosis of intracranial and spinal lesions • To rule out intracranial lesions as the cause of dementia • To evaluate for neurologic abnormalities • To detect diffuse axonal and brain stem injuries • To help determine the cause of seizures	• This test evaluates the condition of the brain or spinal cord. It takes about 1 hour and causes no discomfort. It won't expose him to radiation; however, it exposes him to a strong magnetic field. He should report any metal objects in his body (such as a pacemaker, aneurysm clips, hip prosthesis, bullet fragments, or an implanted infusion pump) that may make him ineligible for the test. • The patient lies on a table that slides into a large cylinder housing the MRI magnets. His head, chest, and arms are restrained to help him remain still. Lying still prevents blurring of the images. A technician can see and hear him from an adjacent room. He'll hear a loud knocking noise while the machine is running. If the noise bothers him, he may be given earplugs or pads for his ears. A radio encased in the machine or earphones may help block the sound (but he will still hear some noise). He may feel some discomfort from being enclosed within the large cylinder. • After the test, he can resume his usual activities
Positron emission tomography (PET) scan (positron emission transaxial tomography) • To evaluate cerebral perfusion • To evaluate cerebral glucose metabolism and thus aid diagnosis of tumors and disorders that alter cerebral metabolism, such as Alzheimer's disease, Parkinson's disease, multiple sclerosis, and cerebrovascular accident	• A PET scan evaluates brain-cell function by measuring how rapidly brain tissue consumes radioactive isotopes. The test takes about 1 hour, is painless, and involves minimal radiation exposure. • The patient lies on a moving table with his head immobilized and placed inside a ring-shaped opening in the machine. He's given a radioactive tracer either by inhalation or by I.V. injection. If he must inhale a radioactive tracer through a mask, he should breathe normally. If the tracer is administered I.V., the patient may feel a warm sensation during the tracer's injection and should report any discomfort to the technician. Next, a dome-shaped hood is placed over his head and face to prevent the exhaled tracer from circulating in the room. He must lie still to avoid blurring the images. • If the I.V. method is used, the doctor removes the needle after the test and collects a blood sample. • After the test, the patient can resume his usual activities.

and antidepressants control behavioral changes, and neuroleptics control seizures. Tacrine hydrochloride (Cognex) may improve cognitive functioning. Tell family members to check with the doctor before giving the patient any over-the-counter drugs (especially sedatives) because drug action may be enhanced in patients with Alzheimer's disease.

Tough to swallow

If the patient has trouble swallowing, advise crushing tablets or opening capsules and mixing them with a semi-

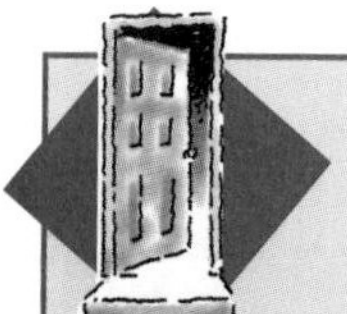

No place like home

Making mealtime manageable

Provide family members with the following guidelines to help make mealtimes more manageable for a patient with Alzheimer's disease.

Limiting decisions
Recommend limiting the number of foods on the patient's plate so that he won't have to make decisions. If the patient puts almost anything in his mouth, whether it's food or not, encourage the family to keep preferred foods handy.

Hand to mouth
If the patient has coordination problems, advise family members to cut his food and to provide finger foods, such as fruit and sandwiches. To prevent injury, suggest using plates with rim guards, built-up utensils, and cups with lids and spouts.

Easy to swallow
If the patient has difficulty swallowing, advise the family to serve semisoft foods. Suggest freezing liquids to a slush or mixing them with other foods. If the patient can't swallow or has no interest in food, nasogastric or gastrostomy tube feedings may be necessary; instruct the family accordingly.

soft food. Caution the family always to check with the pharmacist before crushing tablets or opening capsules because specially formulated drugs shouldn't be altered. Mention that flavored oral suspensions that ease administration problems may be available.

Cerebrovascular accident

Also called stroke, cerebrovascular accident (CVA) is the third leading cause of death in the United States and the leading cause of disability and neurologic deficits.

What is it?

CVA is commonly, but not necessarily, associated with atherosclerosis, a condition that interrupts the blood supply to the brain. A blood clot or plaque can block an artery, producing tissue ischemia (decreased blood supply) and infarction (death of tissue to the affected area from lack of blood supply).

If an internal carotid artery in the neck becomes blocked because of atherosclerosis, a clot may form, halt-

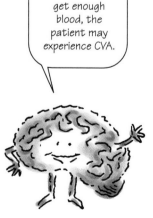

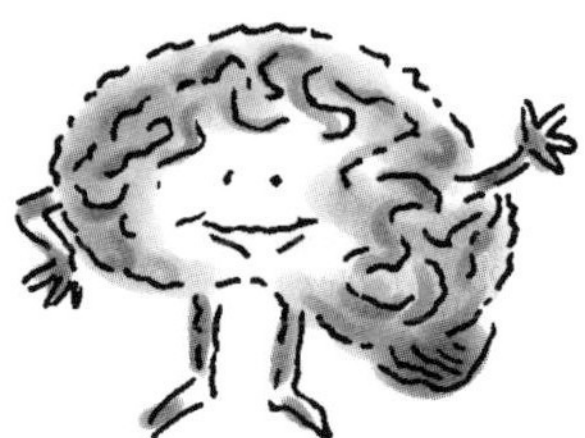
Yikes! If I don't get enough blood, the patient may experience CVA.

ing oxygen flow to the brain. Alternatively, a vessel may rupture, causing increased intracranial pressure from hemorrhage and, possibly, brain herniation.

What's the rush?

To be most effective, decreased blood supply to the brain must be treated within 90 minutes to 6 hours after the onset of CVA symptoms. Explain that CVA treatment seeks to limit the extent of brain injury and prevent or treat complications.

Teaching about tests

Diagnosis involves a complete neurologic workup, beginning with a detailed history and physical examination. Blood tests may be performed to evaluate clotting. Scanning tests may include computed tomography (CT) scans, positron emission tomography (PET), single-photon emission computed tomography, and MRI.

Evaluating flow

Angiography and other tests may be conducted to identify abnormalities and evaluate cerebral blood flow. Additional tests may include cerebral blood flow studies, oculoplethysmography, neuropsychological tests, and transcranial Doppler studies. (See *Teaching patients about neurologic tests,* pages 83 to 86.)

Rehabilitation techniques in CVA

- Physical agents, such as heat, cold, light, and water
- Occupational therapy
- Assistive devices or braces
- Muscle strengthening and conditioning exercises
- Swallowing exercises
- Speech therapy
- Gait training

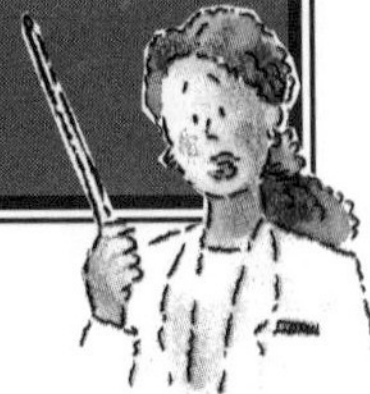

Teaching about activity and lifestyle

Instruct the patient and family members to follow the prescribed exercise program. Teach them how to perform passive range-of-motion (ROM) exercises. Reinforce the need to take well-timed rest periods and to use protective devices to prevent injury and promote safety. Also, discuss strategies to boost the patient's self-sufficiency as well as ways to prevent another CVA. (See *Life after CVA.*)

Take a stab at rehab

Help the patient and his family establish a rehabilitation program. (See *Rehabilitation techniques in CVA.*)

Why risk it?

Teach the patient and family about correcting risk factors for CVA. For example, if the patient smokes, refer him to a

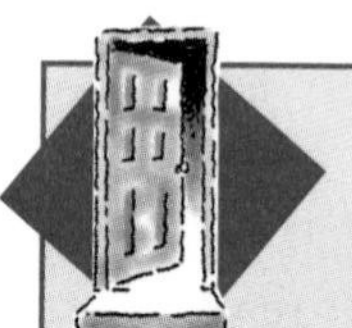

No place like home

Life after CVA

Before your patient who has experienced a cerebrovascular accident (CVA) goes home, provide the following pointers to him and members of his family.

Day by day
To help the patient manage daily activities, pass along the following advice:

- To help distinguish left from right, urge the patient to wear a watch or bracelet on the left wrist as a reminder, mark the left shoe sole with an *L*, or tag the inside left trouser leg or sweater sleeve with colored tape to differentiate left from right.
- If the patient has problems with spatial relations, suggest using maps or colored dots to mark a daily route. Advise the family to keep the environment as uncluttered as possible; for example, keep only a few items on the nightstand. Also suggest pointing to objects to give verbal clues, such as "in the wastebasket" or "under the desk."
- If the patient has difficulty dressing, recommend buttoning shirts (or blouses) from the bottom up. Some patients find it easier to match buttonholes that way.
- Whatever the task, urge family members to praise the patient's efforts. Discouragement can be disabling in itself. A patient with a right-sided lesion will understand encouraging words; a patient with a left-sided lesion may respond to nonverbal encouragement such as a pat on the back.

Beyond words
For a patient with a speech deficit, recommend other communication methods, such as writing or using a picture board. Review prescribed speech and language therapy.

Instruct the family to speak slowly to the patient in normal tones. If the patient has receptive aphasia (difficulty understanding speech), recommend that the family use gestures to clarify their message. If he has expressive aphasia (difficulty forming words and putting sentences together), encourage them to take their time and not rush his response or jump in and finish his sentences. Tell them to give him short, simple directions, cues, and lists.

Trying time
Inform the family that the patient may overestimate his abilities, claiming that he can perform tasks (for example, driving a car) that, in fact, he can't. Explain the importance of carefully monitoring his abilities without frustrating his efforts for independence. Tell them to let him try most activities short of those that could injure him.

Also inform the family that the patient may be emotionally labile — crying or laughing at seemingly inappropriate times. Explain that he can't control these reactions.

Stay safe
Recommend installing grab bars near the toilet and bathtub, removing throw rugs, and securing carpets or removing them entirely if the patient uses a walker or wheelchair. If he has sensory losses, suggest lowering the water heater's temperature to prevent burns.

It's a habit
The patient may benefit from following established routines. To prevent confusing the patient who has difficulty generalizing, advise the family to follow a routine and minimize changes.

One sided
If the patient has a one-sided deficit, encourage him to bathe and dress the affected side first. Suggest calling attention to that side with a watch or a ring. If the patient has homonymous hemianopia (vision loss in the same half of the visual field of each eye), tell him to scan his environment by carefully looking from side to side.

Maintain morale
Keep up the patient's and family's morale, which may flag if the patient's rehabilitative progress fluctuates. Remind them that response to CVA treatment varies among patients. Encourage them to contact a local support group and to obtain additional information from an organization such as the National Stroke Association.

Identify yourself
Urge the patient to obtain a medical identification bracelet or necklace if he's taking anticoagulants or antiplatelet drugs.

smoking cessation program. As appropriate, teach him to maintain his ideal weight; follow his prescribed diet, exercise, and stress-reduction program; and check with the doctor before taking any nonprescription drugs. If the patient is a woman of childbearing age, tell her to avoid using oral contraceptives.

Walk the walk

If the patient needs to use a cane or walker, provide instruction. (See *Using a walker* and *Using a cane.*)

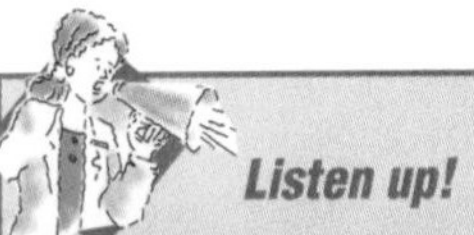

Listen up!

Using a walker

Help your patient become familiar with his walker. Advise him to put on the shoes he'll be wearing when he uses his walker. Then instruct him to stand up straight with his feet close together, relax his shoulders, and put the walker in front of and partially around him.

Watch those elbows

Next tell the patient to grasp the sides of the walker and look at the position of his elbows — they should be nearly straight. If they're not, instruct him to adjust the walker's height by pushing in the button on each of the walker's legs and sliding the tubing up or down as appropriate. Make sure that the button locks back into place and that the patient has adjusted the legs to the same height.

Try it

Now, instruct the patient to try the walker. He should be able to move it without bending over. If he still doesn't feel comfortable, help him to adjust the height again.

Teaching about diet

Reinforce a weight-loss diet or one low in saturated fats if appropriate. If the patient experiences one-sided facial weakness, advise him to eat semisoft foods and to chew on the unaffected side of his mouth.

Instruct the patient to sit upright when eating and to tilt his head slightly forward. Recommend that his family or other caregiver prepare solid foods in a blender and freeze liquids to a slush or mix them with other foods. If the patient has partial arm paralysis, suggest that he use feeding aids, such as specially adapted plates with rims and built-up utensils.

Teaching about medication

Teach the patient about the goals of drug therapy:

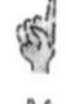 preventing further thrombus formation

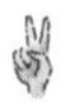 enhancing blood flow to the brain

 protecting brain cells.

Names, dosages, effects

Medications may include antiplatelet drugs, such as aspirin, dipyridamole, and ticlopidine. A thrombolytic agent and other medications may be prescribed. Make sure that the patient, family members, and other caregivers know the names of all prescribed drugs, their proper dosages, and possible adverse effects. (See *Medications for CVA,* page 92.)

Teaching about surgery

Depending on the cause and extent of the CVA, the patient may undergo carotid endarterectomy to remove atherosclerotic plaques. Explain that, after surgery, dressings will cover the incision and that he may experience a tran-

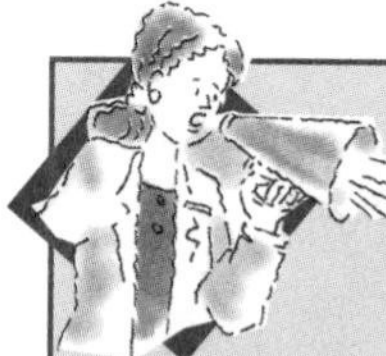

Listen up!

Using a cane

Give your patient the following instructions for walking with a cane if his *left* leg is weaker. If his *right* leg is weaker, start with the cane on his left side, and adapt the instructions. The dotted foot represents the weaker leg.

Preparation

• Wear nonskid, flat-soled, supportive shoes, and check that they fit securely (loose laces can be hazardous). Avoid wearing sandals or clogs because they won't support weight properly. Next, check the cane's rubber tip to make sure that it has no cracks or tears and is wearing evenly. Also, make sure that the tip fits securely and evenly on the cane's end.

• Remove throw rugs and avoid walking on slippery, wet, or waxed floors or on gravel driveways. Also, try to walk close to a wall so that there is something to lean against if the cane is dropped.

Procedure

1. Distribute weight evenly between the feet and cane.
2. Position the cane about 4" (10 cm) to the front and side of the stronger leg, as shown. Then move the weaker foot forward so that it's even with the cane.
3. Shift weight to the weaker leg and the cane and move the stronger leg forward, ahead of the cane. If this step is performed correctly, the heel will be slightly beyond the tip of the cane.
4. Next, move the weaker foot forward so that it's even with the stronger foot. Then move the cane about 4" forward.

Repeat these steps, keeping head erect, shoulders back, and back straight. The abdomen should be drawn in, with knees slightly flexed.

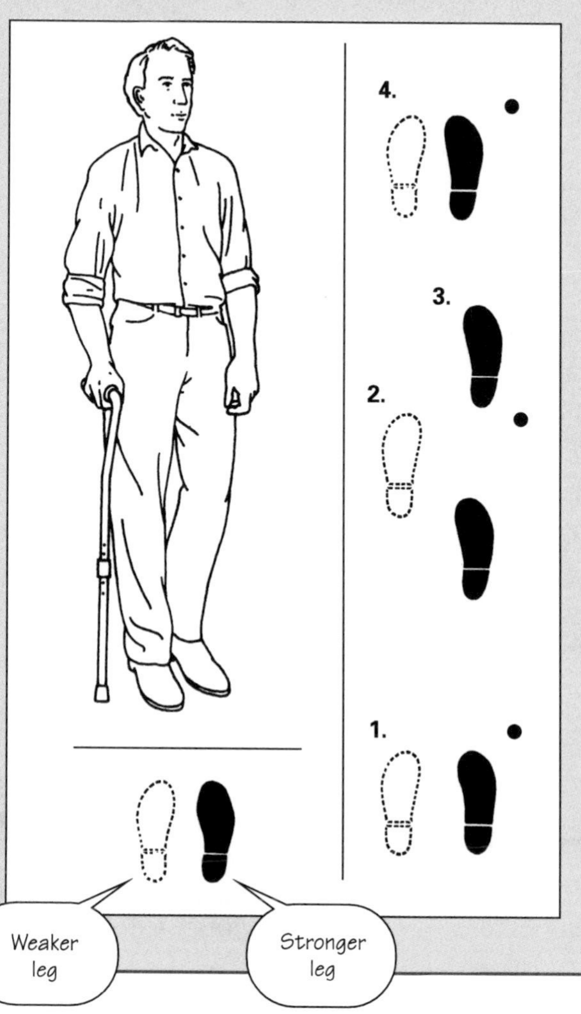

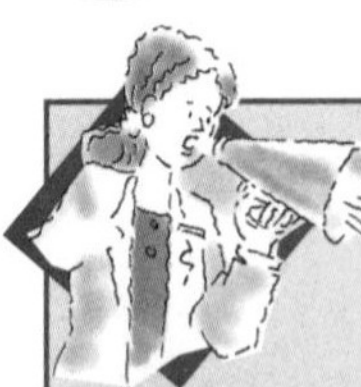

Listen up!

Medications for CVA

Teach the patient and his caregivers about all prescribed medications for cerebrovascular accident (CVA). Make sure that they're familiar with each drug's adverse effects.

Aspirin

The doctor may prescribe aspirin because it helps prevent CVA recurrence by hindering blood clotting.

Adverse effects

If the patient will be taking large doses of aspirin for a prolonged period, tell him to watch for adverse effects, such as unusual bleeding, bruising, rashes, tinnitus, hearing loss, nausea, vomiting, stomach upset, bleeding gums, and bloody or black, tarry stools.

Dipyridamole

If the doctor prescribes dipyridamole (Persantine), tell the patient that this drug prevents blood clotting.

Adverse effects

Instruct the patient to stay alert for adverse effects, such as bleeding, bruising, rash, tinnitus, hearing loss, nausea, vomiting, diarrhea, headache, dizziness, weakness, flushing, and fainting.

Ticlopidine hydrochloride

Ticlopidine hydrochloride (Ticlid), a newer antiplatelet agent, has been shown to reduce CVA recurrence by up to 50% in the first year.

Adverse effects

Teach the patient taking this drug to stay alert for the adverse effects listed previously for aspirin. Stress that he must undergo blood studies for the first 3 months of therapy to check for serious adverse reactions.

Thrombolytic agents

The doctor may prescribe a thrombolytic agent such as alteplase (Activase) to promote neurologic recovery and reduce the chance of lasting disability. For maximal effectiveness, such therapy must begin within 3 hours of symptom onset. Also, the patient's history must be carefully evaluated for contraindications, such as intracerebral hemorrhage, other evidence of bleeding, recent head injury or surgery, and uncontrolled hypertension.

Other agents

The doctor may prescribe a calcium channel blocker such as nifedipine (Procardia) within 18 hours of onset of symptoms. Tell the patient that this drug can reduce neurologic deficits by aiding circulation and easing brain ischemia.

sient numbness and tightness in the incision area and soreness or a lump in his throat. Reassure him that these effects of swelling should disappear in a few days. Inform him that he'll be able to resume his usual daily activities the day after surgery, barring complication. Another procedure — such as hematoma evacuation, embolectomy, or angioplasty — may be used to remove plaques.

Guillain-Barré syndrome

A frightening disease, Guillain-Barré syndrome (GBS, also known as acute inflammatory demyelinating polyneuropathy) can alter the patient's mobility and disrupt his life. GBS progresses rapidly but, in many cases, it can be reversed. The effects of GBS range from mild muscle weakness to complete paralysis.

What is it?

GBS is thought to be an autoimmune response; it typically follows a viral illness or an immunization. The illness or immunization may stimulate a T-cell attack on the nerve's myelin sheath. This prevents the normal transmission of electrical impulses along sensorimotor nerve routes and results in paresthesia, weakness, and motor dysfunction.

What are its symptoms?

Tell the patient and members of his family that GBS causes inflamed, swollen peripheral nerves, producing numbness, tingling, and burning sensations. It also causes bilateral muscle weakness and possible paralysis.

What happens?

GBS progresses through three stages:

 acute

 plateau

 recovery.

In the acute stage, symptoms usually begin in the lower legs and progress upward for 2 to 3 weeks before they peak. As the disease enters the plateau stage, which lasts from several days to 2 weeks, his symptoms may not change. Then gradually, during the recovery stage, he may experience some pain and discomfort, resulting from neural edema or regeneration of peripheral nerve tissue. Explain that recovery can take 2 to 3 years.

What's at risk?

Explain that the patient's inability to use his muscles, if left untreated, can result in serious complications. (See *GBS can lead to....*)

GBS can lead to...

- Thrombophlebitis
- Pulmonary embolus
- Pressure sores
- Contractures
- Muscle wasting
- Respiratory infections
- Life-threatening respiratory and cardiac compromise
- Syndrome of inappropriate antidiuretic hormone secretion

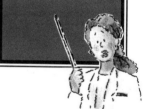

Teaching about tests

Explain that no definitive test can detect GBS. A diagnosis is based on the patient's muscle weakness and progressive symptoms. The doctor also checks for a precursor disease or event, such as a flulike illness, an immunization, or surgery.

To confirm the diagnosis and rule out other neurologic diseases, the doctor may order CSF analysis, electromyography, and nerve conduction studies. (See *Teaching patients about neurologic tests,* pages 83 to 86.)

Teaching about activity and lifestyle

Stress the benefits of a prescribed exercise program, explaining that normal daily activity isn't enough to challenge the GBS patient's muscles.

Everybody in the pool

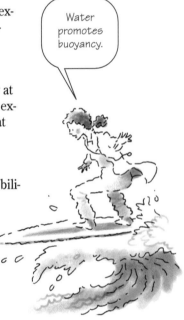

The physical therapist may recommend hydrotherapy at first because water promotes buoyancy, which makes exercising easier and more effective. Also, the moist heat soothes pain and promotes circulation.

Splint stint

During the acute GBS stage, the patient's range of mobility is monitored. As his muscles grow weaker (and possibly progress to paralysis), frequent position changes and ROM exercises are performed to help maintain muscle tone, preserve joint and muscle function, prevent contractures, and relieve pain. Explain that he may have splints applied to his arms and legs to maintain joint function, provide support, promote rest, prevent contractures, and ensure proper body alignment.

Bedridden but mobile

The patient may lie in a movable bed (Rotobed) that allows frequent repositioning and turning from side to side to maintain joint and muscle function. If his vital signs are stable and his condition permits, he'll be allowed out of the bed to sit in a chair for some time each day. Depending on the patient's progress and needs, show him how to use a walker or a cane to increase and support his mobility.

Stronger but achy

During the recovery stage, an exercise program is prescribed to strengthen and retrain weakened muscles. Advise the patient to follow instructions precisely because overdoing the exercise can enhance demyelination and worsen his symptoms or cause a relapse. Tell him to expect aching joints and muscles as his strength increases.

One day at a time

If the patient feels discouraged with his progress, remind him that strengthening and retraining muscles is always slow and tedious. Cite the progress that he's already made. And suggest that he take 1 day and 1 step at a time.

Teaching about diet

As GBS progresses the patient may need tube feeding, especially if he loses his gag reflex or can't swallow enough food by mouth. During recovery, encourage him to consume a high-calorie diet to help restore his strength.

Have some more calories!

Five small meals

The dietitian may recommend five small meals daily rather than three larger ones to ensure that he gets the required number of calories. She may also suggest that he start with thicker fluids, such as pudding or yogurt. To avoid choking, recommend resting before meals, eating slowly, and remaining upright rather than reclining.

Teaching about medication

The doctor may prescribe high-dose immunoglobulin, which may improve GBS symptoms by enhancing the immune response. Pain medication may help to decrease neural inflammation and swelling.

Before it becomes intolerable

Teach the patient to take pain medication before pain becomes intolerable. If aspirin or acetaminophen is recommended, explain possible adverse reactions, including abnormal bleeding, itching, rash, ringing in the ears, and stomach upset.

Watching dosages

Caution the patient against exceeding the recommended dosage or using alcohol with medications because it may cause or increase central nervous system (CNS) or respiratory depression. Describe adverse reactions, such as arrhythmias, hypersensitivity, or seizures. Other reactions include constipation, dizziness, drowsiness, headache, indigestion, light-headedness, minor visual disturbances, nausea and vomiting, rashes, and weakness.

Teaching about procedures

Plasmapheresis accelerates recovery by removing harmful antibodies and myelinotoxic substances from the blood. Doctors suspect that these antibodies attack the nerves and cause muscle weakness.The process takes several hours and is performed every 2 to 3 days for 2 to 4 weeks. Reassure the patient that the entire process causes only minimal discomfort. Mention that the procedure can't reverse symptoms that are already present.

Be prepared

Depending on the severity of GBS, prepare the patient for intensive care, mechanical ventilation, and nonverbal communication and entertainment. (See *GBS care measures*.)

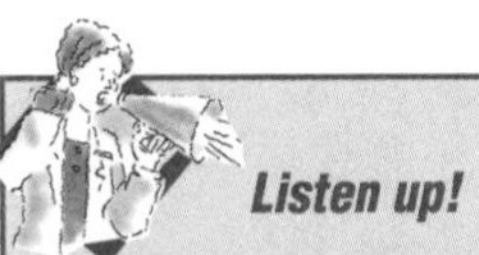

Listen up!

GBS care measures

Teach your patient about the care measures described below.

Intensive care
Describe the intensive care environment as needed. Tell him that he may hear and see unfamiliar sights and sounds.

Mechanical ventilation
Should the patient's muscles become so weak that he can't breathe adequately, describe how he'll breathe through a endotracheal tube.

Nonverbal communication
Because he won't be able to talk, help the patient develop another way to communicate while he has a tracheostomy. For example, suggest that he can answer questions by blinking once for yes and twice for no.

Entertainment
Encourage the patient's family to help him stay mentally alert. Suggest they borrow videos or books on tape from the library if the patient likes films or reading.

Multiple sclerosis

Multiple sclerosis (MS) is a major cause of chronic disability in young and middle-aged adults, affecting more women than men. It's thought to result from a genetic trait that causes susceptibility to autoimmune dysfunction, viral infection, or both.

What's at stake?

Like other progressive degenerative disorders, MS may affect physical, emotional, and psychosocial functioning. Although most patients lead active, productive lives and enjoy prolonged remissions, a minority see the disease progress so rapidly that they have little time to adjust to their loss of abilities.

What is it?

MS destroys myelin, a substance that speeds electrical impulses along nerve pathways to the brain for interpretation. This disrupts the conduction of nerve impulses in the

CNS, sending either partial impulses or no impulses at all to the brain.

Yikes! Without myelin, I can't conduct electrical impulses properly.

What happens?

MS causes unpredictable and spontaneous remissions and exacerbations. Problems may come and go in no predictable pattern. Such problems may include:
- mood swings
- speech, hearing, and visual disturbances
- sensory losses
- bowel, bladder, and sexual dysfunction
- muscle tremors, weakness, and spasms.

Teaching about tests

To distinguish MS from other neurologic disorders and to monitor its course, tests may include CSF analysis, CT scans, MRI, PET, and evoked potential studies (visual, auditory, and somatosensory). Other tests may include nerve conduction studies and neuropsychological tests. Blood tests are ordered to detect antibodies, enzyme deficiencies, and by-products of muscle breakdown and atrophy. Tests of CSF may be used to detect antibodies. (See *Teaching patients about neurologic tests,* pages 83 to 86.)

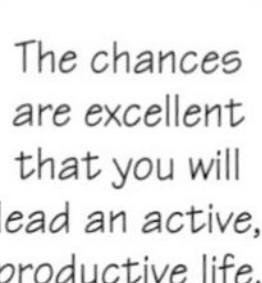

The chances are excellent that you will lead an active, productive life.

Teaching about activity and lifestyle

Discuss the benefits of moderate exercise, including:
- decreasing calcium loss from bones
- preventing renal calculi
- maintaining muscle tone and joint mobility
- promoting circulation.

A slow, gentle stretch

Advise the patient to perform slow, gentle, stretching exercises throughout the day to help diminish spasticity. Fatigue, stress, and overexertion may trigger or intensify MS symptoms, so emphasize the importance of rest periods during activities and working hours.

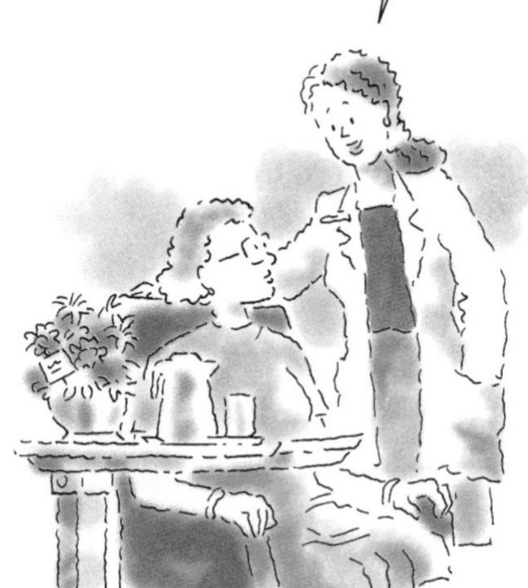

A matter of mobility

If coordination problems interfere with the patient's mobility, teach her to walk with a wide-based gait or to use a weighted cane or walker, if necessary. Also suggest ways to make her home safe for daily living. (See *Walking with a wide-based gait,* page 108.)

If appropriate, teach the patient how to use a wheelchair to maintain her mobility and independence. Instruct her or her caregiver on how to perform safe transfers from the wheelchair to a bed or car. If the patient is immobile, teach her caregiver how to perform proper turning techniques and passive ROM exercises.

MS triggers

- Stress
- Fatigue
- Temperature extremes
- Infection
- Trauma
- Menstruation
- Pregnancy

By the way

Educate the patient about factors that can exacerbate MS symptoms. (See *MS triggers.*) Also, discuss other steps the patient can take to help cope with MS. (See *Living with MS.*)

Teaching about diet

Discuss the nutritious, well-balanced diet the patient needs to maintain her ideal weight and to prevent constipation. Adequate fluid intake, including warm liquids, prune juice, and coffee, along with high-fiber foods help prevent constipation. To help prevent renal calculi and urinary tract infections, encourage the patient to consume about 2 to 3 qt (2 to 3 L) of fluid daily, including some cranberry or other acidic juice.

Benefits of a blender

If the patient has swallowing difficulties, suggest eating semisolid foods. She can chop or soften foods in a blender and freeze liquids to a slush or mix them with other foods to make swallowing easier. Also, suggest that she sit upright with her head tilted slightly forward while she eats. To stimulate the swallowing reflex, tell her to stroke upward from the base of her throat to her chin.

May I recommend a well-balanced diet filled with high-fiber foods?

Tube talk

If swallowing is extremely difficult or aspiration may occur, show the family how to prepare and administer nasogastric or gastrostomy tube feedings.

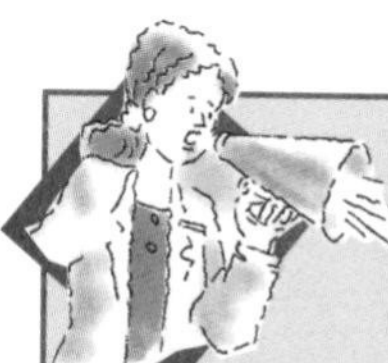

Listen up!

Living with MS

Here are some tips to help your patient with multiple sclerosis (MS) get by.

Activities, etc.

Demonstrate stress-reduction techniques, and encourage the patient to get adequate rest. Also tell her that she may perform activities better and more safely by observing (rather than feeling) her hand and foot movement.

Tremors and spasms

If the patient has head tremors, suggest resting her head against a high-backed chair to give her some stability. Also, teach her how to apply prescribed collars or neck braces. If she has hand tremors, teach her how and when to apply splints.

Show the patient with spasticity how to use a cold pack. Also, tell her how to decrease spasticity in her legs before sexual activity.

Speech, hearing, and visual disturbances

If the patient has speech problems, reinforce the need to perform phonation exercises, if prescribed. Also, if appropriate, explain how to use a communication board and voice amplifier.

Advise the patient with a hearing deficit to always face the speaker. Also, refer her for lip-reading instruction (if available), unless she also has visual disturbances.

Show the patient with diplopia how to use an eye patch or a frosted lens over one eye, alternating the patch every 2 to 4 hours. Discuss ways to adjust to loss of depth perception if the patient has vision in only one eye. Suggest reading books with large print or listening to audiotaped publications. If the patient has corneal sensory loss, show her how to instill eyedrops and use a clear eye shield.

Short-term memory deficit

If the patient has a short-term memory deficit, suggest that she carry a pad and pencil so that she can write down important information right away. She can refer to it later if she forgets something.

Sensory losses

If the patient has sensory deficits, instruct her to be cautious near extremely hot or cold objects. Tell her to use a bath thermometer to test bath water temperature.

Bladder dysfunction

For urinary incontinence or urine retention, advise the patient to drink 2 to 3 qt (2 to 3 L) of fluid daily but to restrict fluid intake about 2 hours before bedtime. If she's incontinent, teach her how to reestablish a normal pattern.

If urine retention becomes a problem, stress methods that the patient can use to completely empty her bladder (to prevent infection). As appropriate, teach her to perform intermittent catheterization. For a male patient, teach him how to catheterize himself. Also, recommend that the patient stimulate voiding by stroking her thighs and vulva (or, for a man, the glans penis).

Bowel dysfunction

For constipation, reinforce dietary guidelines with the patient. Explain that a nutritious, well-balanced diet and physical activity may offer relief. Also discuss a bowel retraining program, for example, using laxatives or suppositories at a prescribed time. Then suggest that she attempt to have a bowel movement about 30 minutes after a meal (usually breakfast), when the gastrocolic reflex is the strongest.

Explain that fecal incontinence usually results from illness, such as the flu, or from irritating substances, such as alcohol, spicy foods, or cigarettes, rather than from MS. Advise the patient to avoid irritating substances and hot liquids, to increase dietary fiber, and to wear incontinence briefs, if necessary.

Other concerns

Discuss any other question the patient may have about disease-related changes in her life such as childbearing concerns.

Teaching about medication

Explain that corticosteroids taken during acute exacerbations can help arrest disabling symptoms. Other medications to help decrease disability may include antispasmodics, anticholinergics, laxatives, antipsychotics, and antidepressants, as needed.

Relax

If muscle spasms become severe, the doctor may prescribe skeletal muscle relaxants, such as baclofen (Lioresal) or dantrolene sodium (Dantrium). Explain that these drugs, which help to relax muscles and relieve spasticity and stiffness, may make her feel confused, dizzy, drowsy, or weak. If these symptoms persist, instruct her to notify her doctor and not to operate machinery or a motor vehicle.

Also, tell her to report constipation, headache, frequent or painful urination, and persistent nausea. Caution her not to discontinue therapy without her doctor's permission. To prevent dizziness, advise her to rise slowly from a sitting or lying position and to avoid hot baths and showers. Suggest that she take the drug with meals or milk to prevent GI distress.

Investigate

If the doctor prescribes an investigational drug for your patient, discuss its potential benefits and risks. Contact the Multiple Sclerosis Foundation for up-to-date information, or consult the Web site (www.infosci.org).

Teaching about procedures

Prepare the patient for plasmapheresis, if appropriate. Explain that although its success rate varies, plasmapheresis may temporarily diminish the severity of symptoms.

Teaching about surgery

If drug therapy doesn't control tremors, the doctor may recommend stereotaxic thalamotomy. (See *Let's talk about stereotaxic thalamotomy.*)

Listen up!

Let's talk about stereotaxic thalamotomy

In this operation, the surgeon creates a surgical lesion in the thalamus on the side of the brain opposite the tremors.

A smooth head
Explain that the patient's head is shaved and cleaned and that a local anesthetic is given. The surgeon then fastens a metal frame to her head to hold it steady while he opens a small hole in her skull.

Sounds like
Describe the drilling sound the patient will hear during surgery. Explain that she'll be awake during surgery so that she can respond to such commands as "Raise your arm" or "Move your hand." This helps the surgeon determine the exact location on the opposite side of the brain.

To be expected
Inform the patient that she may have a headache after surgery.

Other options

Other surgeries may include surgically implanting a pump for delivering baclofen directly into the CSF. This can be helpful when treating severe spasticity.

Myasthenia gravis

Myasthenia gravis (MG) can occur at any age, but is most common in young adults, ages 20 to 30. It strikes more women than men.

Effective teaching can help the patient adjust to progressive fatigue and muscle weakness as well as lifelong treatment. Emphasize that, with adequate treatment, many patients with MG avoid complications and live long, productive lives.

What is it?

MG is thought to be an autoimmune disorder. Muscle weakness and fatigue are caused by a decrease in acetylcholine receptors at neuromuscular junctions resulting from an autoimmune attack. As a result, the patient finds herself working harder and tiring faster when carrying out an ordinary activity. The triggering mechanism of the autoimmune attack is unclear. (See *What happens?*)

> **What happens?**
>
> Tell the patient that myasthenia gravis (MG) is characterized by remissions (sometimes lasting for years) and exacerbations. Signs and symptoms of MG may progress slowly and steadily or rapidly and unevenly. In most patients, MG generalizes, progressing from mild to severe and involving respiratory and skeletal muscles. Tell the patient that MG symptoms usually progress downward from the head (the area served by the cranial nerves).

Teaching about tests

The patient may undergo several tests to rule out a thymoma (a tumor of the thymus), evaluate an enlarged thymus, confirm the diagnosis, measure muscle function and tone, and evaluate respiratory function. (See *Teaching patients about neurologic tests,* pages 83 to 86.)

Chest X-ray

A chest X-ray may rule out thymoma.

Tensilon or neostigmine test

These tests are used to evaluate muscle strength and differentiate between myasthenic and cholinergic crisis.

Respiratory tests

To measure respiratory muscle strength, the doctor may order several breathing tests. Laboratory tests, such as serum thyroxine analysis, serum protein electrophoresis, erythrocyte sedimentation rate, and antinuclear antibody and acetylcholine receptor antibody studies, may also help diagnose and evaluate MG.

Teaching about activity and lifestyle

Advise the patient to avoid repeated or prolonged activity that can cause muscle weakness and fatigue, and stress that regularly scheduled rest periods can conserve her strength.

Tell her to gauge activities according to her tolerance level — planning them for times when her energy peaks — probably coinciding with the time that she takes her medication.

Conserve without complication

Discuss ways to conserve energy but to prevent complications of immobility. For example, if the patient is on bed rest, encourage her to do active ROM exercises to prevent such complications as blood clots or pressure sores.

A lifelong endeavor

Finally, teach MG patients about care measures to help her deal with lifelong treatment. (See *Living with MG.*)

Teaching about diet

If the patient has dysphagia or nasal regurgitation, or both, suggest that she eat semisoft foods (applesauce, mashed potatoes, and pureed foods) and freeze liquids to a slush or mix them with other foods. Inform her that eating semisoft foods will also conserve the energy she would use to chew foods.

Tough to swallow

When the patient has swallowing difficulties, advise her to avoid foods and beverages that stimulate saliva production — milk, for example. Also advise her to avoid substances, such as alcohol, that increase weakness. Mention

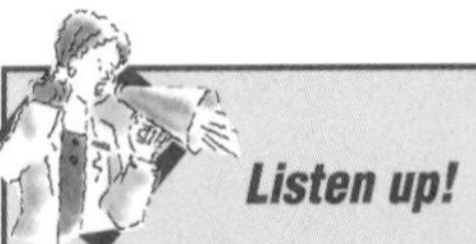

Listen up!

Living with MG

Teach your patient about additional care measures.

One eye at a time
If the patient has diplopia, tell her to use eyeglasses with a frosted lens or an eye patch, alternating the patch every 2 to 4 hours.

Avoid aggravation
Advise the patient to avoid activities or situations that aggravate her condition. Common situations include very hot or cold weather, hot baths, and stress.Tell her to avoid crowds and people with infections and to report any signs of infection to the doctor immediately.

Cough correctly
Teach the patient how to cough productively, using her abdominal muscles. If necessary, instruct her family in suctioning techniques and artificial airway insertion.

Ask for assistance
Tell the patient to keep the number for emergency assistance posted near her phone. Refer her to the Myasthenia Gravis Foundation.

that eating warm (not hot) foods can help ease swallowing, too.

Teaching about medication

The most commonly used medications for MG include anticholinesterase inhibitors and immunosuppressive agents. Advise any patient taking these drugs to wear a medical identification bracelet naming the drug and the disorder.

Enabling impulses

Anticholinesterase inhibitors help build up the body's chemical neurotransmitters, enabling motor nerve impulses to reach the muscles.

These drugs should improve the patient's symptoms, but she may not regain full strength. Suggest keeping a diary to describe the effects of the drug so the doctor can devise a dosage schedule that provides the most relief. Anticholinesterase drugs usually act within 30 minutes, and are effective for about 8 hours.

Be aware

Teach patients the signs of myasthenic crisis. Myasthenic crisis is a medical emergency and the patient should report it to the doctor at once. (See *Signs of myasthenic crisis.*)

Talk about it

The patient should also report adverse reactions to her medications, such as abdominal cramps, diarrhea, frequent urination, GI upset, nausea and vomiting, salivation, and sweating.

Fewer antibodies, more strength

Tell the patient that the doctor may prescribe a corticosteroid, such as prednisone (Orasone), to decrease antibody production and improve strength. Instruct her to take the drug exactly as ordered because suddenly stopping the drug can be life-threatening. Then caution her that the drug may worsen symptoms at first but that muscle strength should gradually improve. A low-maintenance dosage of prednisone on alternating days may be effective for months or years.

Signs of myasthenic crisis

- Worsening symptoms within 1 hour of taking medication
- Respiratory distress or shortness of breath
- Blurred or double vision
- Dizziness
- Faintness
- Increased weakness
- Rapid heartbeat
- Twitching

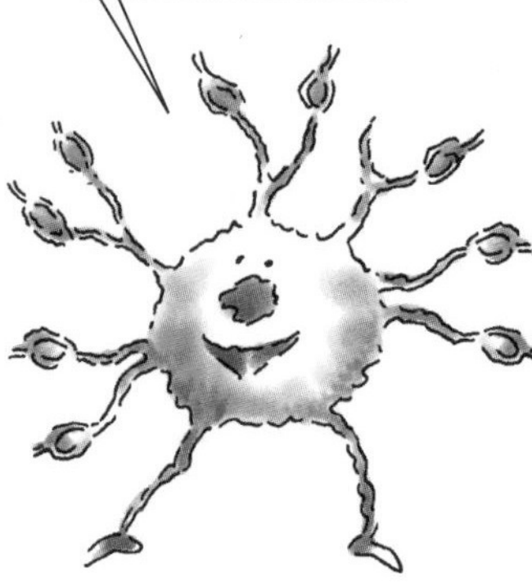
Anticholinesterase inhibitors help my impulses reach muscles.

Avoid and report

Advise taking corticosteroids with food to minimize possible GI distress. For the same reason, the patient should avoid alcohol and aspirin. Instruct her to report adverse effects. (See *Adverse effects of corticosteroids.*)

Immunosuppressive drugs such as azathioprine (Imuran) may also be used, especially if prednisone is unsuccessful or contraindicated. Adverse reactions may include a decrease in bone marrow function, liver failure, and loss of appetite.

Teaching about procedures

If typical treatments prove ineffective and the doctor orders plasmapheresis, explain that this blood-cleaning procedure may help remove harmful antibodies and temporarily ease the patient's symptoms.

Teaching about surgery

Surgical removal of the thymus may be performed. About 85% of patients experience improvement with thymectomy.

Before...

Give the patient general instructions for surgery, and tell her that before the operation her chest will be cleaned and shaved and that she'll receive a general anesthetic.

...and after

Warn the patient that she may awaken from surgery to find a chest tube or drain in place or that she may require intubation and mechanical ventilation after surgery. How soon she recovers depends on how soon she regains muscle strength and breathes without assistance.

Parkinson's disease

An estimated 1 million Americans — most over age 55 — suffer from Parkinson's disease. Effective teaching can help the patient retain control over his life for as long as possible. For instance, you can help the patient learn how

Adverse effects of corticosteroids

Cushingoid signs and symptoms

- Easy bruising
- Edema
- Facial changes
- Humpback
- Vision changes
- Weight gain

Other effects

- Acne
- Bloody or tarry stools
- Dizziness
- Extreme personality changes
- Hypertension
- Indigestion
- Insomnia
- Leg swelling
- Irregular menses
- Mild mood swings
- Nausea, vomiting
- Nervousness
- Restlessness
- Sweating
- Unusual appetite
- Unusual fatigue
- Nonhealing wounds

to perform daily activities despite motor deficits that disrupt coordination and movement.

What is it?

Parkinson's disease is a progressive, degenerative disorder of the CNS. It affects the brain centers that regulate movement; a dopamine deficiency affects the area of the brain that's responsible for control of voluntary muscle movement and posture. As a result, most symptoms relate to problems with posture and movement.

What are the signs?

The signs of Parkinson's disease usually develop gradually and vary in severity from one patient to another. The characteristic signs (typically at rest) include:
- tremors
- bradykinesia (slowness of movement)
- rigidity (increased muscle tone, masked face, stooped posture, and shuffling gait).

Point out that Parkinson's disease initially affects one side of the body but eventually involves both sides. Tremors begin in the fingers, increase during stress or anxiety, and subside with purposeful movement and sleep. (See *Signs of Parkinson's disease.*)

What's parkinsonian crisis?

In your teaching, discuss parkinsonian crisis, a medical emergency that causes a sudden and severe increase in bradykinesia, muscle rigidity, and tremors. The patient may experience increases in his heart rate and respirations, fever, and muscle paralysis that impedes swallowing or breathing.

What's oculogyric crisis?

If Parkinson's disease results from encephalitis, the patient may experience oculogyric crisis, a fixation of the eyes in one position, generally upward, for minutes or even hours.

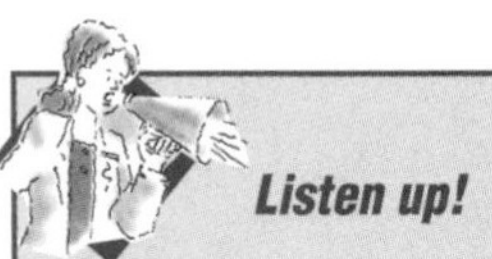

Listen up!

Signs of Parkinson's disease

Discuss with the patient the signs and symptoms that may develop as his disease progresses.

Gait way
Describe the propulsive, shuffling gait in which the body tilts forward while the arms remain at the sides (instead of swinging with walking). The patient may also notice muscle rigidity when performing any activity.

Stiff and masked
As Parkinson's disease progresses, facial expressions become masked and the patient stops blinking. He may drool because of difficulty with swallowing.

Slow speech
Tell the patient that his speech may become slow and monotonous, with poor articulation.

Other signs
Explain that other signs and symptoms, such as oily skin, increased perspiration, insomnia, and mood changes are part of the disorder.

Teaching about tests

Parkinson's disease is diagnosed from clinical findings. The doctor may order a CT scan or MRI to rule out abnormalities such as tumors. The patient may also undergo PET or single-photon-emission computed tomography to detect tumors and disorders that alter cerebral metabolism. (See *Teaching patients about neurologic tests,* pages 83 to 86.)

Urinalysis may be ordered to measure dopamine levels, which are reduced in Parkinson's disease. Cineradiographic swallowing studies may show an abnormal pattern and delayed relaxation of the muscles used in swallowing.

Rule it out

MRI is usually used to rule out small-vessel vascular disease. To help rule out disorders that mimic Parkinson's disease, the doctor may observe the patient's response to dopaminergic drugs and check the patient's medication history for drugs that can cause parkinsonian symptoms.

What exercise can do

- Improve the patient's mobility
- Reduce the risk of contractures
- Promote respiration and circulation
- Aid bowel function
- Lessen muscle rigidity
- Increase strength

Teaching about activity and lifestyle

Moderate daily exercise can have several benefits for a patient with Parkinson's disease. (See *What exercise can do.*)

If possible, encourage the patient to perform active ROM exercises. Otherwise, teach a caregiver how to perform passive ROM exercises.

Encouraging exercise

Tell the patient to exercise when he feels rested and movement seems easiest, such as in the late morning or soon after taking medication. Provide a checklist to help structure an exercise routine. (See *One, two, three, stretch.*)

Enlist the family's help in encouraging the patient to exercise. Caution the patient not to exercise excessively to avoid fatigue.

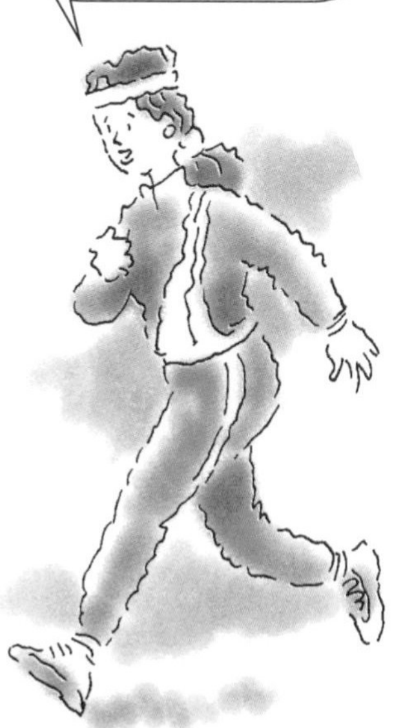
Exercise when you feel rested and it's easy to move. Try the late morning or soon after you take your medication.

Have a seat

Tell the patient that sitting in a chair with arms makes it easier to support himself. Also, elevating the back of a favorite chair by shortening the front legs 1″ to 2″ (2.5 to 5 cm) makes it easier to get up. Suggest tying a sheet to the foot of the bed to help the patient pull himself into a sitting position. Remind him to rise slowly to avoid lightheadedness.

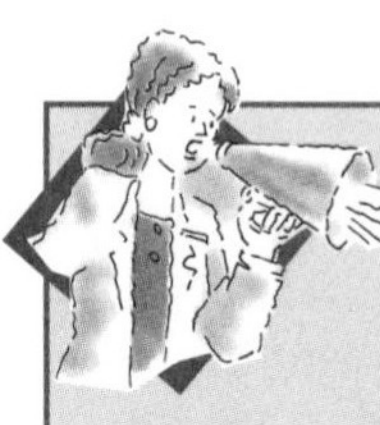

Listen up!

One, two, three, stretch

The doctor may prescribe exercises to help your patient maintain flexibility and muscle strength. Tell him to do each exercise 1 to 5 times daily at first, and then to gradually increase to 10 to 20 times daily. If he's unable to do these exercises standing up, he can do most of them sitting down.

Facial muscle exercises
Instruct the patient to raise his eyebrows and then lower and squeeze them together. Next, tell him to open his eyes wide and then close them tight.

Then tell him to wrinkle his nose and then open his mouth wide in a big "O" and close it tight. Instruct him to shift his jaw from side to side. Finally, tell him to give a big smile and then purse his lips as though trying to whistle.

Instruct him to repeat the exercises.

Neck exercises
Have the patient begin by turning his head from side to side. Next, tell him to bend his head down and back.

Instruct him to repeat the exercises.

Shoulder exercises
Tell the patient to raise his shoulders toward his ears as high as he can. Then tell him to lower them.

Have him repeat this a few more times.

Arm and shoulder exercises
Tell the patient to raise his arms over his head. Then have him swing his arms down, extending them behind his back. Repeat.

Trunk exercises
Instruct the patient to place his hands on his hips, and then twist his body at the waist from side to side, keeping his hips and legs in place. Repeat.

Hip and knee exercises
As the patient holds onto a counter or a sturdy piece of furniture, instruct him to raise his right knee toward his right shoulder. Then have him lower it and then raise his left knee toward his left shoulder. Instruct him to lower the knee and repeat these movements.

Next, have the patient stand facing a wall, about 8" (20 cm) away. Tell him to place his hands on the wall until they're above his head and then raise his right leg up behind him, keeping his knee straight. Instruct him to do the same with the left leg. Repeat.

Knee exercises
Have the patient sit and straighten his right knee, extending his right leg out in front of him. Then have him bend his right leg back under the chair as far as he can. (Tell him to keep his ankle flexed to avoid a muscle spasm.) Have him repeat with the left leg. Tell him to perform this exercise several times.

Ankle and foot exercises
With the patient sitting, tell him to make circles with his right foot — first in one direction and then in the other. Have him repeat with the left foot. Tell him to do this a few more times.

Ankle and toe exercises
With the patient sitting, tell him to extend his leg and point his toes toward the floor. Then have him point them up toward his nose. Tell him to try this several more times.

Maintaining forward momentum

To help the patient maintain balance and forward momentum, teach him to walk with a wide-based gait and to swing his arms. (See *Walking with a wide-based gait,* page 108.) If appropriate, show him how to use a weighted cane or a walker. (See *Using a walker,* page 90, and *Using a cane*, page 91.)

Unstuck

Teach the patient how to "unlock" a position if he gets stuck in one. Common unlocking techniques include:
- turning the head
- opening the mouth
- placing an arm behind the back or across the chest
- tapping a leg with the hand
- bending the knees slightly
- raising the toes.

Tell the patient to use unlocking movements cautiously to avoid losing his balance and falling.

Widen the path

To prevent falls, recommend removing throw rugs and unstable furniture and moving furniture against the walls to widen traffic paths. Also, tell the patient to wear sturdy shoes with good support and traction.

Help the patient preserve his independence by teaching him how to adjust daily activities to his current ability. (See *Living with Parkinson's disease.*)

Listen up!

Walking with a wide-based gait

Walking with a wide-based gait and swinging the arms helps patients maintain balance and keep moving forward. Instruct the patient to follow these step-by-step guidelines to practice this technique.

Walk this way

1. Have the patient start by positioning his feet 8″ to 10″ (20 to 25 cm) apart. Tell him to stand as straight as he can.

2. Next, instruct him to lift his foot high with his toes up, taking as large a step as possible.

3. As he brings his foot down, tell him to place his heel on the ground first and roll onto the ball of his foot and then his toes. Instruct him to perform the same steps with the other foot.

4. Instruct the patient to swing his right arm forward when moving his left leg. Have him swing his left arm forward when moving his right leg.

Teaching about diet

Teach the patient about the importance of maintaining a stable protein level. Excess protein can affect the action of levodopa, an amino acid used to treat Parkinson's disease.

Coffee is out, fluid and fiber are in

Tell the patient to avoid caffeine, which may worsen symptoms. Because intestinal motility may decrease, advise drinking plenty of fluids and eating high-fiber foods, especially if he's troubled by constipation.

If the patient has difficulty chewing or swallowing, recommend semisoft foods (applesauce, mashed potatoes, or solid foods prepared in a blender) to help ensure adequate nutrition and minimize the risk of aspiration.

Sit, tilt, swallow

To prevent choking, suggest freezing liquids to slush or mixing them with other foods such as cereals. Instruct the patient to sit up straight, tilt his head slightly forward, and then swallow.

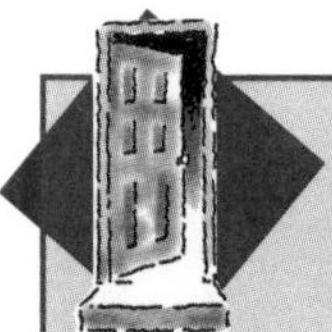

No place like home

Living with Parkinson's disease

Teach the patient with Parkinson's disease about the following additional care measures.

Combating oily skin and increased perspiration
Explain to the patient the importance of daily bathing. Instruct him to avoid oil-based soaps or lotions, and tell him to use an antiperspirant deodorant on his hands if he has sweaty palms.

Dealing with urinary urgency
Tell the patient to stay near a bathroom or to keep a urinal nearby. If he has difficulty sitting and standing, suggest that he install a raised toilet seat and grab bars.

Making dressing easier
Advise the patient to wear clothing with zippers rather than buttons or to use Velcro strips. Loafer-style shoes or elastic shoelaces solve the problem of tying and untying shoes.

Speaking up
Instruct the patient to take his time pronouncing each word. If his voice is too soft, tell him to breathe deeply before beginning each sentence. Tell him that reading aloud (especially poetry) and singing can help his articulation.

Reducing stress
Teach the patient to explore a relaxation technique compatible with his lifestyle. Avoid recommending progressive muscle relaxation, which may increase rigidity and tremors. Simple techniques, such as deep breathing and visualization, can be used spontaneously throughout the day.

Teach a family member simple massage techniques to help reduce the patient's stress at the end of the day. Point out that stress may result from excessive intake of sugar and caffeine and from prolonged exposure to loud noise, bright lights, or extreme temperatures.

Teaching family members
Instruct the family to be alert for signs of depression in the patient, such as anorexia, insomnia, and disinterest in his surroundings. Tell them to encourage the patient's participation in family discussions, even though facial rigidity may cause him to look disinterested.

The emotional or financial crises brought on by the illness may severely strain family relationships. Encourage family members not to neglect themselves. Don't hesitate to suggest counseling, and encourage them to draw on community resources as well as family and friends. Refer both the patient and family to a local group or national organization, such as the National Parkinson's Foundation and Parkinson's Support Groups of America. Finally, urge the patient to wear a medical identification bracelet or necklace at all times.

If the patient eats slowly, advise eating small, frequent meals. Instruct an obese patient about a weight-reduction diet to improve his mobility and absorption of medications.

Teaching about medication

The goal of drug therapy is to control the patient's symptoms. (See *Drug therapy for Parkinson's disease,* page 110.)

Don't stop

Caution the patient never to abruptly discontinue his medication. Doing so may bring on a parkinsonian crisis, intensifying his symptoms. Also, tell the patient that the doctor may increase the dosage as the disease progresses. However, emphasize that the patient must not increase medication dosages on his own because this may lead to drug toxicity.

After meals

Drug therapy may cause nausea and vomiting at first. Reassure the patient that this will subside in a few months. Suggest taking medications after meals to decrease nausea.

Helping the medicine go down

If the patient has difficulty swallowing, suggest that he crush pills or open capsules (unless he's taking a sustained-release form of medication) and then mix the medication with a food that's easy to swallow, such as applesauce.

Teaching about surgery

If medication fails to relieve unilateral tremors, surgery may be performed. Tell the patient who is to undergo stereotaxic thalamotomy that the surgeon creates a lesion in the thalamus to block the transmission of nerve impulses that cause tremors.

Adrenal gland alternative

If your patient is scheduled for adrenal medullary autologous transplant (a procedure that's under research), follow your hospital's protocol for teaching him. The surgery involves removal of one of the adrenal glands (usually the left) and implantation of a section of the adrenal medulla into the brain tissue.

Drug therapy for Parkinson's disease

- Levodopa or levodopa-carbidopa to replace the neurotransmitter dopamine
- Anticholinergics, such as trihexyphenidyl and benztropine, and antihistamines, such as diphenhydramine, to increase inhibition of central motor neurons
- Bromocriptine, an ergot derivative, which acts as a dopamine agonist
- The antiviral agent amantadine, which promotes dopamine synthesis and release

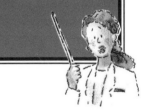

Seizures

Seizures can take a significant toll on the patient and his family. Despite advances in monitoring and treatment, a cure for seizures remains elusive, and myths and misconceptions about seizures and epilepsy still abound.

What is it?

Explain to the patient that a seizure is a sudden change in normal brain activity caused by an abnormal, uncontrolled electrical discharge from brain cells. The seizure results in distinct changes in behavior and body function, which may take the form of alterations in sensation, behavior, movement, perception, or consciousness.

A onetime event or a chronic condition

Some people experience a onetime seizure following an acute CNS disorder (for instance, a head injury) or as a result of fever, drug or alcohol withdrawal, or metabolic disturbances (such as a low blood glucose or sodium level). In contrast, the term epilepsy indicates a chronic condition characterized by recurrent seizures.

What happens?

Explain that the cause of seizures can't always be determined and that the patient's signs and symptoms depend on the site of increased brain activity. There are several types of seizure: generalized convulsive, generalized nonconvulsive, simple partial, complex partial, and partial, secondarily generalized. (See *Let's talk about seizures.*)

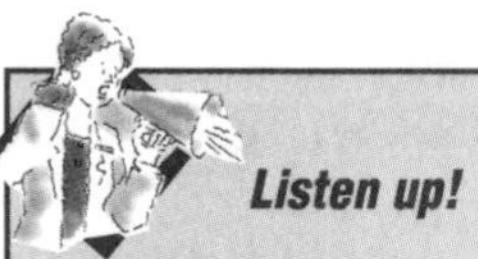

Listen up!

Let's talk about seizures

Help the patient understand his type of seizure. Also, inform the patient that he may experience more than one type of seizure.

In general

A *generalized convulsive* seizure such as a tonic-clonic (or grand mal) seizure involves the entire brain and, therefore, the entire body in convulsive activity.

Partial truths

In a partial seizure, the abnormal activity occurs in one part of the brain. A *simple partial* seizure usually has one associated manifestation, such as a jerking motion of a leg. A *complex partial* seizure has more than one manifestation, such as a jerking motion of an arm and loss of consciousness.

Seeing stars

During the initial seizure phase, the patient may notice an *aura* — a sensory phenomenon, such as seeing stars and smelling roses.

Teaching about tests

Tests used to determine the underlying cause of seizures may include skull X-rays, EEG, closed-circuit television EEG, CT scan, PET, single-photon emission tomography scan, MRI, cerebral blood flow studies, and Wada's (amobarbital) test. (See *Teaching patients about neurologic tests,* pages 83 to 86.)

Periodic blood tests

The patient who is taking anticonvulsant medications undergoes periodic blood testing to monitor blood levels and possible adverse effects of the prescribed drug. Serum electrolyte tests may be ordered to rule out metabolic disorders associated with seizures, such as hypoglycemia and hypocalcemia.

Teaching about activity and lifestyle

Educate the patient and his family about seizure triggers and how to avoid them. (See *Let's talk about triggers.*)

Suspect a seizure?

Encourage the patient to pursue normal activities if possible but to keep safety in mind. Tell him what to do if he suspects a seizure is coming on. Also, make sure that the family knows what to do if a seizure occurs. (See *Helping a seizure patient.*)

It can still happen

Because the patient may experience seizures even if he takes anticonvulsants as prescribed, teach the patient and family members about other care measures for the patient at home. (See *Living with seizures.*)

Teaching about diet

Instruct the patient to eat regular meals and to check with the doctor before dieting. Maintaining adequate blood glucose levels provides the energy needed for neurons to work normally. Teach the patient to recognize the signs and symptoms of hypoglycemia so that he can eat a snack when needed.

Teaching about medication

The patient needs to adhere strictly to the prescribed drug regimen. Point out that complying with therapy may help prevent status epilepticus, a state of continuous or rapidly recurring seizures. Status epilepticus can result in cerebral anoxia, aspiration, hyperthermia, exhaustion, serious injury (such as fractures), and even death.

One drug

Many doctors prefer monotherapy — use of a single medication — to manage epilepsy. Such therapy minimizes potential drug interactions and limits adverse reactions. It also promotes compliance through its simplicity and is cheaper than multidrug therapy.

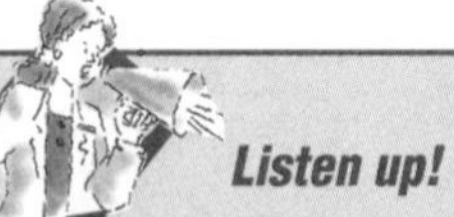

Listen up!

Let's talk about triggers

To help the patient control factors that can trigger a seizure, encourage him to:

- take the exact dose of medication at the times prescribed. Missing doses, doubling doses, or taking extra doses can cause a seizure.
- eat balanced meals. Hypoglycemia (low blood glucose levels) and inadequate vitamin intake can lead to seizures.
- limit alcohol intake. Alcohol can reduce the seizure threshold.
- get enough sleep. Excessive fatigue can bring on a seizure.
- treat a fever early during an illness and avoid hyperthermia because it may lead to seizures.
- control stress. Suggest relaxation techniques such as deep-breathing exercises.
- avoid factors that may trigger seizures—for example, flashing lights and loud noises.

Helping a seizure patient

Provide family members with the following instructions.

During the seizure

Tell the family to turn the patient on his side and remove hard or sharp objects from the area. They should loosen restrictive clothing, and place something soft and flat under the patient's head. Remind them *never* to force anything into the patient's mouth, especially fingers.

After the seizure

Advise the family to allow the patient to lie quietly. As he awakens, they should gently call him by name, and reorient him. Instruct the family to write down the seizure's duration and what the patient was doing before and during the seizure. They should then notify the doctor.

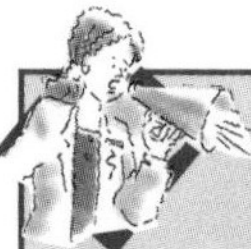

Listen up!

Living with seizures

To help the patient cope teach him the following.

Getting there

Point out that, in many states, patients with uncontrolled seizures aren't permitted to drive . Stress the serious consequences of violating laws designed to protect the patient and others in the community. Provide information on community services that offer alternative methods of transportation.

Everyone needs a helping hand

Patients with epilepsy commonly confront psychosocial challenges. The unpredictability of seizures can create problems at home, at work, or in interpersonal relationships.

Encourage the patient's family to provide emotional support to help the patient adjust to epilepsy without making him feel dependent. Refer the patient and family to appropriate associations such as the Epilepsy Foundation of America.

Not a cure-all

Make sure the patient understands that anticonvulsant drugs can't cure seizures, but will control them. Advise him to take the medication exactly as ordered; both undermedication and overmedication can cause seizures. Explain that the prescribed dosage may periodically change — for example, with age or illness.

No misses

If illness prevents the patient from taking his oral medication, tell a family member or other caregiver to contact the doctor immediately. The doctor may decide to administer medication by another route. Warn the patient that he may have withdrawal seizures if he abruptly stops taking his anticonvulsant medication.

Teaching about surgery

A patient with disabling, medically intractable epilepsy may be a candidate for surgical intervention. The most common procedure is a temporal lobectomy to remove the part of the brain where seizures originate without causing neurologic or cognitive deficits.

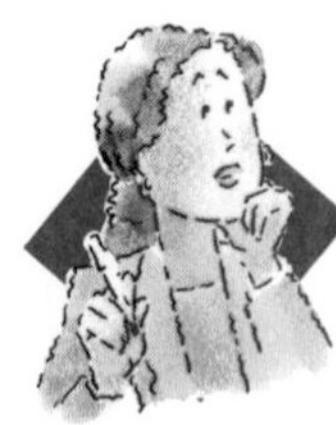

Quick quiz

1. The signs and symptoms by which relatives of a patient with Alzheimer's can recognize the progress of the disorder are:

A. flu, aching back, chest pain, tension.
B. forgetfulness, activity decline, confusion, total deterioration.
C. fluid imbalance, chewing difficulty, muscle weakness.

Answer: B. These signs and symptoms typically mark the progression of Alzheimer's disease.

2. CVA patients who have difficulty eating should:

A. sit upright and use special plates and utensils.
B. avoid caffeine.
C. lean back and eat only liquids.

Answer: A. Sitting upright can prevent choking. Feeding aids can help patients with partial arm paralysis feed themselves.

3. If the seizure patient is a child, teach the parents to do all of the following except:

A. notify the day-care or school authorities of their child's condition.
B. have the child wear a medical identification bracelet or necklace at all times.
C. restrict the child's participation in day-to-day activities.

Answer: C. The parents should encourage their child to pursue normal activities, if possible, but should remind him of safety considerations.

Scoring

☆☆☆ If you answered all three questions correctly, good going! The transmission of electrical impulses along your sensorimotor nerve routes is accurate and effective.

☆☆ If you answered two questions correctly, nice job. Your neuroceptors are in fine form.

☆ If you answered fewer than two questions correctly, don't lose your nerve. Moderate, daily review of this chapter is guaranteed to kick those electrical impulses back into high gear.

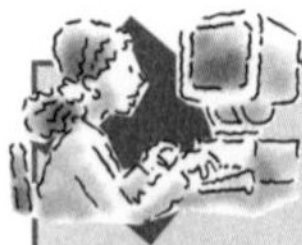

Getting connected

Asking about Alzheimer's

For more information about Alzheimer's disease, direct the patient or his family to the following Web sites:

- Alzheimer's Association (www.alz.org)
- Alzheimer's Disease Education and Referral Center (www.alzheimers.org).

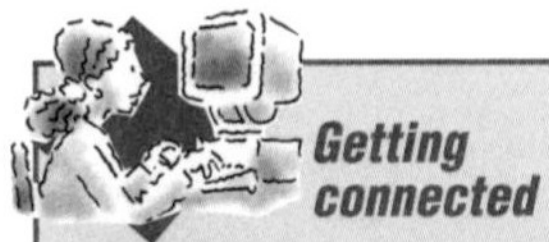

Getting connected

Posing questions about Parkinson's

For more information about Parkinson's disease, direct the patient or his family to the following Web sites:

- National Parkinson's Foundation, Inc. (www.parkinson.org)
- Parkinson's Information (www.parkinsonsinfo.com)

Gastrointestinal disorders

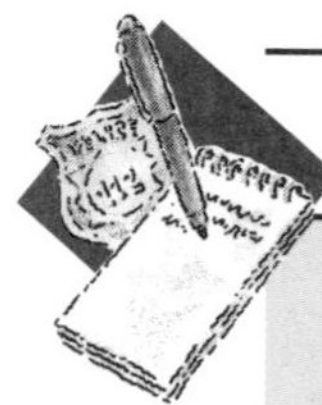

Just the facts

In this chapter, you'll learn how to teach patients with the following GI disorders:

- cirrhosis
- gallstones
- hepatitis
- inflammatory bowel disease
- irritable bowel syndrome
- chronic pancreatitis
- peptic ulcer disease.

Cirrhosis

Tell the patient that cirrhosis is a chronic disorder in which liver cells are irreversibly damaged. Explain that the healthy liver plays a major role in vitamin storage, blood clotting, toxin elimination, and carbohydrate, protein, fat, and steroid metabolism. When these functions are impaired, the result may be nutritional deficiencies, increased susceptibility to infection, and greater potential for bleeding.

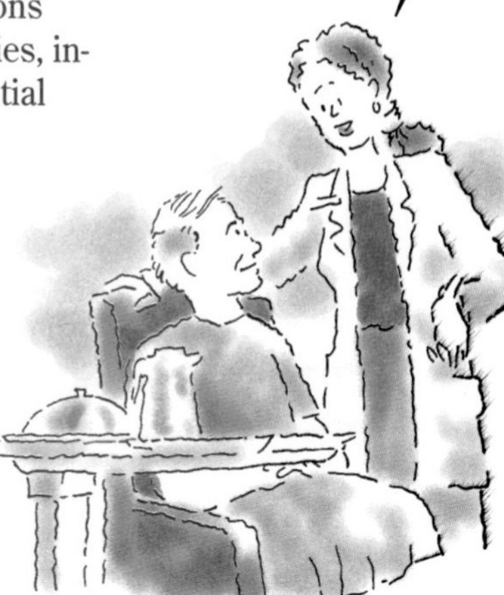
Your condition puts you at risk for nutritional deficiencies, infection, and bleeding.

What causes it?

Of all the possible causes of cirrhosis, alcohol and drug abuse are the most common.

What's the prognosis?

Emphasize that once major signs and symptoms occur, cirrhosis can't be cured. Inform the patient that although the liver has remarkable regenerative powers if he abstains from alcohol and follows his treatment plan, new tissue doesn't function as effectively. Nonetheless, with proper treatment, he may gain long-term remission of symptoms.

What's at risk?

Discuss the danger of failing to comply with the prescribed diet and medication therapy. (See *Complications of cirrhosis.*)

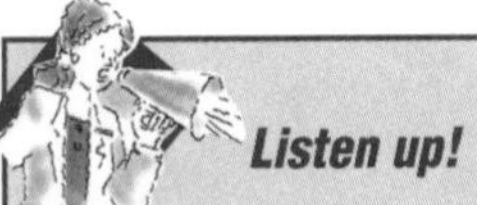

Complications of cirrhosis

Discuss with your patient the dangers of a failure to comply with therapy.

One thing leads to another
Progressive liver cell damage may lead to portal hypertension and hepatic encephalopathy. Portal hypertension can lead to esophageal varices. If varices rupture, massive bleeding may occur, requiring emergency treatment.

Less acute but ominous
Ascites (accumulation of fluid and albumin in the peritoneal cavity) is a less acute but still ominous complication. Uncontrolled ascites can compromise respiratory and renal function.

Teaching about tests

Inform the patient that the doctor will perform routine tests of liver function. However, because the results may be normal in cirrhosis, the patient may need to undergo a liver biopsy and a liver scan to confirm or evaluate cirrhosis.

The best bet: A biopsy

Explain that a liver biopsy is the definitive test for cirrhosis and that it detects destruction and fibrosis of liver tissue.

Also mention that blood samples (electrolytes, bilirubin, ammonia, blood sugar, and prothrombin levels), urine specimens, and stool samples may be collected to test liver function. (See *Teaching patients about gastrointestinal tests,* pages 118 to 122.)

Teaching about activity and lifestyle

Encourage the patient to change harmful habits that may interfere with his recovery. Above all, stress the need to abstain from alcohol. (See *Home care measures for cirrhosis.*)

Teaching about diet

Because cirrhosis is linked partly to nutritional deficiencies, stress the importance of following the doctor's dietary instructions to achieve remission of symptoms. Instruct the patient to take the supplemental vitamins recommended by the doctor. Typically, these vitamins include A, B complex, D, and K to compensate for the liver's inability to store them, and vitamin B_{12}, folic acid, and thiamine to correct anemia.

Teaching about medication

Because the patient's liver doesn't detoxify substances as well as it should, urge the patient to take medications carefully, following instructions on when to take doses and taking the exact dosage prescribed.

Relieve, reduce, decrease

As appropriate, teach the patient about any drugs prescribed to relieve nausea, reduce swelling, and decrease the risk of GI bleeding. If the doctor prescribes lactulose (Cephulac), explain that this medication helps to reduce the ammonia-forming bacteria in the GI tract and the blood. This, in turn, may reverse some of the harmful effects of liver failure on the central nervous system. Mention that diarrhea is the desired effect of this drug.

Teaching about surgery

If the patient will undergo portosystemic shunting to treat portal hypertension and prevent massive bleeding, tell him that the shunt diverts blood flow from the portal vein into the vein that empties directly into the vena cava.

Nothing to rush into

Inform the patient that preparation for surgery may take 4 to 6 weeks. During that time, he'll be placed on a regimen that includes adequate rest, a nutritious diet, supplemental vitamins, and adequate protein to relieve abdominal fluid buildup and improve liver function. He'll receive neomycin, an antibiotic, for 1 week to clean the bowel.

Tubes and drains

Explain that, after surgery, the patient will probably be sent to the intensive care unit with several tubes and drains in place. For example, he'll have a nasogastric (NG) tube, which prevents abdominal swelling by draining the GI tract, and a drain or chest tube at the incision site to remove accumulated fluid.

(Text continues on page 122.)

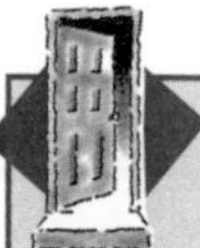

No place like home

Home care measures for cirrhosis

Inform the patient that impaired prothrombin production by the liver may cause a bleeding tendency. Tell him to watch for and report signs of bleeding, such as weakness, coughing up blood, and blood in the stools and urine. To help him minimize this risk, advise him to avoid aspirin, bruising, and straining during defecation. Instruct the patient to avoid contact with people who are ill, get adequate rest, and contact the doctor right away if he becomes ill.

Counseling options
If appropriate, encourage him to seek counseling for alcohol or drug dependency. Provide him with the address and telephone number of the Alcoholics Anonymous group in his area or of the organization's national headquarters. Spouses of alcoholics can find support in Al-Anon, another self-help group; children, in Alateen.

Teaching patients about gastrointestinal tests

Test and purpose	What to teach the patient
Barium enema study • To examine the large intestine	• Pretest procedures focus on completely cleaning the intestine. • During the test, a small, lubricated tube is inserted into the patient's rectum. As soon as the tube is inserted, the barium slowly fills the bowel while X-rays are taken. • He should keep his anal sphincter tightly contracted against the tube to hold it in position and prevent barium leakage. Accurate test results depend on adequately coating the large intestine with barium. • If he feels cramps or the urge to move his bowels as the barium or air fills the large intestine, he should breathe slowly and deeply through his mouth to ease the discomfort. • After the test, he can expel the barium into a bedpan or toilet. Then he receives another laxative and an enema to flush any remaining barium from the intestine, where it could harden, causing intestinal obstruction or impaction. • He may resume eating and taking medications, as ordered. He should drink plenty of fluids to prevent dehydration from bowel preparation and the test. Also, he should rest because the test is tiring.
Barium swallow (esophagography) • To help diagnose hiatal hernia, diverticula, and varices • To detect strictures, tumor, ulcers, or polyps in the pharynx and esophagus	• This test examines the pharynx and esophagus through X-ray films taken after a barium swallow, which clearly outlines these structures. • The patient shouldn't eat or drink for 6 to 8 hours before the test and shouldn't smoke on the morning of the test. • He should remove jewelry, dentures, hair clips, and other objects that may obscure details on the X-ray films. • During the test, he lies on an adjustable table and swallows thick and thin mixtures of barium sulfate. Barium has a chalky taste, but can be flavored to make it more palatable. As the barium outlines his pharynx and esophagus, the table is adjusted so the doctor can take films from several angles. • After the test, he resumes his normal diet and medications, as ordered, and receives a laxative to help expel the barium. Retained barium may harden, causing obstruction or impaction. He'll have chalky stools for 1 to 3 days as the barium passes through the bowel. He should call the doctor if his stools aren't chalky.
Basal gastric secretion test • To evaluate epigastric pain	• This test helps evaluate stomach pain by measuring the stomach's acid secretion when the patient is fasting. It takes about 90 minutes. • For 24 hours before the test the patient must refrain from taking, as ordered, antacids, anticholinergics, cholinergics, cimetidine, reserpine, adrenergic blocking agents, and adrenocorticosteroids. He must also refrain from eating and smoking. • During the test, a flexible tube is passed through the patient's nose into his stomach. He may feel some discomfort and may cough or gag as the tube is advanced. He then lies in various positions as his stomach contents are suctioned through the tube for analysis. • After the test, the patient may have a sore throat. He may resume his normal diet and, as ordered, his medications.

Teaching patients about gastrointestinal tests *(continued)*

Test and purpose	What to teach the patient
Cholangiography (percutaneous and postoperative) • To determine the cause of upper abdominal pain that persists after cholecystectomy • To evaluate jaundice • To determine the location, extent, and often the cause of mechanical obstruction	• This radiographic test examines the biliary ducts after injection of a contrast medium ("dye"). It takes about 30 minutes. • He must fast for 8 hours before the procedure, but should continue any prescribed drug regimen. Because the test may be uncomfortable, he'll receive medication to help him relax. • During the test, the doctor drapes and cleans an area on the patient's abdomen and injects a local anesthetic to minimize discomfort from the test. The injection will sting briefly. The patient should hold his breath as the contrast medium is injected into the liver. (If he undergoes this test postoperatively, the dye is injected through a T tube inserted into the common bile duct after surgery.) This injection may cause a sensation of pressure and right upper back discomfort. He should report immediately any adverse effects: dizziness, headache, hives, nausea, and vomiting. • He should lie still, relax, breathe normally, and remain quiet as X-ray films are taken of the biliary ducts. • After the test, the patient's vital signs are checked frequently for several hours, and he must remain in bed on his right side for at least 6 hours. He may resume his normal diet.
Colonoscopy or proctosigmoidoscopy • To aid diagnosis of inflammatory, infectious, and ulcerative bowel disease	• This test allows the doctor to see inside the lower GI tract with an endoscope, a flexible fiberoptic tube inserted into the rectum. It takes about 30 minutes. • Dietary restrictions and intestinal preparation are essential to clear the lower GI tract for an unobstructed view, so the patient takes a laxative the afternoon before the test. • During the test, an I.V. line is inserted into his hand or arm to administer a sedative to help him relax. • The doctor inserts a flexible tube into the patient's rectum. The patient may feel some lower abdominal discomfort and the urge to move his bowels as the tube advances. To control the urge to defecate and ease the discomfort, he may breathe deeply and slowly through his mouth. • Air may be introduced into the intestines through the tube. If he feels the urge to expel some air, he shouldn't try to control it. He may hear and feel a suction machine removing any matter that obscures the doctor's view. • After the test his vital signs are checked frequently for 8 hours. He can eat after recovering from the sedative, in about 1 hour. If air was introduced into the intestine, he may pass large amounts of gas. He should report any blood in his stool.
Computed tomography scan of the biliary tract, liver, or pancreas • To detect abnormalities of the biliary tract, intestines, liver, or pancreas, such as tumors, abscesses, cysts, and hematomas	• This test examines the biliary tract, intestines, liver, or pancreas through computerized X-rays. It's painless and takes about 1½ hours. • The patient must not have food or fluids after midnight before the test, but should continue any drug regimen as ordered. • During the test, the patient lies on a table while X-rays are taken. He should lie still, relax, breathe normally, and remain quiet because movement will blur the X-ray images and prolong the test.

(continued)

Teaching patients about gastrointestinal tests *(continued)*

Test and purpose	What to teach the patient
Computed tomography scan of the biliary tract, liver, or pancreas *(continued)* • To detect or evaluate pancreatitis • To determine the cause of jaundice	• If the doctor is using an I.V. contrast medium, the patient may experience discomfort from the needle puncture and a localized feeling of warmth on injection. He should report immediately any adverse effects: nausea, vomiting, dizziness, headache, or hives. However, these reactions are rare. • The patient may resume his normal diet after the test.
Endoscopic retrograde cholangiopancreatography • To evaluate tumors and inflammation of the pancreas, gallbladder, or liver • To locate obstructions in the pancreatic duct and hepatobiliary tree • To help determine the cause of jaundice	• This test examines the liver, gallbladder, and pancreas through X-ray films. Films are obtained with a flexible tube passed through the mouth into the intestine. The test takes 30 to 60 minutes. • The patient must refrain from food and fluids after midnight before the test, but should continue prescribed drugs as ordered. Although the test is uncomfortable, he'll receive a sedative to help him relax. • During the test, the patient lies on an X-ray table, and an I.V. line is inserted into his hand or arm to administer medication. • Before tube insertion, the patient's throat is sprayed with a local anesthetic. The spray tastes unpleasant and will make the patient's mouth and throat feel swollen and numb, causing difficulty swallowing. He should let the saliva drain from the side of his mouth. A mouth guard is provided to protect his teeth from the tube. He should have no difficulty breathing. • After the tube is inserted, the patient receives I.V. medication to relax the small intestine. As soon as the small intestine relaxes, he's asked to assume various positions to advance the tube to the pancreas and hepatobiliary tree. He may experience warmth or flushing when the contrast medium is injected. • After the test, the patient's vital signs are checked frequently. He'll be allowed to eat when his gag reflex returns, usually in about 1 hour. He may have a sore throat for several days.
Gastric acid stimulation test • To aid diagnosis of duodenal ulcer, Zollinger-Ellison syndrome, pernicious anemia, and gastric cancer	• This test determines if the patient's stomach is secreting acid properly. It takes about 1 hour. • The patient should stop taking antacids, anticholinergics, cholinergics, cimetidine, reserpine, adrenergic blockers, and adrenocorticosteroids, as ordered, 24 hours before the test. He should restrict food, fluids, and smoking after midnight before the test. • During the test, a flexible tube is passed through the patient's nose into his stomach. He may feel some discomfort and may cough or gag as the tube is advanced. Then he receives a subcutaneous injection of a medication (pentagastrin) to stimulate stomach acid secretion. Next, the doctor obtains several samples of stomach contents for analysis. • After the test, the patient may have a sore throat. He may resume his normal diet and medication as ordered.

Teaching patients about gastrointestinal tests *(continued)*

Test and purpose	What to teach the patient
Liver-spleen scan • To detect abnormalities of the liver and spleen • To help diagnose diseases of the liver • To demonstrate enlargement of the liver or spleen	• This noninvasive test examines the liver and spleen through pictures taken with a special scanner or camera. It takes about 1 hour. • During the test, the patient receives an injection of a radioactive substance (usually technetium Tc 99m) through an I.V. line in his hand or arm; this allows better visualization of the liver and spleen. The injection contains only trace amounts of radioactivity and rarely produces adverse effects. • He may hear a soft, irregular, clicking noise as the scanner moves across his abdomen. He may feel the camera lightly on his abdomen. He should remain still, relax, and breathe normally. He may be asked to hold his breath briefly to ensure clear pictures.
Oral cholecystography • To detect abnormalities of the gallbladder, such as gallstones, tumors, and inflammation	• This test examines the gallbladder through X-rays taken after ingestion of a contrast medium. It takes 30 to 45 minutes. • If ordered, the patient eats a low-fat breakfast and lunch the day before the test and a fat-free meal that evening. After the evening meal, he can have only water, but should continue any ordered drug regimen. He's given a cleansing enema, and 2 to 3 hours before the test, he's asked to swallow six tablets, one at a time, at 5-minute intervals. The enema and tablets help outline the gallbladder on the X-ray film. • During the test, the patient lies in a supine position on an X-ray table while films are taken of his emptying gallbladder and the patency of the common duct. • After the test, the patient should drink plenty of fluids to help eliminate the dyelike substance in the tablets.
Percutaneous liver biopsy • To help diagnose cirrhosis, metastatic diseases, and granulomatous infection	• This test diagnoses liver disorders through examination of liver tissue. The doctor obtains a small liver specimen by inserting a needle. It takes about 15 minutes. • During the test, the patient is awake, but will be given medication to help him relax. The doctor drapes and cleans an area of the patient's abdomen and injects a local anesthetic, which may sting and cause brief discomfort. Then the patient is asked to hold his breath and lie still as the doctor inserts the biopsy needle into the liver. The needle may cause a sensation of pressure and some discomfort in his right upper back. • After the test, the patient's vital signs are checked frequently for several hours. He must remain on his right side for 2 hours and on bed rest for 24 hours. He may resume his normal diet.

(continued)

Teaching patients about gastrointestinal tests *(continued)*

Test and purpose	What to teach the patient
Ultrasonography of the gallbladder, biliary system, liver, spleen, or pancreas • To help diagnose disorders of the gallbladder and biliary system (such as cholelithiasis and cholecystitis), liver (such as cirrhosis and hepatitis), and pancreas	• This test examines body structures using sound waves. It takes 15 to 30 minutes. • The patient must restrict food and fluids for 8 to 12 hours before the test. The doctor may order a special diet the day before the test. • As the patient lies on a table, a technician applies conductive gel or oil to his abdomen. Then the technician moves the transducer across the patient's abdomen. This doesn't cause discomfort. The patient should lie still, relax, breathe normally, and remain quiet. Any movement will distort the picture and prolong the test. He may also be asked to hold his breath or inhale deeply. • If he's having ultrasonography of the gallbladder, he may receive an injection of a drug (sincalide) to stimulate gallbladder contraction. He should report immediately any adverse effects: abdominal cramping, nausea, dizziness, sweating, or flushing. • After the test, the patient may resume his normal diet.
Upper GI endoscopy (esophagogastroduodenoscopy) • To identify abnormalities of the esophagus, stomach, and small intestine, such as esophagitis, inflammatory bowel disease, Mallory-Weiss syndrome, lesions, tumors, gastritis, and polyps	• This test examines the esophagus, stomach, and duodenum using a flexible tube inserted into the intestine through the mouth. It takes about 30 minutes. • He must not eat or drink for 6 hours before the test, but should continue any prescribed medications as ordered. • During the test, he lies on an X-ray table and an I.V. line is inserted into his hand or arm to administer medications, if needed. He'll receive a sedative to help him relax. • Before tube insertion, his throat is sprayed with an anesthetic. The spray tastes unpleasant and will make his mouth feel swollen and numb, causing difficulty swallowing. He should let the saliva drain from the side of his mouth. A mouth guard is provided to protect his teeth from the tube. • As the doctor advances the tube, the patient may be asked to assume various positions. He can expect to feel abdominal pressure and fullness or bloating as the doctor gently introduces air for a better view of internal structures. • After the test, the patient's vital signs are checked frequently for 8 hours. He can resume eating when his gag reflex returns—usually in about 1 hour. He may have a sore throat for several days.

From clear liquids to solid foods

Also tell him that several catheters will be in place to monitor hemodynamic pressure. Tell him that, after bowel sounds return and the NG tube is removed, his diet will consist of clear liquids and will progress gradually to solid foods.

Turn, cough, breathe deeply

Pulmonary complications are common after portosystemic shunting because the incision line is close to the diaphragm. To help prevent these complications, instruct the patient to turn in bed and to cough and breathe deeply at least once every hour.

Getting back on your feet

Explain to the patient that, to enhance his recovery, the doctor may prescribe a low-protein, low-salt diet; vitamin supplements; and adequate rest. Urge the patient to comply with all instructions.

Gallstones

About 25 million Americans (mostly women) have cholelithiasis (gallstones), making it the most common biliary tract disorder in the United States. Less than half of these people develop symptoms. Between 500,000 and 700,000 cholecystectomies (gallbladder removals) are performed each year.

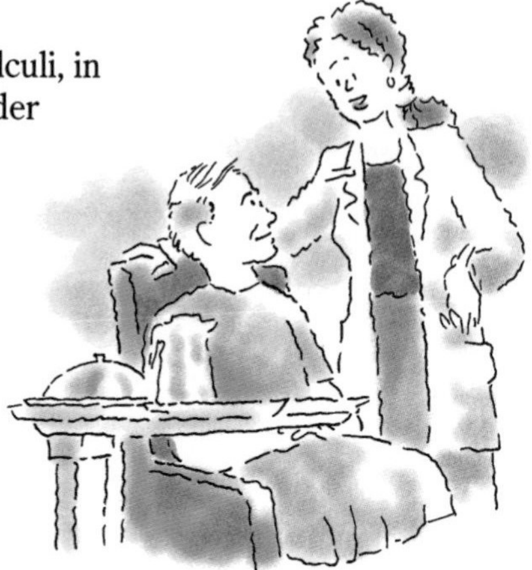
Gallstones may be as small as the head of a pin or as large as the egg of a hen.

What are they?

Inform the patient that gallstones are stones, or calculi, in the gallbladder. Gallstones signal that the gallbladder has become sluggish, giving cholesterol, calcium bilirubinate, or a mixture of cholesterol and bilirubin pigment a chance to settle and crystallize. The resulting stone is usually pea-sized, but can be as tiny as a pinhead or as large as a hen's egg.

Who's at risk?

Point out that although no one knows for sure what causes gallstones, certain contributing factors set the stage for stone formation. At highest risk for gallstones are women — especially obese women over age 40 who have had several pregnancies.

Are they always painful?

Explain that about half the patients with gallstones are asymptomatic and learn of their condition only when an X-ray or ultrasonography is performed for other reasons. The other half suffer the severe, episodic pain of acute cholelithiasis (also called gallbladder attack or biliary colic). This pain begins in the middle of the abdomen or the right upper quadrant and commonly spreads to the back and right scapula. It lasts up to several hours, and walking or changing position offers no relief.

Where does pain come from?

Inform the patient that the pain results from a stone becoming lodged in the gallbladder's neck or in the cystic duct. The pain diminishes when the stone dislodges and either slips back into the gallbladder or passes into the intestine. Emphasize that untreated gallstones can cause life-threatening complications.

> **Seize the moment**
>
> Take time to answer questions as soon as possible. Satisfy the patient's immediate need for information, and augment your teaching with more information later.

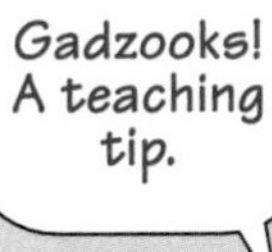
Gadzooks!
A teaching
tip.

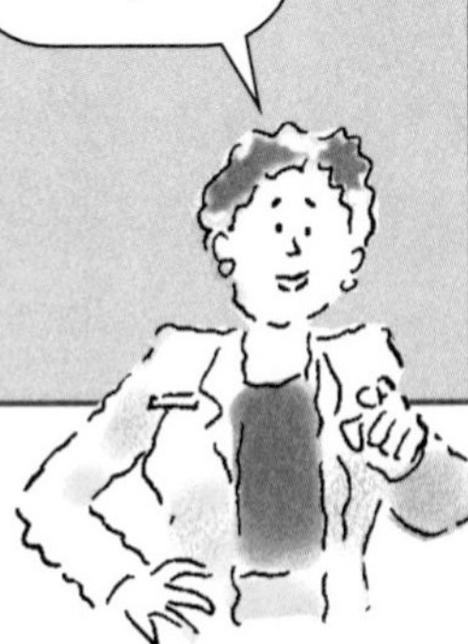

Teaching about tests

Tell the patient that several diagnostic studies can detect gallstones in patients who suffer the symptoms. The most commonly performed tests are biliary ultrasonography and oral cholecystography. If these tests fail to reveal gallstones, the doctor may order endoscopic retrograde cholangiopancreatography (ERCP) or percutaneous transhepatic cholangiography. Routine laboratory tests of blood samples and urine specimens may also support the diagnosis. (See *Teaching patients about gastrointestinal tests,* pages 118 to 122.)

Teaching about diet

If the patient asks whether a special diet (such as a fat-free diet) can relieve symptoms, tell her that clinical findings no longer support the effectiveness of diet therapy.

Teaching about medication

Treatment for gallstones doesn't begin until the patient has symptoms. Medications to treat gallstones may include analgesics to relieve pain, antibiotics to prevent infection, and drugs to dissolve the stones.

Analgesics

A narcotic analgesic such as meperidine (Demerol) may be prescribed for the patient with episodic biliary colic or for the hospitalized patient with gallstones complicated by acute cholecystitis. Tell the patient that pain and inflammation usually subside in 2 to 7 days.

Antibiotics

For the patient with gallstones and acute cholecystitis, the doctor may prescribe a broad-spectrum antibiotic, such as tetracycline, to prevent infection — especially if the patient is elderly, has gallstones in the common bile duct, or has diabetes mellitus or another serious disorder.

Oral dissolution therapy

If the patient's gallstones are noncalcified and contain mainly cholesterol, the doctor may recommend oral dissolution therapy.

Shrink, dissolve, and prevent new ones

Explain that the bile salts chenodiol (Chenix) and ursodiol (Actigall), alone or in combination, can shrink or dissolve existing gallstones and prevent new formations. Inform the patient that this therapy will continue for about 2 years and that the patient's progress will be monitored by ultrasonography.

You will undergo oral dissolution therapy for about 2 years. Your progress will be monitored by ultrasound testing.

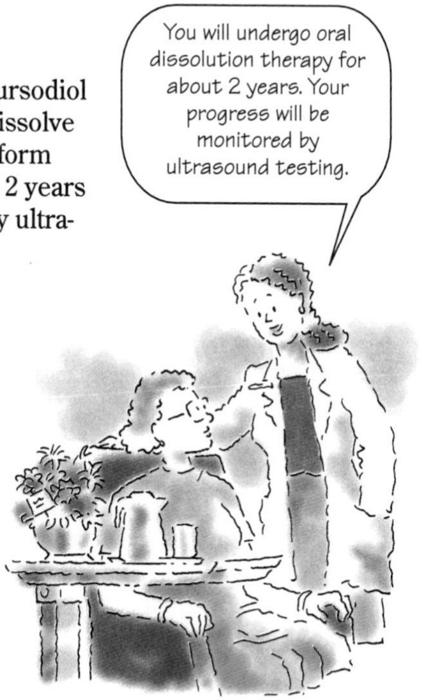

Making it work

Teach the patient how to take these drugs. Because the dosage is based on weight, tell her to weigh herself at the same time daily and to alert the doctor about significant weight loss. Urge her to keep scheduled appointments for laboratory tests that will monitor how the therapy affects her liver function. Tell her to report immediately diarrhea, severe abdominal pain, nausea, or vomiting.

Topical solvents

The topical solvent methyl *tert*-butyl ether (MTBE) dissolves cholesterol stones. Point out that the solvent is instilled through a catheter inserted either into the abdomen or through the nose to the hepatic duct, depending on the gallstones' location. Explain that the procedure usually requires a local anesthetic and takes place in the hospital outpatient department.

They may be back

Explain that this drug can dissolve any size or number of cholesterol stones within hours; however, the stones may recur later.

Teaching about procedures

The choice of treating gallstones surgically versus treating them nonsurgically depends on several factors. (See *Treatment for gallstones.*) If the doctor recommends a nonsurgical intervention, the patient may undergo one of the treatments discussed below. Explain the treatment the patient will undergo, and also review care measures to take after the procedure. (See *Advice for nonsurgical gallstone patients.*)

Therapeutic ERCP

If gallstones are detected during diagnostic ERCP, the doctor may attempt to remove them at the same time. Explain to the patient that the doctor will insert a basket-like device through an endoscope to secure and retrieve the stones.

Endoscopic sphincterotomy

If the doctor schedules this procedure, tell the patient that an endoscope and special devices are used to remove gallstones in the common bile duct. Tell her to fast after midnight before the day of the procedure.

Explain that she'll receive medications to relax her, and an I.V. line will be inserted in her hand or arm to administer medication. A local anesthetic is given to ease endoscope insertion. During the procedure, she'll assume various positions to help advance the endoscope for proper placement.

No gag

Tell the patient that afterward, her vital signs are monitored until they're stable. She can eat and drink when the gag reflex returns, but will remain in bed for 6 to 8 hours (or overnight in the hospital). Warn her that she may have abdominal discomfort for 1 to 2 weeks.

Listen up!

Treatment for gallstones

Treatment for gallstones depends on signs and symptoms. If the patient is asymptomatic, she won't require treatment. If she has had at least one gallbladder attack and test results confirm gallstones, the doctor may recommend gallstone removal.

Surgery or not?
The doctor will likely choose to perform surgery if one or more of the following factors exist:

- frequent, severe symptoms, such as pain, that interfere with the patient's daily routine
- a history of prior complications of gallstone disease, such as cholecystitis, pancreatitis, or gallstone fistula
- the presence of underlying conditions that increase the risk of gallstone complications.

Extracorporeal shock-wave lithotripsy

Extracorporeal shock-wave lithotripsy uses high-energy shock waves to shatter gallstones.

Explain that extracorporeal shock-wave lithotripsy (ESWL) is a noninvasive, painless procedure that uses high-energy shock waves to shatter gallstones, thereby allowing them to be eliminated naturally. The 30- to 60-minute procedure works best for patients with mild to moderate symptoms and only a few small-diameter stones consisting mainly of cholesterol. For the procedure, the patient may receive I.V. narcotics or, occasionally, a general anesthetic.

Shock waves

Tell the patient that immediately before ESWL begins, the doctor locates the stones precisely by ultrasonography. Then the machine's hydraulic stretcher lowers her into a water tank until the shock-wave generator can focus directly on the gallstones. Next, the lithotriptor discharges serial shock waves through the water to shatter the stones without damaging surrounding tissue. Ultrasonic or fluoroscopic devices monitor the process until the gallstones disintegrate — usually in 1 to 2 hours.

No pain but...

Reassure the patient that she won't feel pain but may feel a fluttering sensation or mild blows. If a catheter was inserted, the doctor may also inject monooctanoin through the catheter to decrease the stones' size.

Monitoring for shock-wave damage

Tell the patient that her vital signs are monitored during ESWL, and she'll undergo liver function studies to make sure her liver sustained no damage from the shock waves. Instruct her to report without delay posttreatment abdominal pain, fever, nausea, or vomiting.

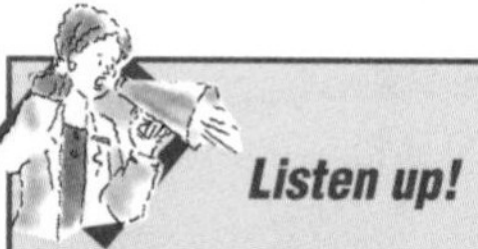

Listen up!

Advice for nonsurgical gallstone patients

Inform the nonsurgical patient that repeated episodes of biliary colic caused by gallstones may warrant hospitalization, nasogastric tube insertion, and I.V. therapy for hydration and antibiotic administration. Explain that treatment to remove the stones usually begins soon after the episode subsides.

Countering complications

Encourage the patient to keep follow-up appointments and to take medications as directed to help prevent recurrent biliary colic and other complications.

From the gallbladder to the intestine

In the days immediately after ESWL, most of the stones travel from the gallbladder to the intestine, and are excreted naturally. (See *Post-ESWL warning.*)

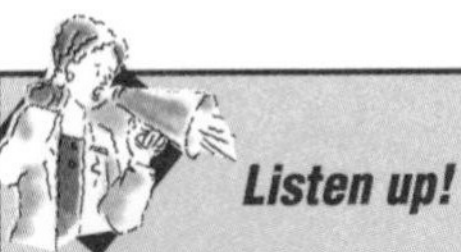

Listen up!

Post-ESWL warning

Because incompletely pulverized stones can lodge in the biliary tract or pancreas or develop into new calculi, urge the patient to keep scheduled follow-up appointments.

Teaching about surgery

Cholecystectomy (gallbladder removal) is the most common surgery for gallbladder disease. Other types of surgery include cholecystotomy (incision of the gallbladder) and choledochostomy (formation of an opening into the common bile duct). Laparoscopic cholecystectomy, a relatively new procedure, may also be performed.

Cholecystectomy, cholecystotomy, and choledochostomy

Tell the patient that most gallbladder operations require a general anesthetic before surgery. Advise her to consume only clear liquids the day before surgery and nothing after midnight before the operation.

Talkin' 'bout the T tube

Warn the patient that she'll have an NG tube in place for 1 to 2 days after surgery and a drain at the incision site for 3 to 5 days. She may also have a T tube inserted into the common bile duct to drain excess bile and allow removal of retained stones.

If appropriate, explain that the T tube may remain in place for up to 2 weeks, depending on the type of surgery, and that she may be discharged with the tube. Teach her how to perform coughing and deep-breathing exercises to help prevent postoperative atelectasis, which can lead to pneumonia. (See *Take care of your T tube.*)

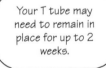

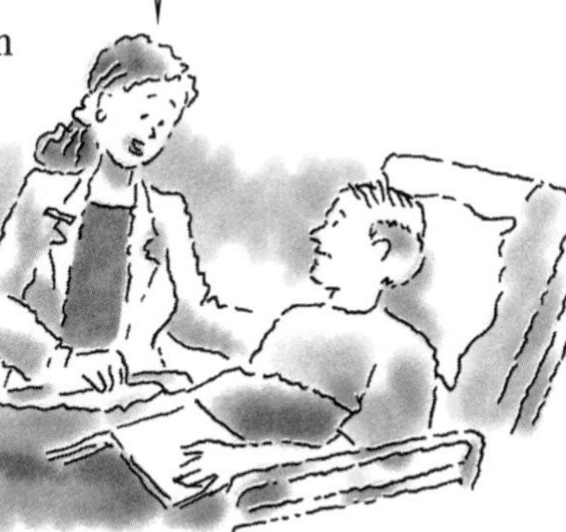
Your T tube may need to remain in place for up to 2 weeks.

Laparoscopic cholecystectomy

Inform the patient that the surgeon may remove her gallbladder through one of four small abdominal incisions. The surgery takes about 90 minutes and requires a general anesthetic.

Overnight stay

Tell the patient that she may be admitted to the hospital on the day of surgery and be discharged the same day or the next day. Instruct her to fast after midnight the day before surgery. Explain that the surgeon will use a laparoscope to visualize her gallbladder, and other tools to excise the gallbladder and remove it through a small incision.

After surgery

Advise the patient that she may experience minor discomfort at the site where the surgeon inserts the laparoscope and mild shoulder pain for up to 1 week — either from diaphragmatic irritation caused by abdominal stretching or from residual carbon dioxide. Oral analgesics or anti-inflammatory agents can be ordered to relieve these symptoms.

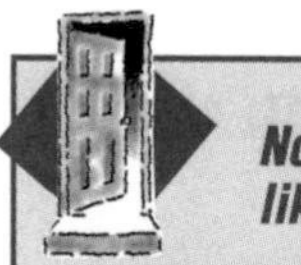

No place like home

Take care of your T tube

If a patient is going home with a T tube in place, make sure that she knows how to perform tube care. Explain to her how to care for her incision, and direct her to report signs or symptoms of infection, such as redness, tenderness, or drainage at the incision site. Also advise her to report signs or symptoms of biliary obstruction: fever, jaundice, itching, pain, dark urine, and clay-colored stools.

Hepatitis

Hepatitis is an inflammation of the liver that interferes with normal liver function. Initial symptoms of hepatitis include malaise, fever, chills, aching muscles, photophobia, anorexia, nausea, headache, and abdominal pain.

As the disease progresses, jaundice — a yellowish discoloration of the skin and the whites of the eyes — usually develops. The patient may also experience dark urine, light-colored stools, hepatomegaly, and enlarged lymph nodes.

What causes it?

Explain that the term "viral hepatitis" means hepatitis caused by a virus — most commonly hepatitis virus A, B, C, D, E, and possibly G (although A, B, C, and D are the most common). Other viruses that cause hepatitis include Epstein-Barr virus and cytomegalovirus.

What's at risk?

Emphasize that strict adherence to the treatment plan is essential for liver regeneration. Incomplete regeneration can lead to cirrhosis — progressive destruction of the liver characterized by scarring, fibrosis, and fatty deposits. Point out that cirrhosis can, in turn, lead to conditions that may bring on hemorrhage, coma, and even death.

Teaching about tests

Inform the patient that a diagnosis of hepatitis hinges on the signs and symptoms and the results of a number of studies, such as liver function tests and, possibly, a liver biopsy. (See *Turn to the side, please,* and *Teaching patients about gastrointestinal tests,* pages 118 to 122.)

Turn to the side, please

If viral hepatitis is suspected, tell the patient that the doctor will order a hepatitis profile. A blood sample will be analyzed to identify the specific virus responsible for his disorder.

Teaching about activity and lifestyle

In the early stages of hepatitis, the patient will suffer from fatigue. Although rest remains important, as the patient begins to feel better, he may be reluctant to comply with activity restrictions. Therefore, stress the importance of curtailing unnecessary activity. For instance, help him find ways to minimize job demands, food shopping, child care, and stair climbing.

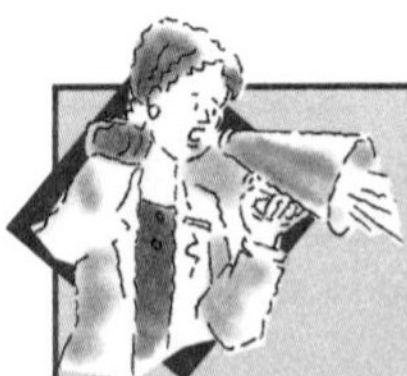

Listen up!

Preventing the spread of hepatitis

To prevent the patient from transmitting hepatitis to others, educate him about how the disease is spread.

Hepatitis A

Hepatitis A is spread when fecal matter from an infected person contaminates food or water. Common sources of such contamination include infected restaurant workers, sewage leaks into a water supply, and raw shellfish from polluted waters.

Explain that when the patient has a bowel movement, some of the hepatitis virus passes out of his body in his stool. This infected fecal matter will contaminate any food or water it comes in contact with. In turn, anyone who eats or drinks the contaminated food or water can develop hepatitis A. Oral-anal sexual relations can also transmit hepatitis A.

Advise the patient to wash his hands thoroughly after every bowel movement and before handling food or preparing meals. Warn him not to share food, eating utensils, or toothbrushes.

Hepatitis B, C, or D

Hepatitis B, C, or D may be spread parenterally or through sexual relations. Point out that the hepatitis virus is present in the patient's blood and in any of his body fluids.

If any of the patient's blood enters another person's bloodstream (for example, by sharing intravenous needles), that person can catch hepatitis from the patient.

Also inform him that if his blood or body fluids come in contact with a break in another person's skin or with the mucous membranes of another person's mouth, vagina, or rectum, that person can develop hepatitis.

Instruct the patient to wash his hands thoroughly and frequently. Articles soiled with feces should be disinfected. Clothing should be laundered separately in hot water. The patient shouldn't prepare food for others, nor should he share food, eating utensils, or toothbrushes. If he injects drugs, tell him not to share the needle. Also instruct him not to have unprotected sex with anyone and not to donate blood.

No sharing

If the patient has viral hepatitis, explain that anyone exposed to the disease through contact with him should receive immune globulin or the hepatitis B vaccine as soon as possible after exposure. Help him to identify those at risk, and teach him and his family to avoid spreading the disease. (See *Preventing the spread of hepatitis* and *Before you say goodbye.*)

Teaching about diet

Inform the patient that good nutrition promotes liver regeneration. Because the patient may experience anorexia, nausea, or vomiting, help him build an appealing meal plan based on frequent, small meals encompassing a low-fat, high-carbohydrate, high-calorie diet. Inform him that a well-balanced diet can meet his nutritional needs. If appropriate, refer him to a dietitian.

Teaching about medication

Inform the patient that there's no specific drug therapy for hepatitis, but because some drugs are metabolized by the liver, advise the patient to check with the doctor before taking any medication, including nonprescription drugs.

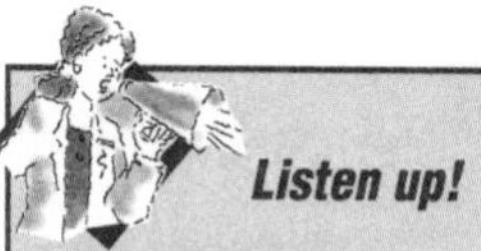

Listen up!

Before you say goodbye

Stress the importance of continued medical care for the patient with hepatitis.

About 2 weeks
Advise the patient to see the doctor again about 2 weeks after being diagnosed. At this time, the doctor will determine if the patient's fluid intake is adequate and will perform additional blood tests to evaluate liver function.

Follow-up, follow-up, follow-up
After this, the patient will need a follow-up appointment once a month for up to 6 months. Then, if chronic hepatitis develops, the patient must visit the doctor at regular intervals to monitor the course of the disease.

More info
Finally, refer the patient to the American Hepatitis Association or the American Liver Foundation for further information.

Inflammatory bowel disease

The patient who has inflammatory bowel disease faces the need to cope with a chronic disorder. Although interruption of daily activities and possible lifestyle changes may frustrate the patient, emphasize that he can lead a normal life.

What is it?

Inform the patient that inflammatory bowel disease involves chronic inflammation of the GI tract lining. Explain that this disease has two forms: ulcerative colitis and Crohn's disease. (See *Comparing ulcerative colitis and Crohn's disease,* page 132.)

Comparing ulcerative colitis and Crohn's disease

Review the information in this chart to help you focus your teaching on the patient's type of inflammatory bowel disease — ulcerative colitis or Crohn's disease.

Characteristic	Ulcerative colitis	Crohn's disease
Usual site	Colon and rectum	Commonly terminal ileum and right colon; may be anywhere from mouth to anus
Depth of involvement	Mucosal, submucosal	Transmural
Distribution	Continuous	Segmental
Bowel lumen size	Normal	Narrow
Rectal bleeding	Common	Unusual
Anorectal fistulas	Rare	Common
Anal abscesses	Rare	Common
Crypt abscesses	Common	Rare
Cobblestoned mucosa	Rare	Common
Inflammatory masses	Rare	Common, extensive
Toxic megacolon	May occur	May occur
Pseudopolyps	Common	Rare
Granulomas	Absent	Common
Strictures	Absent	Common
Bowel shortening	Common	Rare
Mesenteric fat and lymph involvement	Absent	Common
Carcinoma	High risk after 10 years	Risk increases with age
Diarrhea	Common	Common
Tenesmus	Severe	Rare
Abdominal pain	May occur	Common
Weight loss	Common	Common

Age and stage

In your teaching plan, consider the patient's emotional, psychological, and cognitive development as well as physical growth and development.

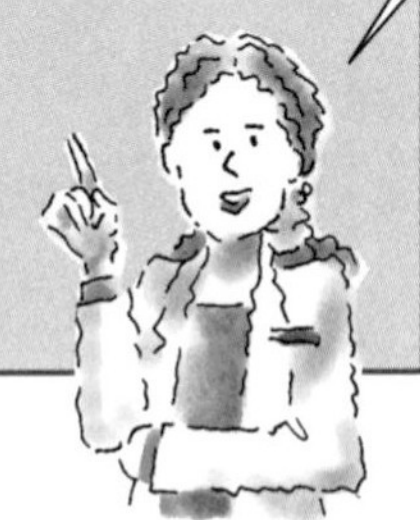

What's at risk?

Crohn's disease may lead to complications, such as fibrous scarring, obstructions, abscess with sepsis, fistula formation, and perforation.

Tell the patient with ulcerative colitis that he may be at risk for cancer, especially if the disease has persisted for more than 10 years.

What's changed?

Encourage the patient to report any changes in his condition so the doctor can tailor the treatment plan most effectively. Although inflammatory bowel disease doesn't have an emotional origin, warn the patient to avoid excessive stress.

Get it?

Look for signs of understanding and adjust your teaching to the patient's cognitive abilities.

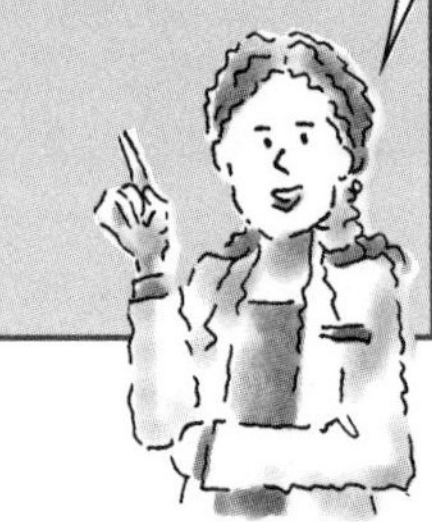
Surprise! A teaching tip.

Teaching about tests

Teach the patient about the various tests that diagnose inflammatory bowel disease and monitor its course. In addition to undergoing routine blood, urine, and stool studies, he'll usually have a barium enema, barium swallow, lower and upper GI endoscopy, and an upper GI series. If appropriate, inform the patient that the doctor may schedule a computed tomography (CT) scan to confirm a suspected abscess. (See *Teaching patients about gastrointestinal tests,* pages 118 to 122.)

Teaching about activity and lifestyle

Explain to the patient the importance of adequate rest. To decrease intestinal motility during an attack, advise him to reduce physical activity. If his attack is mild, suggest that he rest more during the day.

When nature calls

Urge the hospitalized patient with severe diarrhea to use the call light whenever he needs help going to the bathroom. If he can use the bathroom unassisted, instruct him to tell the nurse when he has a bowel movement so she can record the number of stools, their consistency, color, and volume, and the presence of bleeding. (See *Living with inflammatory bowel disease,* page 134.)

Teaching about diet

Explain that dietary changes allow the bowel to heal by decreasing its activity while providing the calories and nutrition necessary for healing. Stress the importance of following the prescribed diet to help decrease symptoms. Make sure he understands his prescribed diet, which will be high in protein, calories, and vitamins.

Steer clear

Advise him to avoid foods that irritate his intestines or that require excessive intestinal activity, such as milk products, spicy or fried high-residue foods, raw vegetables and fruits, whole-grain cereals, monosodium glutamate, and sugarless gum and mints containing sorbitol.

Discourage carbonated, caffeine-containing, and alcoholic beverages because they increase intestinal activity. Also discourage extremely hot or cold food and fluids because they cause gas.

Explain that he may need supplemental vitamins to compensate for the bowel's inability to absorb them.

Eat little and often

Advise eating small, frequent meals. If anorexia is a problem, reinforce the importance of an adequate diet to pro-

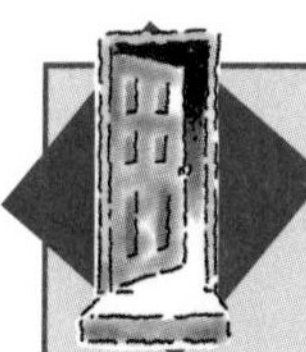

No place like home

Living with inflammatory bowel disease

Here are some tips for helping your patient cope with inflammatory bowel disease.

Do's and don'ts

Discourage smoking; it contributes to altered bowel motility. If diarrhea is severe, teach the patient proper skin care. Because persistent diarrhea and vomiting may lead to serious metabolic complications, instruct him to report signs of dehydration (confusion, lethargy, dry skin and mucous membranes, dry mouth, weakness, and reduced urine output).

Don't keep it a secret

Instruct the patient to notify the doctor if he experiences signs and symptoms of complications: fever, fatigue, weakness, or a rapid heart rate, along with abdominal cramping, vomiting, and acute diarrhea. Abdominal pain and cramping can signal progressive inflammatory bowel disease, indicating stricture or obstruction. Fatigue and weakness, accompanied by pallor and dizziness, can indicate anemia.

Ileostomy insights

If the patient has an ileostomy, tell him to avoid laxatives, enteric-coated pills, and timed-release capsules, because they won't be fully absorbed. Urge him to contact the doctor if he acquires an infection or experiences diarrhea or vomiting because they can lead to life-threatening metabolic complications. Also arrange for follow-up examinations by a health care professional. Emphasize the importance of wearing a medical identification bracelet or necklace at all times. Advise him to see the doctor regularly for checkups.

In addition to teaching the patient about ostomy care, you'll need to help him learn how to adapt his lifestyle. Be prepared to answer questions on a range of issues.

Support suggestions

Refer the patient and his family to the local chapter of the National Foundation for Ileitis and Colitis to provide them with support. Tell the family that many patients feel that their problems are unique. Encourage both patient and family to express their feelings. For the patient with an ostomy, contact the United Ostomy Association to provide guidance and support.

mote healing. Suggest snacks, favorite foods (if permitted), good mouth care (to enhance taste), and a pleasant dining atmosphere.

Teaching about medication

Explain that medications aim to decrease inflammation and control or relieve symptoms.

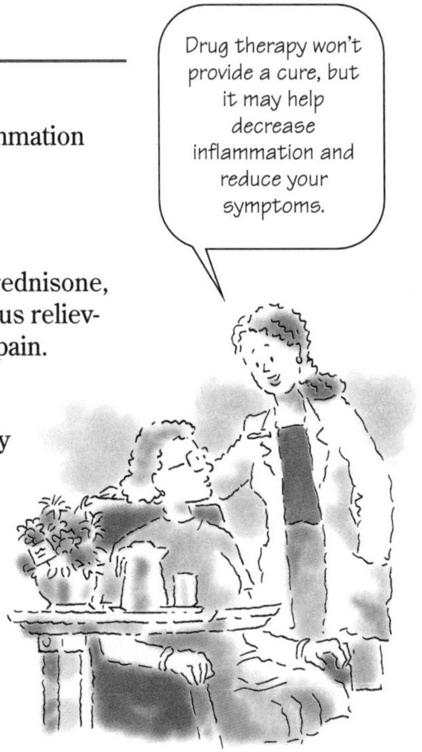

Drug therapy won't provide a cure, but it may help decrease inflammation and reduce your symptoms.

Corticosteroids

If the doctor orders a corticosteroid, such as prednisone, explain that this drug reduces inflammation, thus relieving such symptoms as diarrhea, bleeding, and pain.

To the letter

Teach the patient to take corticosteroids exactly as prescribed and not to stop taking them abruptly. Stress that after long-term use, stopping the drug suddenly can cause adrenal crisis. Warn about possible adverse effects of corticosteroids, including osteoporosis, increased susceptibility to infection, fluid retention, and mood swings.

Sulfasalazine

Explain that the doctor may prescribe sulfasalazine to reduce inflammation. Tell the patient to take it with a full glass of water, after food intake.

Don't keep it a secret

Advise him to report aching joints and muscles, dizziness, fever, hematuria, itching, jaundice, low back pain, photosensitivity, rash, abdominal pain, or unusual bruising or bleeding. Also, instruct him to report if he loses weight, feels nauseated, or vomits. The doctor may alter the dose because many of these reactions are dose-related.

Immunosuppressants

Tell the patient with ulcerative colitis that the doctor may order an immunosuppressive drug, such as azathioprine, to alter the body's response to antigens. This drug increases the risk of serious infection by diminishing production of white blood cells and platelets. Advise the patient to report bleeding tendencies, chills, fever, and sore throat.

Narcotics

If the doctor orders narcotics, explain that these drugs may control pain and diarrhea. Warn the patient to contact the doctor or go to an emergency center immediately if he has difficulty breathing or decreased respirations. Caution him about the risk of addiction with long-term use.

Listen up!

Which surgery?

Based on the patient's particular disorder and symptoms, explain which surgery he's likely to have.

Coping with Crohn's
Explain to the patient that surgery for Crohn's disease depends on the affected area and the type of complications. Inform him that surgery may result in resection with a primary anastomosis, or a temporary or permanent colostomy or ileostomy. Tell him that surgery won't cure the disease, and it may recur.

Conquering colitis
Explain to the patient with ulcerative colitis that surgery usually involves removal of the rectum and large bowel, with creation of a permanent ileostomy.

Teaching about surgery

Surgery may be needed if inflammatory bowel disease doesn't respond to treatment, if premalignant or malignant changes appear in the bowel, or if complications become unmanageable. (See *Which surgery?*)

Colostomy

Tell the patient that a colostomy is a surgically created opening between the colon and the surface of the abdomen, through which he'll excrete body wastes. Show the patient drawings of the colon before and after surgery.

Stoma story

Inform him that the stoma is normally red, moist, and swollen postoperatively, but that swelling will subside. Explain that the stoma won't hurt when touched because it has no nerve endings. He may be able to learn to control his bowel movements by irrigating the colostomy (if this isn't contraindicated because of his Crohn's disease). In the meantime, he'll need to wear a colostomy pouch to collect any wastes that drain from the stoma. Ask a representative of the United Ostomy Association to help the patient adjust to having a colostomy.

As soon as possible

After surgery, encourage the patient to look at his stoma and to participate in colostomy care and irrigation as soon as possible. Teach him how to remove, empty, and reapply his colostomy pouch.

Clean, dry, and free from irritation

Stress the importance of proper skin care, and show him how to keep the skin around the stoma clean, dry, and free from irritation.

There to help

Instruct the patient to notify the doctor or enterostomal therapy nurse if he repeatedly has trouble inserting the irrigation cone or if he develops persistent diarrhea or constipation, bloody or abnormal drainage, unusually colored or foul-smelling stools, or skin irritation around the stoma.

Ileostomy

If the patient is scheduled for an ileostomy, use diagrams to show him what will be removed. Stress that the small bowel remains intact and that his digestion should remain normal.

Prepare for preparation

Inform the patient that preoperative preparation is usually done the day before surgery (or 3 to 4 days before, depending on the disease's severity), and that he'll receive oral laxatives as well as antibiotics to reduce the risk of postoperative infection.

Prepare for what's next

Inform the patient that he'll return from surgery with a pouch covering his stoma. Also describe the color and consistency of the drainage, and explain that it will change as his diet changes.

Tell him that he'll have an NG tube in place for several days to prevent distention by draining the GI tract. Also explain that he won't eat for several days after surgery. Once he resumes his diet, he'll begin with clear liquids and gradually include solid foods.

Turn, cough, and breathe deeply

To prevent pulmonary complications, instruct the patient to turn in bed, cough, and deep breathe at least once every hour, and use incentive spirometry. Assure him that he'll receive medication if movement and coughing cause pain. To minimize abdominal pain when turning and coughing, show him how to splint his surgical site. Also

Why reinvent the wheel?

National associations, pharmaceutical companies, and foundations usually have large supplies of patient-teaching materials. Many are provided free of charge or for a nominal cost.

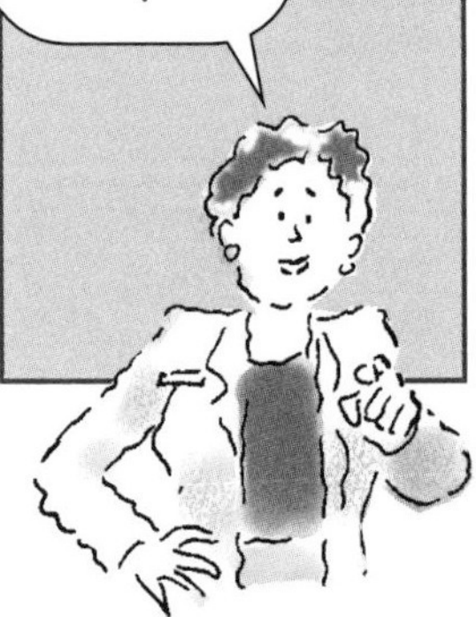
Gadzooks! A teaching tip.

explain important measures for posttreatment care at home. (See *After an ileostomy.*)

Continent ileostomy

Depending on the extent of bowel disease, the doctor may form a continent ileostomy. With a continent ileostomy, a pouch wouldn't be needed to collect stool.

Pros

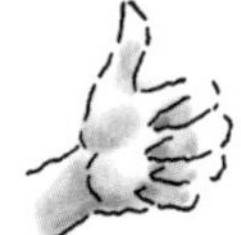

Many patients welcome continent ileostomies over traditional ostomies because the reservoir is internal and preserves the patient's body image.

Cons

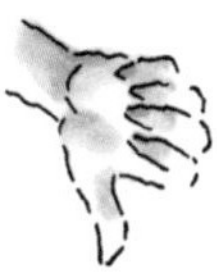

However, the procedure does have disadvantages. It's difficult to perform, and should be done only by a surgeon experienced in the procedure. The patient may have difficulty differentiating among gases, fluids, and solids in the rectum. In addition, he may experience fecal urgency, nocturnal incontinence, diarrhea, frequent bowel movements, and perianal skin denudation.

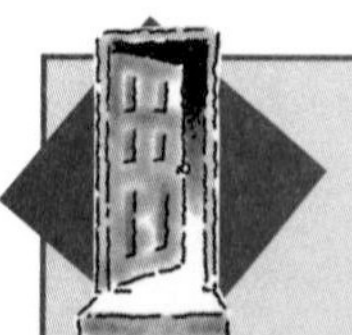

No place like home

After an ileostomy

Here's advice for helping a patient live with an ileostomy.

Don't forget the family
Include a family member in discharge teaching to assist the patient if he can't care for himself — for example, because of severe viral infection or a broken wrist.

Show, instruct, teach
Show the patient how to care for the skin around his stoma site to prevent breakdown and infection. Instruct him to contact the doctor or enterostomal therapy nurse if he observes redness, rash, or swelling or if he experiences itching, warmth, pain, elevated temperature, or unusual drainage. Teach him how to manage his ostomy equipment.

Speaking of smell
Assure the patient that odor shouldn't be a problem because newer pouches are odor-proof. Instruct him to notify the doctor of any marked decline in ostomy output or spurting or squirting of drainage from the stoma. This may signal stoma stricture and require medical intervention. Also tell him to report any unusually foul odor; it may indicate infection or may be only diet-related.

Pouch practicalities
To prevent gas from filling his pouch, advise him to avoid gas-producing foods, such as cabbage and broccoli. Also, he may want to use a pouch with a filter. Inform him that he may wear his pouch when taking a bath or shower, because water won't loosen the pouch seal. He may also remove the pouch if desired because water won't hurt the stoma.

Irritable bowel syndrome

Irritable bowel syndrome usually develops as a response to stress. Patients may have trouble changing the ingrained responses that caused the syndrome, and may be frustrated with symptoms that have no organic cause and treatment that doesn't produce a cure. You'll need to emphasize the positive, helping the patient trust the treatment regimen so that he can positively affect his condition.

Good news and bad news

Caution the patient that he'll probably experience recurring bouts of irritable bowel syndrome if he doesn't follow the prescribed treatment. However, assure him that despite being chronic, irritable bowel syndrome doesn't progress to other disorders or affect his life span. There is also no evidence linking it to cancer (although constipation may result from a low-fiber diet, which *is* associated with colon cancer and diverticular disease).

What is it?

Inform the patient that irritable bowel syndrome, also called spastic or irritable colon or mucous colitis, is usually chronic and marked by relapses and remissions. In this syndrome, the intestines function abnormally, producing chronic, excessive contractions. Explain that these abnormal contractions, or spasms, usually lasting for 3 months or more, cause cramping and discomfort, altered stool frequency and consistency, and altered stool passage (straining, urgency, and feeling of incomplete evacuation).

Where does it come from?

Tell the patient that the exact cause of irritable bowel syndrome remains unknown. It's thought to be caused by abnormal neuromuscular function. Contributing or aggravating factors include anxiety and stress, diet (fiber, fruits, alcohol, and highly seasoned, cold, or laxative foods), hormones, laxative abuse, and allergy to certain foods, beverages, and drugs. Initial episodes usually occur early in life; anxiety or stress probably causes most exacerbations. (See *Good news and bad news.*)

Teaching about tests

Inform the patient that tests can't specifically diagnose irritable bowel syndrome, but they can rule out other disorders. It's only by this process of elimination that the doctor can identify irritable bowel syndrome.

Knowing what it's not

Explain to the patient that to rule out inflammatory bowel disease, a disorder with signs and symptoms that are similar to irritable bowel syndrome, the doctor might order:

• a stool culture, to eliminate an infectious process. (See *Preparing patients for a stool culture.*)
• a barium enema study, to detect intestinal spasms, ruling out inflammatory bowel disease, diverticula, tumors, and polyps.

To detect and evaluate lower GI tract inflammation and abnormalities, the doctor might order a colonoscopy or proctosigmoidoscopy.

An upper GI and small-bowel series helps detect motility disorders, abnormal structures, esophageal reflux, pylorospasm, gastric retention, decreased gastric emptying, and small-bowel spasm. (See *Teaching patients about gastrointestinal tests,* pages 118 to 122.)

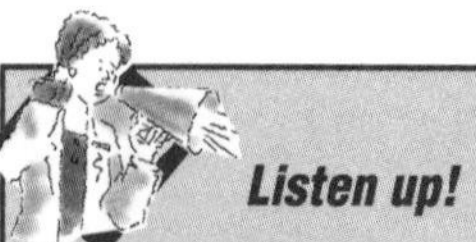

Listen up!

Preparing patients for a stool culture

Tell the patient that he'll be asked to provide a stool sample for laboratory analysis. To ensure the best results, instruct him that, for 48 hours before the collection period and during it, he should follow a high-fiber diet and avoid red meats, poultry, fish, turnips, and horseradish. As ordered, instruct him to stop taking medications for this period.

Teaching about activity and lifestyle

Since significant lifestyle changes are necessary to manage irritable bowel syndrome, discuss these important changes with the patient. (See *Living with irritable bowel syndrome.*)

Teaching about diet

Emphasize that a diet planned to prevent or relieve irritable bowel syndrome can decrease the patient's pain, con-

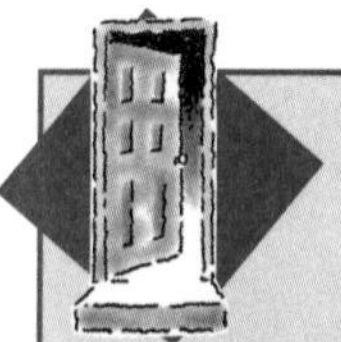

No place like home

Living with irritable bowel syndrome

Here are some guidelines for helping your patient live with this disorder.

Easy does it

Teach the patient that effective treatment may require lifestyle alterations to control emotional tension. Be sure to help him set priorities by pinpointing the activities he enjoys, scheduling more time for rest and relaxation and, if possible, delegating responsibilities. If appropriate, encourage him to seek professional counseling for stress management.

Do's and don'ts

Remind the patient that regular physical exercise helps eliminate anxiety and promotes good bowel function. Discourage smoking because it contributes to altered bowel motility. Also help him establish a regular bowel routine.

Check it out

Stress the need for regular physical examinations. For patients over age 40, emphasize the need for colorectal cancer screening, including annual proctosigmoidoscopy and rectal examinations.

stipation, and diarrhea. (See *Managing irritable bowel syndrome with diet.*)

Teaching about medication

Inform the patient that drugs are prescribed only to relieve severe symptoms. Anticholinergic antispasmodic drugs, such as propantheline bromide, may be used to reduce intestinal hypermotility; antidiarrheal drugs and laxatives may be tried as well.

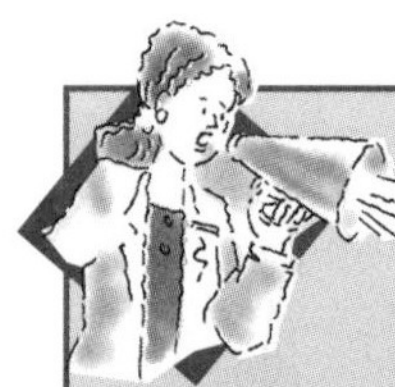

Listen up!

Managing irritable bowel syndrome with diet

Advise the patient to follow the dietary recommendations listed below to help relieve symptoms of irritable bowel syndrome.

Protect against pain, reflux, and esophagitis
Instruct the patient to follow a low-fat diet and to avoid substances that irritate the gastric and esophageal mucosa, including alcohol, caffeinated beverages, chocolate, peppermint, tomatoes, and orange juice.

Defend against diarrhea
Instruct the patient to eliminate, one by one, citrus fruits, coffee, corn, dairy products, tea, and wheat from his diet. This will help him determine if his symptoms result from food intolerance.

Warn the patient to avoid sorbitol, an artificial sweetener that may cause diarrhea. Advise him to consume more products that contain bran. Explain that adding dietary bulk increases the time the stool remains in the bowel, allowing it to become more solid.

Battle abdominal distention and bloating
Tell the patient to avoid lactose- and sorbitol-containing foods and nonabsorbable carbohydrates, such as beans and cabbage. Explain that these products increase flatulence.

Combat constipation and abdominal pain
Advise the patient to increase dietary bulk using such sources as wheat bran, oatmeal, oat bran, rye cereals, prunes, dried apricots, and figs. Unless contraindicated, tell him to drink eight glasses of water daily.

Establish a schedule
Explain that the GI tract works best on a schedule. To promote regularity, the patient should eat three meals daily of about the same volume and at about the same time, and avoid between-meal or late-night snacks. Advise the patient to eat slowly and carefully to prevent swallowing air and consequent bloating.

For the record
Suggest that the patient keep a daily record of food intake and symptoms, including number and type of stools and the presence, severity, and duration of pain. He should also note all foods that appear to trigger symptoms. Then he can proceed to eliminate them one at a time, thereby discovering which symptoms occur with certain foods.

A lack of lactase?
Note that a lactase deficiency can cause symptoms similar to irritable bowel syndrome. If the patient must exclude milk products from his diet, remind him to include other calcium-rich foods, such as green, leafy vegetables.

Other possibilities

Other possible medication choices include antacids, antiemetics, simethicone and, occasionally, tranquilizers or antidepressants. Advise your patient always to consult his doctor before treating constipation or diarrhea with over-the-counter medications because many irritate the bowel.

Chronic pancreatitis

Chronic pancreatitis is usually the result of damage to the biliary tract from infectious disease, trauma, alcohol, or drugs. Biliary tract disease and alcoholism are the two most common associated factors.

Because this disorder is of long duration, damage may have occurred before you noticed symptoms.

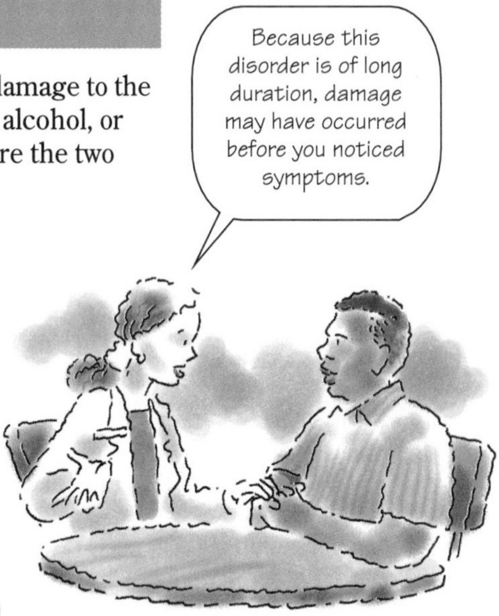

What is it?

Define chronic pancreatitis for your patient as an inflammatory condition of the pancreas.

What are the signs and symptoms?

Point out that chronic pancreatitis is of long duration and that damage may have occurred well before any signs or symptoms appear. Tell the patient that continuous or intermittent stomach pain is the hallmark of the disease. Additional signs and symptoms include frothy, foul-smelling stools and weight loss.

Teaching about tests

Describe the diagnostic studies used to confirm chronic pancreatitis and detect complications, including abdominal X-ray or CT scans to reveal pancreatic calcification, ultrasonography or CT scans to evaluate the size of the pancreas and pseudocysts, and ERCP to visualize the pancreatic ducts. Pancreatic blood analysis may be performed to assess endocrine and exocrine functions.

We'll need to make a few adjustments...

If the doctor wants to evaluate exocrine function, teach the patient how to collect a stool sample to check for steatorrhea and fecal blood. Tell him to watch for stools that are greasy or oily (possibly with a silver sheen), foul-smelling, and difficult to flush down the toilet. Tell him to eat a fat-restricted diet for 2 to 3 days, then to collect stool samples for 3 days. Explain that the presence of steatorrhea may indicate the need for adjustments in enzymatic and dietary therapy.

Teaching about activity and lifestyle

Explain that the patient may have less energy than usual because of malabsorption of calories and nutrients. Advise him to conserve energy by resting frequently between activities. Also instruct him to rest after meals to aid digestion.

As things get better...

Assure the patient that he may be able to tolerate more activity as his condition improves. Even so, instruct him to check with the doctor or a nutritionist before making major changes. (See *Living with chronic pancreatitis.*)

Teaching about diet

Tell the patient that diet therapy aims to reduce gastric secretion. Usually, the doctor prescribes a low-fat, high-pro-

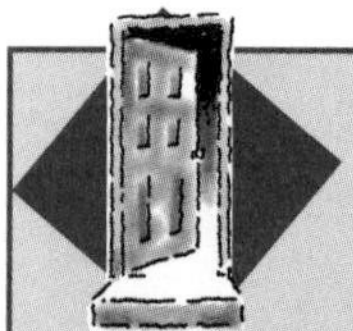

No place like home

Living with chronic pancreatitis

Here are some guidelines for helping your patient cope with chronic pancreatitis.

Against infection
Stress the importance of avoiding infection by hand washing, getting adequate rest, and avoiding crowds and people with known infections. Tell the patient to contact the doctor immediately if he becomes ill.

Without drugs
To reduce the patient's need for narcotics, teach him about relaxation techniques to manage pain.

Put out the cigarette
Discourage smoking. Explain that smoking changes pancreatic secretions that neutralize gastric acid in the duodenum.

More help
If the patient needs help abstaining from alcohol, encourage him to contact Alcoholics Anonymous; if he's a diabetic, refer him to the American Diabetes Association.

tein diet, free from alcohol and gastric stimulants (such as coffee) to decrease the demand for pancreatic enzymes.

Let me recommend a low-fat, high-protein, alcohol-free, coffee-free diet.

Lesser amounts, greater frequency

Encourage the patient to eat small, frequent meals to minimize the secretion of pancreatic enzymes. Remind the patient that he must abstain from alcohol.

Teaching about medication

Inform the patient that drug treatment relieves signs and symptoms of chronic pancreatitis and prevents complications. Teach about prescribed drugs, such as histamine-2 (H_2) receptor antagonists or antacids (to reduce the flow of pancreatic juice) and narcotics to relieve pain.

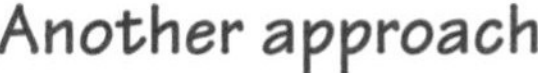

Another approach

Instead of using narcotics to reduce pain, a newer approach is to administer high doses of oral pancreatic enzymes (pancrelipase) with each meal.

Teaching about surgery

Explain that surgery aims to relieve chronic pain, treat complications, and preserve functioning pancreatic tissue. Surgical options fall into two categories: pancreatic resection and decompression of the ductal system.

Relief, but at what price?

Unfortunately, although pancreatic resection often provides excellent pain relief, it may cause immediate diabetes mellitus and other major complications. Also, decompression of the ductal system isn't feasible for many patients. Those with ducts too small to decompress may not experience pain relief. Advise the patient to discuss with the doctor the risks and benefits of surgery, then weigh his decision carefully.

Peptic ulcer disease

Peptic ulcer disease affects more than 10% of the American population. Although peptic ulcer disease can lead to serious complications, most patients achieve a good outcome if they comply with prescribed treatment.

Acceptance of teaching and compliance with treatment depend largely on the patient's understanding of his responsibility for managing the disease.

What is it?

Although the patient already knows that a peptic ulcer causes intense pain, he may not know that an ulcer is an erosion of the stomach lining. Inform him that a peptic ulcer may occur in the duodenum (the first part of the small intestine) or the stomach.

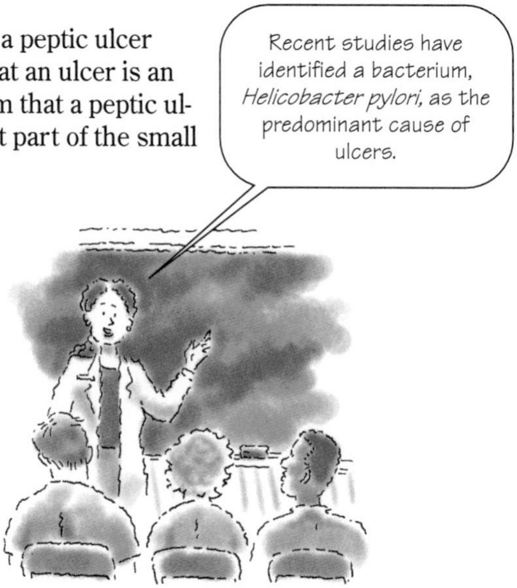

Recent studies have identified a bacterium, *Helicobacter pylori,* as the predominant cause of ulcers.

What causes it?

For many years this erosion was thought to result from contact with acidic gastric secretions (pepsin or hydrochloric acid). Recent studies have identified a bacterium, *Helicobacter pylori,* as the predominant cause of ulcers.

What happens?

Point out that peptic ulcers usually have a chronic, recurrent course. Not all patients exhibit signs and symptoms; some experience them only when complications occur. The pain from an ulcer may feel like a burning, gnawing, or aching sensation as well as soreness, an empty feeling, or hunger.

What's at risk?

Caution the patient that an unchecked, unhealed ulcer can cause life-threatening complications, such as hemorrhage, perforation of the stomach wall, peritonitis, abdominal or intestinal infarction, and shock.

Teaching about tests

Explain to the patient that the doctor diagnoses peptic ulcer disease based on signs and symptoms and the results of diagnostic tests. These tests may include a basal gastric secretion test, an upper GI endoscopy, a gastric acid stimulation test, and an upper GI and small-bowel series. (See *Teaching patients about gastrointestinal tests,* pages 118 to 122.)

Teaching about activity and lifestyle

Help the patient identify stressors in his life and formulate new coping methods or plans to eliminate stress. Advise the patient to avoid the use of aspirin and NSAIDs that can irritate the GI mucosa. If the patient smokes, encourage him to quit, as there is an increased incidence of peptic ulcers among people who smoke.

To help the patient cope with lifestyle changes, refer him to the Digestive Disease National Coalition, the National Digestive Disease Information Clearinghouse, or the National Ulcer Foundation.

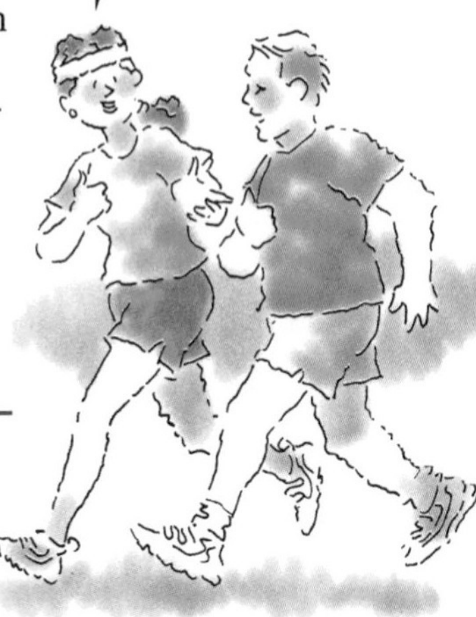
I'm going to help you find ways to reduce stress.

Teaching about diet

Point out that no firm evidence proves that a particular diet speeds ulcer healing or prevents ulcer recurrence. Therefore, the doctor is likely to recommend that the patient eliminate only those foods that cause distress (such as fruit juices or spicy or fatty foods). (See *Treatment for peptic ulcer.*)

Hold the pepper, hold the coffee

Advise the patient to avoid pepper and coffee. Pepper is the only food that objective studies suggest is harmful; coffee (even decaffeinated coffee) may produce ulcer-like stomach upset in some persons.

Hold the soda and other stuff

The doctor may also instruct the patient to avoid caffeinated soft drinks, tea, chocolate, nicotine, and alcohol. Encourage the patient to snack between meals.

Treatment for peptic ulcer

- Resting the stomach
- Dietary changes
- Medication
- Stress reduction or lifestyle changes
- Possible surgery

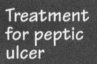

Teaching about medication

Inform the patient that in light of the recent studies identifying *H. pylori* as the main cause of peptic ulcers, doctors are still debating which drugs to use for treatment. However, most believe the best approach is a combination of traditional antiulcer medications, antibiotics, and bismuth compounds.

Suppress or shield

If the doctor prescribes traditional medications, explain to the patient that these either suppress gastric acid production or shield the GI tract lining. Drugs that suppress gastric acid secretion — proton pump inhibitors and H_2-receptor antagonists — are the most widely prescribed. The doctor may also prescribe antianxiety drugs to promote rest and relaxation.

Antacids

Inform the patient that antacids relieve pain by neutralizing gastric acid. Warn him not to take systemic antacids, such as sodium bicarbonate, because they're absorbed into the circulation and can cause acid-base imbalance.

H_2-receptor antagonists

Inform the patient that H_2-receptor antagonists, such as cimetidine (Tagamet) and famotidine (Pepcid), work by inhibiting the production of histamine, thus decreasing gastric acid secretion. Caution him that over-the-counter formulas of H_2-receptor antagonists have much lower dosage levels than the prescribed version and may not be effective.

Proton pump inhibitors

Inform the patient that proton pump inhibitors, such as omeprazole (Prilosec), are more potent than H_2-receptor antagonists. Explain that these drugs block the formation of gastric acid. Before prescribing one of these agents, the doctor, pharmacist, or nurse practitioner reviews the patient's current medications closely because proton pump inhibitors can interact with certain medications.

Other drugs

If the patient will take sucralfate (Sulcrate), tell him that this drug combines with proteins to form a protective coating in the base of the ulcer, thus relieving symptoms and promoting ulcer healing. Instruct him to take sucralfate with a full glass of water, 1 hour before meals. If he's also taking cimetidine, instruct him to take sucralfate 2 hours before or after cimetidine. Advise him not to take sucralfate with an antacid.

Protecting the GI lining

If the patient will take misoprostol (Cytotec), inform him that this medication helps protect the GI lining by decreasing acid secretion. Tell the patient to take this drug with food. (See *Caution for women taking misoprostol.*)

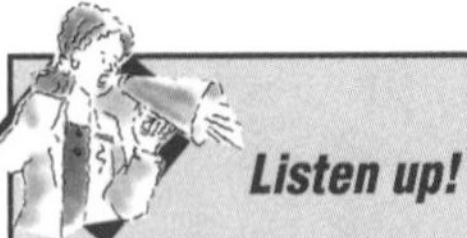
Listen up!

Caution for women taking misoprostol

Caution women of childbearing age that misoprostol may induce miscarriage. To prevent miscarriage, advise the patient to have a serum pregnancy test 2 weeks before starting medication, to use an effective contraceptive during therapy, and to tell her doctor if she is pregnant or plans to become pregnant. If pregnancy is suspected, she should discontinue the medication immediately.

Double whammy

Recently, the Food and Drug Administration approved a combination drug for treating peptic ulcer: omeprazole plus the antibiotic clarithromycin (Biaxin). This drug combination is designed to eradicate *H. pylori*.

More ways to protect that lining

Advise the patient with an ulcer to avoid taking preparations that contain corticosteroids, aspirin, or other NSAIDs such as ibuprofen (Motrin). Explain that these drugs inhibit mucus secretion and leave the GI lining vulnerable to injury from gastric acid. Recommend using an alternative, such as acetaminophen (Tylenol), to relieve pain.

Teaching about surgery

Surgery may be necessary if conservative treatments fail or if complications develop. Explain the type of surgery the patient will undergo. In *vagotomy*, the surgeon severs the vagus nerve that stimulates gastric acid secretion. Vagotomy may be accompanied by removal of part of the stomach or removal of the ulcerated area.

Before surgery...

If the patient will be undergoing planned surgery, inform him that he'll receive cleansing laxatives and enemas the evening before surgery and undergo the insertion of an NG tube the next morning. Explain that both measures prevent complications during surgery.

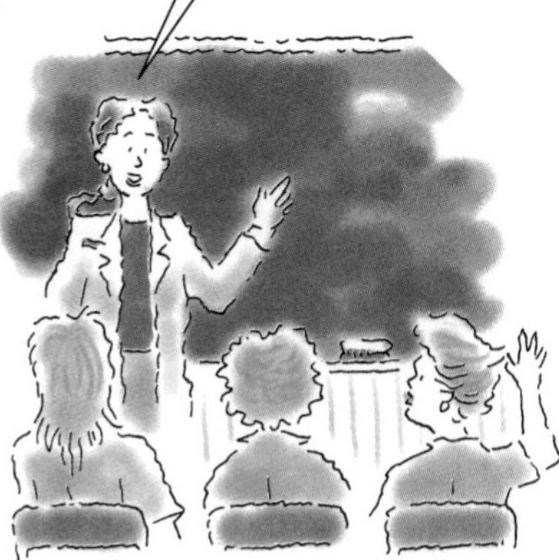
Be aware that misoprostol may induce miscarriage.

...and after

Also inform the patient that he'll have a drain at the incision site for 1 to 2 days after surgery to remove any accumulated fluid, and he may be fed through a gastrostomy tube. He'll probably resume eating several days after surgery, starting with clear liquids and gradually advancing to solid foods.

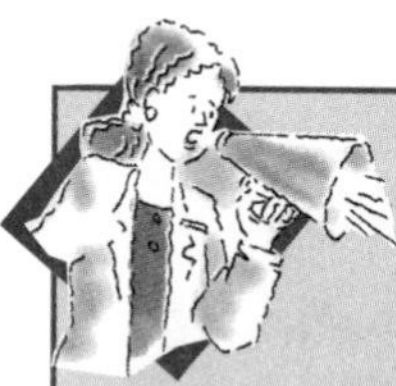

Listen up!

Dealing with dumping syndrome

If your patient has had a gastric resection with pyloric removal, prepare him for dealing with dumping syndrome, which may begin about 2 weeks after surgery and typically occurs between 15 and 30 minutes after eating.

Yikes! Diarrhea, palpitations, fainting

Lasting about 1 hour, the syndrome causes abdominal cramps, diaphoresis, diarrhea, palpitations, fainting, a fast pulse, and weakness.

Here's what to do

To minimize or prevent signs and symptoms, recommend that the patient:

- eat four to six small meals a day
- maintain a normal intake of fats and proteins (they leave the stomach more slowly and attract less fluid into the intestine)
- avoid foods with concentrated carbohydrates (they pull more fluid into the intestine)
- drink fluids between meals, not with meals
- avoid overly hot or cold foods and fluids
- lie down for 30 minutes to 1 hour after eating
- take medication to slow intestinal motility, if prescribed.

Within a year

Reassure the patient that the syndrome usually resolves within 1 year after surgery. However, a few patients may have long-term problems and require reconstructive surgery.

Follow-through

Tell the patient that he can probably resume normal activities a few weeks after discharge. If appropriate, describe the signs and symptoms of dumping syndrome and teach him to minimize or prevent this problem by properly managing his diet. (See *Dealing with dumping syndrome.*)

Stay alert

Instruct the patient to watch for and immediately report signs and symptoms of life-threatening complications, such as hemorrhage, obstruction, and perforation. (See *Hemorrhage, obstruction, or perforation?*)

Hemorrhage, obstruction, or perforation?

Hemorrhage

- Bloody or black, tarry stools (melena)
- Bloody or coffee-ground vomitus
- Chills and sweating
- Dizziness on standing
- Restlessness

Obstruction

- Foul taste in the mouth
- Coated tongue
- Abdominal fullness or distention worsening after meals and at night
- Nausea and vomiting
- Anorexia with weight loss

Perforation

- Rapid, shallow breathing
- Facial flushing, fever, and sweating
- Dizziness
- Swollen abdomen
- Severe pain in the shoulders or stomach

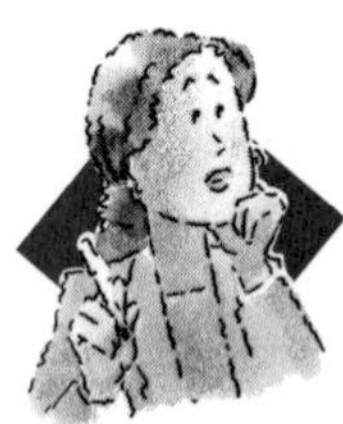

Quick quiz

1. Teach the patient with gallstones that treatment will depend on:

A. severity of signs and symptoms.
B. dietary history.
C. number of gallstones in the gallbladder.

Answer: A. If the patient is asymptomatic, she won't require treatment.

2. If the patient-teaching plan emphasizes extra rest, adequate intake of good nutrition and fluids, and measures to prevent spreading the disorder, your patient probably has:

A. cirrhosis.
B. peptic ulcer disease.
C. viral hepatitis.

Answer: C. These are common general treatments for viral hepatitis.

3. If your patient has a peptic ulcer, tell him the most likely cause is:

A. excessive consumption of rich food, caffeinated drinks, nicotine, or alcohol.
B. *Helicobacter pylori,* a bacterium.
C. stress.

Answer: B. *H. pylori* is the predominant cause of ulcers.

Scoring

☆☆☆ If you answered all three questions correctly, congratulations! Your learning curve is right on tract.

☆☆ If you answered two questions correctly, good job! You've found this material easy to digest.

☆ If you answered fewer than two questions correctly, there's no reason to panic. Remember that stress doesn't improve learning (or help GI disorders).

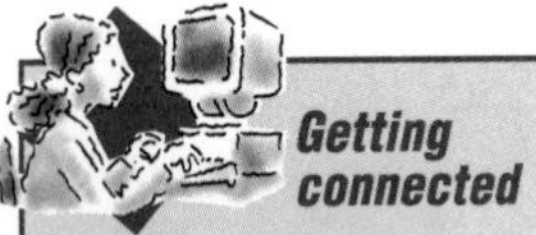

Information to digest

For more information about GI disorders, direct the patient to the following Web sites:

- American Gastroenterological Association (www.gastro.org)
- National Institute of Diabetes and Digestive and Kidney Diseases (www.niddk.nih.gov).

Blood and immune system disorders

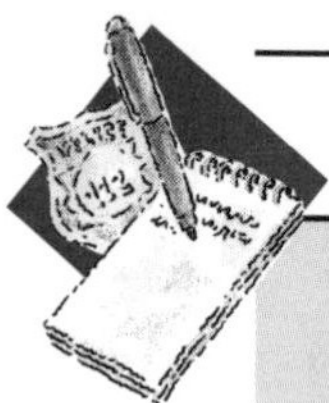

Just the facts

In this chapter, you'll learn how to teach patients with the following blood and immune system disorders:

- ♦ acquired immunodeficiency syndrome
- ♦ hemophilia
- ♦ latex allergy
- ♦ rheumatoid arthritis
- ♦ sickle cell syndrome
- ♦ systemic lupus erythematosus
- ♦ thrombocytopenia.

Acquired immunodeficiency syndrome

Acquired immunodeficiency syndrome (AIDS) results from infection with human immunodeficiency virus (HIV), which impairs the immune system. This virus attaches to specialized white blood cells (WBCs) called T or helper T cells. HIV has two gradual effects on these cells:

 It depletes their number.

 It hinders their response to infection.

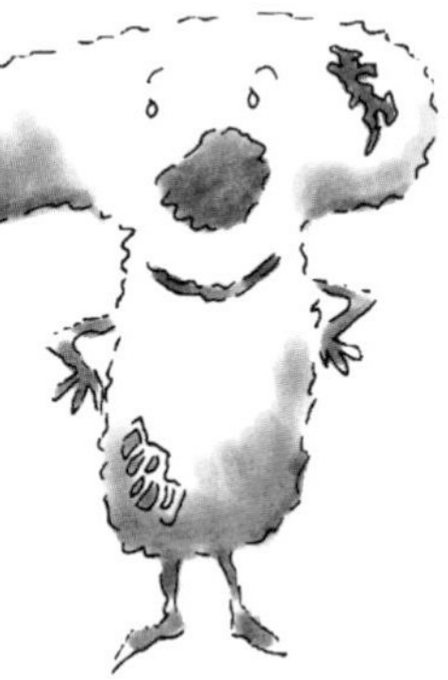
HIV hinders my response to infection.

The crippled immune system leaves the patient vulnerable to opportunistic infections and cancers. (See *Common opportunist,* page 152.)

How does HIV spread?

HIV infection can be transmitted through unprotected vaginal, oral, or anal intercourse; needles contaminated with blood; a blood transfusion; or transplacental contact and breast-feeding (in infants). Body fluids known to transmit HIV include blood, semen, vaginal secretions, and breast milk.

In addition to known transmission fluids, HIV has been found in other body fluids, such as saliva, urine, tears, and feces, but there is no evidence of transmission through these fluids.

When does HIV infection turn into AIDS?

Point out that HIV-infected patients develop AIDS at varied rates. Some remain asymptomatic until they abruptly develop an opportunistic infection, such as *Pneumocystis carinii* pneumonia (PCP), or cancer, such as Kaposi's sarcoma. More often, though, patients develop several concurrent infections after a history of nonspecific signs and symptoms, such as:

- fatigue
- afternoon fevers
- chills
- night sweats
- weight loss
- diarrhea
- enlarged lymph nodes
- cough. (See *AIDS and infection.*)

What's Kaposi's sarcoma?

Kaposi's sarcoma is a common form of cancer in AIDS patients. The disease aggressively compromises the blood vessels, then invades the deeper organs and tissues, especially the GI tract. Small red or purple multicentric lesions can develop over the entire body. In advanced stages, the disease obstructs the lymphatic system, causing swelling of the legs, head, and neck.

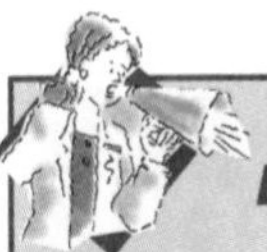

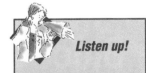

Listen up!

Common opportunist

The most common opportunistic infection associated with AIDS is *Pneumocystis carinii* pneumonia (PCP). It's caused by a one-celled organism (a protozoan) that affects the lungs. When the immune system is suppressed, numerous cysts composed of clumped organisms multiply in the lungs' air spaces and eventually cause obstructive disease. Emphasize that successful management of PCP depends on the early detection of pulmonary involvement.

PCP can be recognized by:

- dry cough
- mild fever
- night sweats
- weight loss
- weakness
- difficulty breathing on exertion
- respiratory failure.

Teaching about tests

HIV antibody tests and other diagnostic studies are used to establish an initial diagnosis of HIV infection and detect opportunistic infections or cancer.

HIV antibody tests

Two blood tests commonly used to detect HIV antibodies are the enzyme-linked immunosorbent assay (ELISA) and the Western blot.

In the ELISA, the patient's blood sample is incubated with live HIV. If HIV antibodies are present, they react with the test solution. If findings are positive, a Western blot assay is performed on the same blood sample to confirm the results and identify specific HIV antibodies.

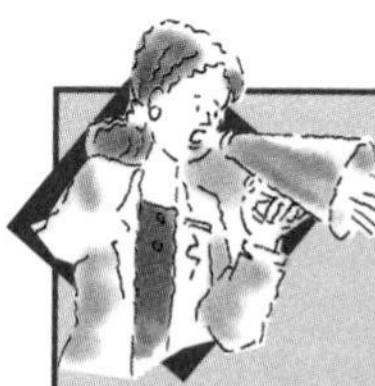

Listen up!

AIDS and infection

One key factor in protecting the acquired immunodeficiency syndrome (AIDS) patient from infections is thorough hand washing by caregivers, visitors, and the patient.

Do's and don'ts

Encourage the patient to adhere to the following guidelines whenever possible:

- Avoid crowds and people with known infections, such as herpes, influenza, mononucleosis, and cytomegalovirus. Even stay away from people who have minor colds.
- Get adequate sleep at night, and rest often during the day.
- Eat frequent, small meals, even if you've lost your appetite and have to force yourself to eat.
- Practice good hygiene, especially good oral hygiene. Use a soft toothbrush. Don't use commercial mouthwashes because their high alcohol and sugar content may irritate your mouth and provide a medium for bacterial growth.
- Don't use unprescribed I.V. drugs.
- Avoid traveling to foreign countries. If you must travel, drink only bottled or boiled water and avoid raw vegetables and fruits to prevent a possible intestinal infection.
- Wear a mask and gloves to clean birdcages, fish tanks, and cat litter boxes.
- Keep rooms clean and well ventilated, and keep air conditioners and humidifiers cleaned and repaired so they don't harbor infectious organisms.
- Use good hand-washing technique.

Looking out for infection

Encourage the patient to contact his doctor immediately if he notices any of the following signs or symptoms:

- persistent fever or nighttime sweating not related to a cold or the flu
- swollen lymph nodes in his neck, armpits, or groin that last more than 2 months and aren't related to any other illness
- profound, persistent fatigue unrelieved by rest and not related to increased physical activity, longer work schedules, drug use, or a psychological disorder
- loss of appetite and weight loss
- open sores
- dry, persistent, unproductive cough
- persistent, unexplained diarrhea
- white coating or spots on his tongue or throat, possibly accompanied by soreness, burning, or difficulty swallowing
- blurred vision or persistent, severe headaches
- confusion, depression, uncontrolled excitement, or inappropriate speech
- persistent or spreading rash or skin discoloration
- unexplained bleeding or bruising.

Is it HIV?

Positive results in both tests establish HIV infection. Stress that this doesn't mean the patient has AIDS, only that he's infected with the virus. On the other hand, a negative result doesn't necessarily mean that he isn't infected. A patient exposed to the virus may carry HIV for up to 6 months before developing detectable antibody levels. Encourage patients with possible exposures or high-risk behaviors to be tested again.

CD4+

A CD4+ count is used to evaluate the patient's immune status. When the count falls below 200/µl, and opportunistic infections occur (caused by normally nonpathogenic organisms), the AIDS diagnosis is confirmed.

Other tests

Direct tests can be performed to detect HIV, rather than the antibody. These tests include antigen tests, HIV cultures, nucleic acid probes of peripheral blood lymphocytes, and a polymerase chain reaction test.

Teach the patient about tests that may be ordered to support the diagnosis and evaluate the severity of immunosuppression. These include bronchoscopy, chest X-rays, arterial blood gas studies, pulmonary function tests, and tissue biopsy. (See *Teaching patients about blood and immune system tests.*)

Teaching about activity and lifestyle

Although AIDS is incurable at this time, treatment measures can suppress HIV, control opportunistic infections, and improve the patient's quality of life. The first step is to prevent further injury to the immune system. The patient can accomplish this by:

- recognizing symptoms
- seeking medical help promptly
- following recommended treatments to limit infection.

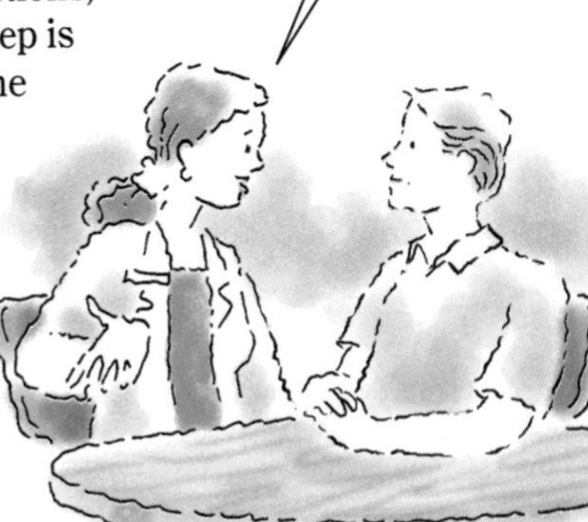
Preventing further injury to your immune system will help maintain your quality of life.

Exercise is excellent

Explain that moderate exercise can be used to:

- maintain muscle mass
- improve circulation
- achieve a feeling of well-being.

Teaching patients about blood and immune system tests

Test and purpose	What to teach the patient
Bleeding time • To assess hemostasis • To detect bleeding disorders such as hemophilia	• This test measures the time it takes to form a clot and stop bleeding. It usually takes 10 to 20 minutes. • The technician cleans the patient's forearm with antiseptic. Then the technician applies a blood pressure cuff to the upper arm and makes two tiny cuts on the forearm. He then uses filter paper to blot drops of blood until a platelet plug forms and oozing stops.
Bone marrow aspiration and biopsy • To assess the number, size, and maturation of megakaryocytes, red blood cell precursors, and white blood cell precursors • To determine if thrombocytopenia, leukopenia, or anemia results from decreased or abnormal production of blood cells and to determine possible cause	• This test evaluates blood cells made in bone marrow and takes 5 to 10 minutes. • During the test, the technician cleans the skin over the iliac crest (the bony protrusion just above the buttock) with antiseptic solution and then anesthetizes the area. After that, a surgeon introduces a hollow needle with a stylet into the bone marrow cavity. He then removes the stylet, attaches a syringe, and aspirates a small volume (0.5 ml) of blood and marrow. For biopsy, the surgeon makes a small skin incision (3 to 4 mm) so he can introduce a larger hollow needle and remove a tiny core of bone marrow. The patient may experience brief discomfort when the marrow is aspirated. • Pressure is applied for 10 to 15 minutes after this procedure. The patient can expect slight soreness over the puncture site but should report bleeding or severe pain.
Skin testing • To confirm allergic sensitivities and help identify their cause	• Skin tests evaluate the immune system after application or injection of small doses of antigens. The patient needn't restrict food or fluids before the test. • During intradermal skin testing, the doctor injects antigens into the patient's skin at spaced intervals on the forearm or interscapular area. At the same time, he injects a control substance (which should cause no reaction). After 15 to 30 minutes, the doctor inspects the injection sites for wheals and surrounding erythema, which indicate a positive reaction. This test can detect allergies to pollen, feathers, animal dander, and dust. • In scratch testing, an alternative to intradermal testing, the doctor cleans areas of the patient's skin with alcohol. When the skin dries, the doctor uses an instrument to make a superficial scratch (about 1 to 4 mm long) on the patient's skin and applies an extract containing the test antigen. After waiting 30 minutes, the site is checked for erythema. • If the doctor suspects allergies to fibers, detergents, perfumes, or cosmetics, he may order patch testing. In this test, a gauze pad is saturated with the suspected antigen and taped to the patient's skin. After 48 hours, the doctor removes the patch, inspects the skin, and grades the response. A plus sign (+) signifies erythema only; ++ indicates erythema and papules; +++ indicates erythema, papules, and vesicles; ++++ signifies erythema, papules, vesicles, and bullae or ulceration.
Synovial fluid analysis • To help diagnose rheumatoid arthritis	• This test helps determine the cause of joint inflammation and swelling and helps identify which type of arthritis the patient has. • During the aspiration process, the doctor inserts a needle into the joint to obtain a fluid sample. Although the patient is given a local anesthetic, he may feel discomfort when the needle penetrates the joint. • He should report increased pain or fever (indications of joint infection) after the test.

All things in moderation

Tell the patient to exercise regularly, avoid overexertion, and alternate periods of activity and rest. Adequate rest is crucial to reduce the risk of infection.

If the patient is well enough to go outdoors, walking is ideal exercise. If he spends long hours in bed, he can lift light hand weights. He should modify his exercise program if his condition deteriorates. He can discuss an exercise program with the doctor or a physical therapist.

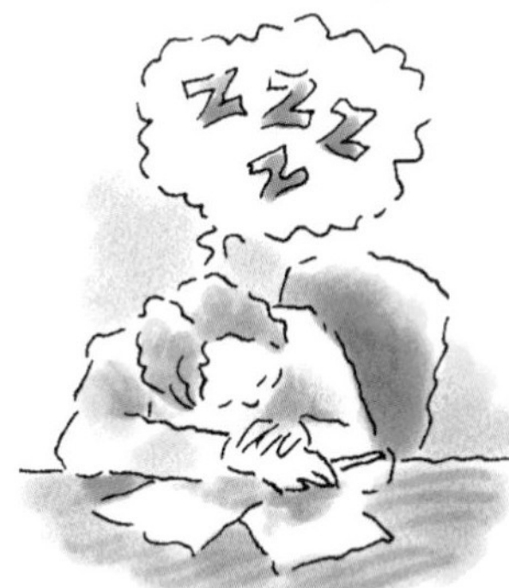
Exercise, yes. But the patient also needs adequate rest to reduce the risk of infection.

There's more

Tell the patient and his caregivers about other measures to help them cope with AIDS, including how to prevent AIDS transmission. (See *Preventing AIDS transmission* and *More teaching points for AIDS.*)

Teaching about diet

Stress the importance of maintaining a healthy diet. It should provide adequate nutrients to prevent infection and weight loss.

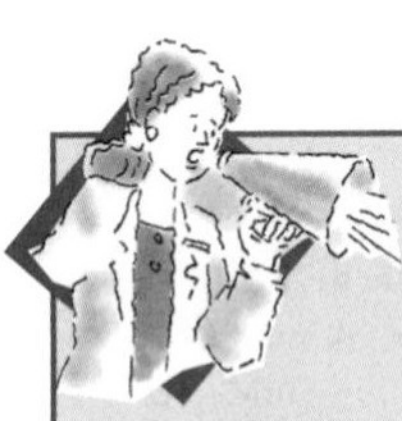

Listen up!

Preventing AIDS transmission

Teach the patient how to prevent transmitting acquired immunodeficiency syndrome (AIDS) to others.

Watching out for others

- Tell him not to donate blood, organs, tissue, or sperm.
- If he uses I.V. drugs, caution him not to share needles and to warn any persons with whom he shared needles in the past that he's infected.
- Stress the need to use precautions in activities of daily living so that friends, roommates, and family members don't contract AIDS.
- Warn him to tell potential sex partners that he has tested positive for the human immunodeficiency virus.

Let's talk about sex

- Stress that sexual practices in which body fluids are exchanged put the patient at high risk for AIDS transmission. Examples include anal or vaginal intercourse without a condom, fellatio without a condom, cunnilingus, insertion of a foreign object into the rectum followed by anal intercourse without a condom, and oral-anal stimulation.
- Discuss safer sexual practices with your patient. These include hugging, kissing, petting, massaging, mutual masturbation, using sex toys (but not sharing them), and having protected sexual intercourse.

Small, frequent, protein-packed, and high-calorie

Encourage the patient to eat small, frequent, high-calorie, high-protein meals and to drink plenty of fluids. Discuss ways to stimulate the appetite and make mealtimes more pleasant.

If the patient continues to lose weight, show him how to keep a calorie count, and teach him about commercial dietary supplements. Teach him to perform good mouth care before meals.

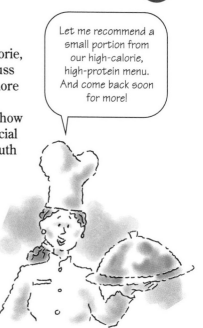

Teaching about medication

Educate the patient about drugs used to modify HIV infection, including antiviral drugs, such as didanosine, saquinavir, and zidovudine (Retrovir, AZT).

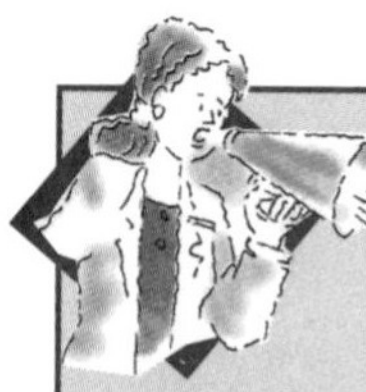

Listen up!

More teaching points for AIDS

Here are a few additional teaching points to pass on to a patient with acquired immunodeficiency syndrome (AIDS):

AIDS in children

If your patient is a child, teach his caregivers about the special concerns and precautions involved. Tell them about programs that can help the child cope with a terminal illness.

AIDS in pregnancy

Caution a pregnant patient that infants may become infected before birth, during delivery, or during breast-feeding, so caution them not to breast-feed. Advise female patients of child-bearing age to postpone getting pregnant until more is known about the AIDS virus and pregnancy.

Trying an alternative

Tell the patient about alternative therapies if he asks. These treatments include:

- acupuncture
- Chinese herbals
- megavitamins
- coenzyme Q
- diets (such as macrobiotic, immune power, or yeast-control).

Have the patient contact local or national AIDS organizations for information and referrals before starting an alternative therapy. Encourage him to continue with his prescribed regimen even if he uses an alternative therapy and to tell the doctor about other therapies he's trying.

Seeking support

Provide information about local and national AIDS organizations and support groups for patients, their partners, and family members. Tell the patient about various services, such as one-on-one volunteer counseling and assistance with medical insurance. Urge him to seek support from these organizations and, if necessary, help him contact them. Also tell him about the AIDS information Web site (www.hivnet.org).

To treat related infections and cancers, the patient may receive co-trimoxazole, pentamidine isethionate, and chemotherapeutic drugs.

Promising results

Point out to the patient that the combination of protease inhibitors and reverse transcriptase inhibitors shows promising results. Protease inhibitors, which help prevent viral proteins from becoming infectious, have been found to reduce HIV in the blood.

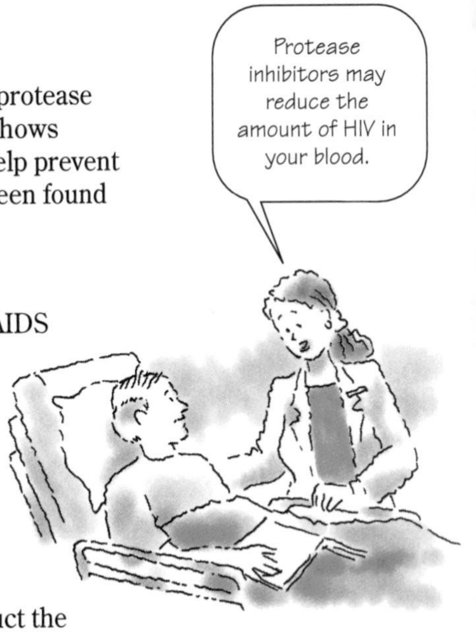

Protease inhibitors may reduce the amount of HIV in your blood.

Hope for the future

There's hope for the future thanks to ongoing AIDS research. Advise the patient to check with the doctor about the availability of investigative drugs.

Pummeling PCP

Co-trimoxazole (sulfamethoxazole and trimethoprim [Bactrim, Septra]) is the drug of choice for PCP. Discuss how and when to take the drug and its possible adverse effects. Instruct the patient to complete the prescribed course of therapy and to take each dose as ordered.

Infusion alternative

If the patient is allergic to sulfa drugs or if co-trimoxazole isn't effective in treating PCP, the doctor may order pentamidine isethionate (Lomidine, Pentam 300). This drug can cause severe hypotension, so instruct the patient to lie down while receiving the I.V. infusion. Tell him that the nurse takes his blood pressure when the drug is being administered and several times afterward until blood pressure stabilizes. (See *Pentamidine problems.*)

Chemo for Kaposi's

Vincristine and vinblastine are the cornerstone of treatment for Kaposi's sarcoma, although etoposide, doxorubicin, and interferon alfa-2a or 2b may also be used. Provide advice on controlling the adverse effects of chemotherapy, such as avoiding people with infections and monitoring the fluid imbalance that HIV can cause.

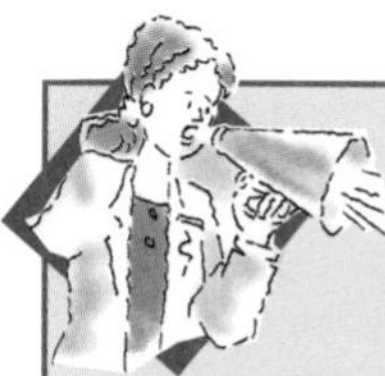

Listen up!

Pentamidine problems

Inform the patient receiving pentamidine of the following potential problems:

- The drug may lower the white blood cell count, increasing the patient's chance of infection.
- It may lower his platelet count, increasing the risk of bleeding.
- It may also cause acute renal failure, pancreatitis, electrocardiogram abnormalities, dizziness, confusion, and hallucinations.

What to do

Tell the patient to avoid people with colds or other infections and to check with the doctor immediately if he thinks he's getting a cold or other infection. He should also contact the doctor if he notices any unusual bleeding or bruising.

Tell him to brush and floss his teeth carefully, to check with the dentist for other ways to clean his teeth and gums, and to contact the doctor before having any dental work done. Instruct him to use an electric shaver instead of a safety razor and to use fingernail and toenail clippers cautiously.

Teaching about procedures

There are two procedures that are often used to treat Kaposi's sarcoma:

1. If the sarcoma affects only small areas of the skin, the lesions may be treated with laser therapy and cryotherapy.
2. If the sarcoma invades deeper tissues, radiation therapy or chemotherapy may be used. If the doctor orders radiation, explain the procedure to the patient.

Hemophilia

Hemophilia is an inherited bleeding disorder that affects mostly males. Fortunately, early recognition and treatment of bleeding episodes can prevent many complications that were common before clotting factor concentrates and home I.V. infusion programs were developed.

What's at risk?

Explain to the patient that most hemophiliacs can expect a normal life span. However, damage from abnormal bleeding does pose a serious threat. For instance, bleeding near nerves may cause nerve inflammation and degeneration, pain, abnormal sensations (such as numbness, tingling, and prickling), and muscle shrinkage.

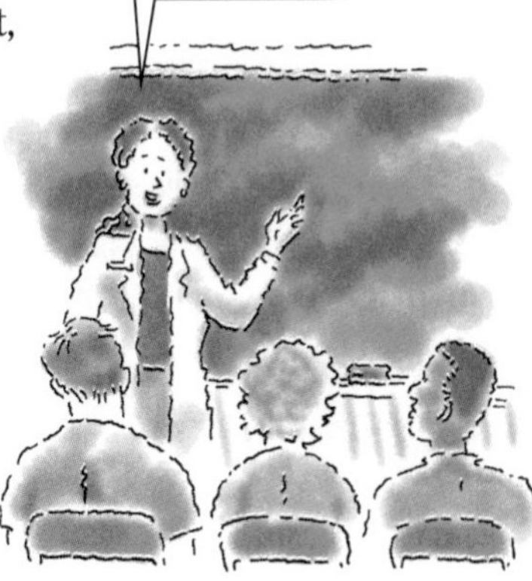
A person with hemophilia doesn't bleed faster than other people, but bleeding may be prolonged.

What happens?

Bleeding typically occurs with injuries to the kidneys, joints, muscles, and subcutaneous tissue. Make it clear that the patient doesn't bleed faster than anyone else but, because of the missing or defective clotting factor, he may have prolonged bleeding or delayed clotting.

What is the difference between hemophilia A and hemophilia B?

Hemophilia A is the most common type and affects about 1 in 4,000 males. It's characterized by a lack of antihemophilic factor VIII. Hemophilia B involves a deficiency of factor IX, and affects both males and females.

Teaching about tests

Explain that a family or personal history of bleeding after trauma or surgery (including tooth extraction) or of spontaneous bleeding into muscles or joints usually indicates a defect. Specific clotting factor assays are used to confirm and identify the type and severity of hemophilia.

The key: Blood studies

Blood studies are the key diagnostic tool for assessing hemophilia. The usual tests for any suspected bleeding disorder are bleeding time, platelet count, coagulation screenings (prothrombin time and partial thromboplastin time), and clotting factor assays. (See *Teaching patients about blood and immune system tests,* page 155.)

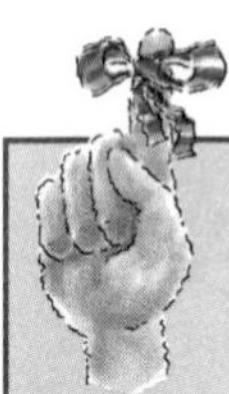

Memory jogger

Patients can remember what to do in case of a major bleeding episode by thinking of the 3 Rs:

React by infusing the clotting factor.

Report the situation to the doctor.

Record the facts of the matter.

Required regularly

Once the diagnosis is confirmed, regularly required tests include clotting factor assays and an occasional inhibitor screen, all of which can be done with one blood sample.

Teaching about activity and lifestyle

The patient may go for years without requiring treatment, depending on the severity of the disorder. Emphasize, however, that he must always act cautiously to prevent injury and, when necessary, receive I.V. clotting factors promptly. (See *Identify, prevent, follow up.*)

Regular and moderate

Advise the patient to get regular, moderate exercise as prescribed by his doctor. Explain that strong muscles may protect the joints and help prevent recurrent joint bleeding.

Gearing up

Encourage the patient to take up swimming, hiking, or bicycling. Review safety precautions with the parents of young patients. For example, the child may require supervision and protective apparel, such as a helmet, elbow and knee pads, and leg guards, to prevent injury.

No roughhousing

Urge the patient to avoid such sports as football, lacrosse, and boxing that obviously increase the risk of serious bleeding. Tell patients with chronic joint disease to avoid such sports as soccer, basketball, skiing, aerobic exercise,

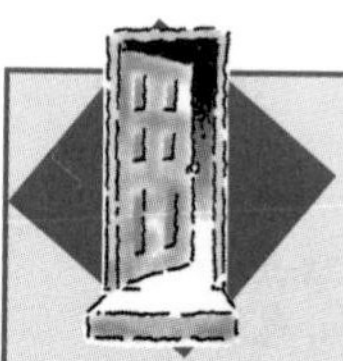

No place like home

Identify, prevent, follow up

Here are a few more teaching points to help patients living with hemophilia.

Identify

Tell the patient to wear a medical identification bracelet or necklace to ensure that he receives clotting factor infusions as soon as possible after a major accident or loss of consciousness.

Prevent

Preventive dental care is especially important for someone with hemophilia. Make sure he understands that he can have cavities filled and teeth extracted, but he'll need clotting factor infusions before some of these procedures. Emphasize that poor dental hygiene can lead to bleeding from inflamed gums.

Those undergoing minor surgical procedures such as tooth extraction may receive desmopressin (DDAVP) before the procedure. This drug stimulates the release of stored factor VIII in the body and can temporarily raise factor VIII levels high enough to control minor bleeding. He may also receive ϵ-aminocaproic acid (EACA). This drug (an antifibrinolytic agent) stabilizes clot formation in the mouth.

Follow up

Because of the patient's extensive home care needs, the doctor or nurse usually refers him to the nearest hemophilia center for evaluation and follow-up teaching. Encourage interested family members to go, too. Explain that these centers typically offer carrier testing, prenatal diagnosis, and other genetic counseling services. Provide the names of organizations that can offer the patient and his family further information and support.

and ice hockey because they stress the joints and carry a high risk of joint injury.

Besides avoiding certain sports, caution the patient to refrain from activities that increase his risk for injury and prolonged bleeding. These include heavy lifting and carrying and using potentially harmful equipment such as power tools.

Teaching about medication

The primary treatment for hemophilia is I.V. administration of the missing clotting factor. The replacement factor or other preparation the patient receives depends on the type and severity of his hemophilia. He may also need blood transfusions and repeated factor infusions because clotting factors have a short half-life. (See *Clotting factor replacement products.*)

Teaching about procedures

Teach the patient or his parents how to:
- give clotting factor infusions
- care for veins
- keep accurate records

Clotting factor replacement products

Products available for clotting factor replacement include:
- cryoprecipitate, a frozen human plasma product containing mostly factor VIII
- prothrombin complex concentrate, which contains factors II, VII, IX, and X
- purified factor VIII
- fresh frozen human plasma, which contains factors VIII and IX
- anti-inhibitor coagulant complex, derived from the plasma of people with factor VIII inhibitor
- factor IX.

Making it minimal
Reassure the patient that products are purified to minimize the risk of passing on communicable diseases, such as hepatitis and human immunodeficiency virus.

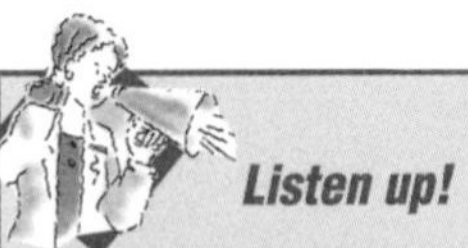

Preserving veins

Teach the patient to take the following steps to keep veins intact:

- Remove the needle after injection without putting pressure on the site.
- Apply firm pressure with one finger (with his arm straight, not bent) for 3 to 5 minutes after removing the needle.
- Remind health care professionals to use stainless steel butterfly needles whenever possible and to remove them after each infusion. (Plastic inside-the-needle catheters may inflame and scar the vein, especially if they're left in place for several days.)
- Tell health care professionals to perform a new venipuncture for each infusion (except when continuous I.V. fluids or antibiotics are needed, or when venipuncture is difficult, as in young children).

• prevent complications
• recognize and manage bleeding.

Self-infusion

Most parents learn to administer clotting factors to their hemophilic child by the time he enters school. Hemophilic children usually learn to perform self-infusion between ages 8 and 12. Reinforce instructions for performing the technique and preventing infection.

Protecting veins

Because of the need for lifelong therapy, the patient must take steps to preserve his veins. (See *Preserving veins.*)

On the record

Advise the patient and his family to keep accurate treatment records, and to send or take this information to the hemophilia treatment center at least once each month. Instruct them to write down the:
• problem that required an infusion treatment
• nature of the treatment
• treatment outcome.

Complications

Describe possible complications, such as internal bleeding and inhibitor development. Also, warn about blood-borne infection. Hepatitis, for example, may be transmitted through blood products. Urge the patient to be immunized against hepatitis B. (No vaccines exist for hepatitis C or D.) (See *So disease doesn't spread.*)

Respond promptly

To prevent serious blood loss and chronic joint disease, teach how to recognize the symptoms of internal bleeding and respond promptly. (See *Recognizing and managing bleeding,* page 164.)

It isn't working

Advise the patient to call the doctor if home treatments don't seem to be controlling bleeding episodes. The patient may be treated with anti-inhibitor coagulant complex. Additional occasional treatment with desmopressin (DDAVP) or aminocaproic acid (Amicar) may help.

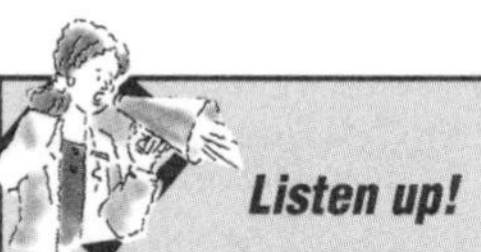

Listen up!

So disease doesn't spread

Tell patients to prevent spreading blood-borne communicable diseases (such as hepatitis) to others by:
• disposing of needles, syringes, and blood-contaminated waste in a hard plastic or cardboard container and returning the container to the hospital or treatment center for disposal.
• placing larger wastes contaminated with blood in an impermeable plastic bag and returning it to the hospital or treatment center.

Recognizing and managing bleeding

Bleeding in hemophilia may occur spontaneously or because of an injury. Tell your patient and members of his family about possible types of bleeding and their signs and symptoms. Advise them when to call for medical help.

Bleeding site	Signs and symptoms	What to teach the patient
Intracranial	Change in personality or wakefulness (level of consciousness), headache, nausea, labored respirations	Notify the doctor immediately and treat symptoms as an emergency.
Joints (generally affects the knees, followed by elbows, ankles, shoulders, hips, and wrists)	Joint pain and swelling, joint tingling and warmth (at onset of hemorrhage), extreme tenderness	Begin antihemophilic factor (AHF) infusions and then notify the doctor.
Muscles	Pain and reduced function of affected muscle; tingling, numbness, or pain in a large area away from the affected site (referred pain)	Notify the doctor. Start an AHF infusion if reasonably certain that bleeding results from recent injury.
Subcutaneous tissue or skin	Pain, bruising, and swelling at the site (Delayed oozing also may occur after an injury.)	Apply appropriate topical agents, such as ice packs or absorbable gelatin sponges (Gelfoam), to stop bleeding.
Kidneys	Pain in the lower back near the waist, decreased urine output, blood in the urine	Notify the doctor. Start an AHF infusion if reasonably certain that bleeding results from recent injury.
Heart (cardiac tamponade)	Chest tightness, shortness of breath, swelling (usually occurs in hemophiliacs who are very young or who have severe disease)	Contact the doctor or go to the nearest emergency department at once.

Rheumatoid arthritis

Rheumatoid arthritis is a chronic, progressive, and painful inflammatory disorder affecting the synovial joints. (See *Joints affected by rheumatoid arthritis.*)

What's at risk?

The good news is that the pain and inflammation of rheumatoid arthritis can be controlled with the right treat-

ment regimen. However, the patient with rheumatoid arthritis may suffer the following difficulties:
- joint deformities
- partial dislocations (subluxations)
- contractures
- pain
- loss of function.

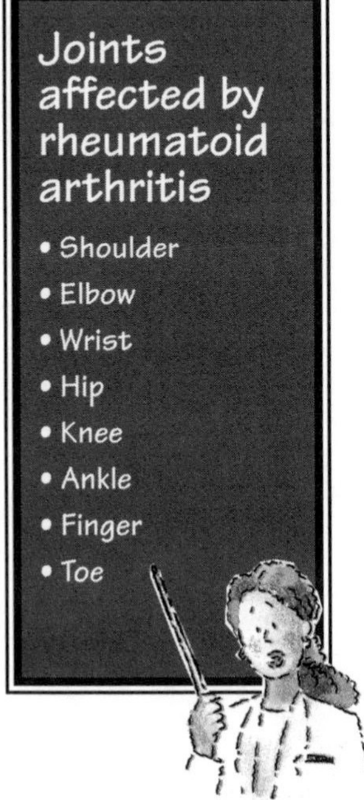

Joints affected by rheumatoid arthritis
• Shoulder
• Elbow
• Wrist
• Hip
• Knee
• Ankle
• Finger
• Toe

What causes it?

The cause of rheumatoid arthritis is unknown, but researchers think it may develop in response to an infectious agent in a susceptible host.

Teaching about tests

Teach the patient about three blood tests, each of which requires a small blood sample: rheumatoid factor (RF), erythrocyte sedimentation rate (ESR), and complete blood count (CBC).

The RF test, which is not specific for rheumatoid arthritis, is positive in about 80% of rheumatoid arthritis patients. The ESR may reflect inflammation. The CBC can be used to detect anemia, a frequent finding in rheumatoid arthritis. No single blood test provides a conclusive diagnosis.

Two telling tests

Explain to the patient that synovial fluid analysis can help doctors determine the cause of joint inflammation and swelling. X-rays are used to assess joint damage and may be taken at intervals to monitor bone erosion and joint deformity. (See *Teaching patients about blood and immune system tests,* page 155.)

Teaching about activity and lifestyle

Because this is an insidious, chronic, and painful inflammatory disorder, the patient can easily become discouraged. Help the patient overcome discouragement by emphasizing that inflammation and joint pain can be controlled. Also, encourage the patient to experiment with self-care measures and assistive devices to find the best way to meet his needs.

Slow down

It's time to slow down when pain or fatigue increases and dexterity progressively decreases in involved joints. If pain lasts for 2 hours or more after completing a task, the patient should do a little less the next time or simplify his effort.

Be adaptable

If a flare-up occurs, encourage the patient to adjust his schedule and ask for help with daily tasks. Suggest ways to conserve his energy. (See *Tips for conserving energy.*)

Pleasant dreams

Recommend sleeping 8 to 10 hours each night and lying down for 1/2 hour twice each day. For the patient who can't sleep well because of pain, discuss methods to aid sleep. (See *Getting Z's.*)

Just do it

Describe the benefits of adding an exercise program to the patient's daily routine. It can:
- make flexing and extending joints easier
- reduce pain and stiffness
- prevent loss of joint function and even help restore joint function.

Before you do it

Remind the patient to check with the doctor or therapist before beginning and to stay within reasonable limits. Caution against performing strenuous exercise during acute inflammatory episodes.

The best time to do it

Encourage exercising when he has the least pain and stiffness and the most energy and when medication achieves its peak. If the patient experiences muscle cramping or pain while exercising, tell him to:

 stop exercising

 gently massage the cramped muscle

 resume activity when symptoms diminish.

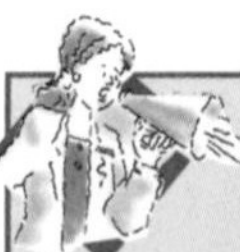

Listen up!

Tips for conserving energy

To help your patient conserve energy, provide the following tips:

- Use dressing aids, including a long-handled shoehorn, a reacher, elastic shoelaces, a zipper pull, and a buttonhook.
- Wear mittens if it's difficult to put fingers into gloves.
- Use helpful household items, such as a handheld shower nozzle, hand rails, grab bars, and easy-to-open drawers.
- Keep needed materials, utensils, and tools organized and handy.
- Sit while performing strenuous activities, such as dressing or cooking, to prevent stress on weight-bearing joints.

Keep up the good work

Warn the patient that if he doesn't follow the prescribed exercise program, muscle strength and joint mobility may diminish. Weakness in hip flexor and quadriceps muscles can also lead to gait problems, demanding extra energy and placing further stress on other joints. (See *More about rheumatoid arthritis.*)

Teaching about diet

Encourage the patient to eat a balanced diet, including foods high in vitamins, proteins, and iron, which can promote tissue building and repair. Also make sure that the patient knows how to select foods from the food pyramid groups to meet daily requirements. In addition, review ways to promote healthy and regular eating habits. (See *Overcoming eating obstacles,* page 168.)

Teaching about medication

Help the patient understand that the goal of drug therapy is to control inflammation and pain and arrest the progress of rheumatoid arthritis. Achieving this may require several types of drugs, including:

- anti-inflammatory drugs to reduce inflammation, thereby diminishing pain

Getting Z's

Equipment
- Firm mattress
- Bed board
- Small, flat pillow

Habits
- Correct body position during rest (joints extended, not flexed)
- Good body mechanics at all times
- Wearing splints (if prescribed) whenever possible

Warning
- Placing pillows under the knees fosters joint deformity.

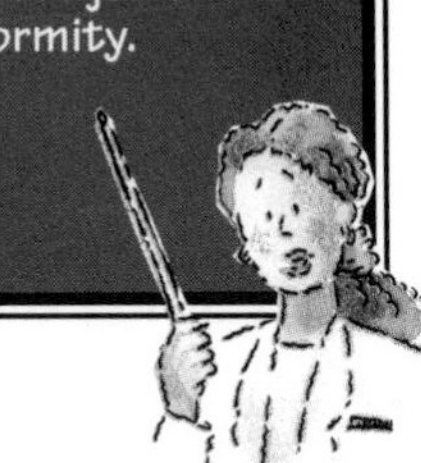

More about rheumatoid arthritis

Here are a few more teaching points to give your patient with rheumatoid arthritis.

Alternative treatments
Make it clear that there are no miracle cures for rheumatoid arthritis, despite claims to the contrary. Encourage the patient to check with you, the doctor, or the local chapter of the Arthritis Foundation before trying any alternative treatment.

Let's talk about sex
Because arthritis changes the way the patient looks and moves, he may need reassurance that he can still enjoy a satisfying sexual relationship.

More info
To help the patient cope with rheumatoid arthritis, refer him to an organization that can offer further information and support, such as the Arthritis Foundation.

• disease-modifying antirheumatic drugs to slow the disease process
• immunosuppressants to inhibit the autoimmune response in rheumatoid arthritis. (Because immunosuppressants heighten the risk of severe infection, teach the patient infection control measures.)

Warning! Warning! Warning!

Warn the patient that improperly treated rheumatoid arthritis can lead to excruciating joint pain. If he fails to follow his drug regimen, irreversible joint damage and severe deformities may occur. Urge him to call the doctor if symptoms worsen during therapy.

Help the medicine go down

Help the patient devise a medication calendar to keep track of his regimen. If he has weak or crippled hands or if moving them hurts, tell him to ask the pharmacist not to use childproof caps.

Advise the woman of childbearing age with rheumatoid arthritis to let her doctor know if she plans to become pregnant. He may adjust her medication dosage.

Overcoming eating obstacles

• Advise eating frequent, small meals if the patient's appetite is poor.
• Teach techniques for making meal preparation easier.
• Tell the patient to plan breaks between cooking chores.
• When symptoms become severe, suggest eating convenience foods.
• Promote the use of assistive devices and appliances for meal preparation and eating.

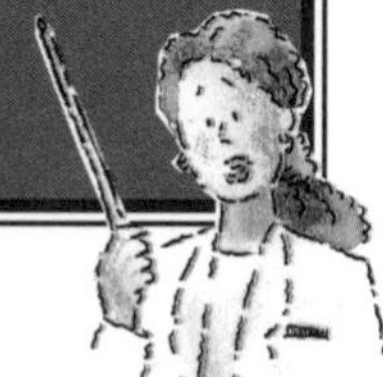

Teaching about surgery

Joint surgery may relieve pain, increase mobility, and improve appearance. Describe relevant surgical procedures, which may include:
• synovectomy — removing synovial membranes (the synovium) from joints to reduce pain and swelling
• osteotomy — cutting and resetting a bone to correct a deformity
• resection — removing a bone or part of a bone; frequently performed on the feet to increase comfort when walking
• arthrodesis — bone fusion to diminish pain (this also decreases mobility)
• arthroplasty — repairing or replacing joints to reduce pain and increase flexibility and mobility.

After surgery

Urge the patient to comply with the prescribed postsurgical regimen, including physical therapy. Tell the patient to expect muscle — not joint — pain early on during therapy. Assure him that this decreases with time. Depending on the type of surgery, he may require several months of therapy.

Latex allergy

Having an allergy — or hypersensitivity — means the body's defenses are exaggerated. (See *Three forms of hypersensitivity.*) Latex allergy is hypersensitivity to the proteins in natural latex rubber (not synthetic latex) or to additives used in manufacturing latex. Latex — the milky sap

Three forms of hypersensitivity

Latex allergy can take one of three forms:

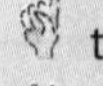 type I (immediate)

 type IV (delayed)

 chemical irritation dermatitis.

Type I reactions

A type I reaction to latex is a reaction that occurs within 2 hours after latex proteins enter the body through the skin, airways, or mucosal membranes. Type I reactions may be further described by four categories based on severity:

 localized urticaria (hives) in the area of contact

 generalized urticaria with angioedema

 urticaria with asthma, watery eyes, runny nose, and orolaryngeal and GI symptoms

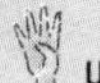 urticaria with anaphylaxis.

About 1% of the general population has type I latex allergy. The incidence is much greater in health care providers (roughly 10% to 15%) and in children with spina bifida (roughly 65%).

Type IV reactions

Type IV reactions are delayed, localized reactions affecting the skin or mucous membranes. They're thought to be triggered by the chemicals added to latex in manufacturing.

Chemical irritation dermatitis

Chemical irritation dermatitis — the most common adverse reaction to latex — is also thought to result from the chemicals used in latex manufacturing. It's usually a mild chemical dermatitis or skin inflammation. Although this reaction doesn't involve the immune system, it may contribute to later development of immunologic reactions to latex. Chemical irritation dermatitis is especially common among people who continually wear latex gloves at work.

of the rubber tree — is used in more than 40,000 industrial, household, and medical products.

How does it happen?

Latex sensitization may result from direct exposure to the proteins in latex or from indirect exposure, as when the protein adheres to the powder in a glove, becomes airborne, and is inhaled. A latex-sensitive person is particularly vulnerable in places where there's a high level of airborne latex such as hospitals.

Is it minor or major?

Although some reactions to latex are relatively minor (such as sneezing and runny nose), others are life-threatening. Some people initially experience mild reactions that eventually progress to more serious ones such as anaphylactic shock.

Latex phobia

Fear of latex exposure can cause a high level of stress in latex-sensitive patients. Some patients are afraid to seek medical help for fear of latex exposure. Provide emotional support to help your patient cope with stress. Also, ask your manager to obtain products made from latex substitutes.

Latex allergy alerts

- Other known allergies (especially to certain foods)
- Hand dermatitis
- Development of hives after using latex gloves
- Allergic conjunctivitis after touching the eye with a recently ungloved hand
- Swelling around the mouth after blowing up a balloon or undergoing a dental procedure
- Vaginal burning after contact with a condom
- Occupational asthma related to latex exposure
- Undiagnosed reactions or complications during surgery, dental work, or anesthesia

Teaching about tests

No single test for latex allergy is widely accepted. To evaluate a suspected latex allergy, the doctor takes a thorough patient history. (See *Latex allergy alerts.*) To aid diagnosis of latex allergy, the patient may undergo a skin prick test, intradermal testing, radioallergosorbent test (RAST), or spirometric flow measurements. (See *Teaching patients about blood and immune system tests,* page 155.)

Teaching about activity and lifestyle

Prevention is the foundation of treatment for latex allergy. Give the patient a list of household items containing latex, and emphasize the importance of avoiding these. Tell him about nonlatex product substitutes. Also teach him about foods and plants associated with cross-sensitivity to latex. (See *Avoiding cross-reactions.*)

Let it be known

Emphasize the crucial need for the patient and family members to tell all health care providers — including emergency medical rescuers — about the patient's latex sensitivity. Stress the importance of wearing a medical identification bracelet that specifies latex sensitivity.

Reacting to reactions

Tell the patient and members of his family to call for emergency medical assistance if the following symptoms of latex exposure occur:
- hives
- wheezing
- coughing
- shortness of breath
- palpitations
- redness, swelling, and itching of the skin.

Also review ways to avoid latex reactions during future health care visits. (See *Additional teaching points for latex allergy patients,* page 172.) Finally, to help the latex-sensitive patient cope with the disorder and its implications, refer him to appropriate resources for further information and support.

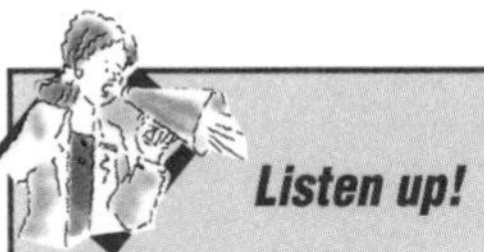

Avoiding cross-reactions

Natural latex is 2% to 3% protein and contains more than 240 polypeptides. Many of these polypeptides are found in fruits and plants, which may explain why persons with latex allergy may experience cross-reactions with certain foods.

Grocery don'ts

Warn patients that cross-reactions can occur after eating foods such as:
- bananas
- cherries
- peaches
- plums
- figs
- papayas
- chestnuts
- tomatoes
- celery
- avocados
- kiwi.

Teaching about medication

For patients with known allergies, prevention is the best medicine. When caring for a latex-sensitive patient, keep him away from known latex products, such as latex gloves, plastic syringes with latex-tipped plungers, and latex nasopharyngeal tubes. If a reaction does occur, discuss medications that may be given.

Mild reactions

For a mild reaction, patients usually receive antihistamines. A patient with hives may also receive antihistamines; if the hives become generalized, oral or systemic steroids may be given.

Serious reactions

A more serious reaction — throat swelling, bronchospasm, wheezing, and shortness of breath — calls for antihistamines, steroids, histamine-2 (H_2) receptor antagonists, bronchodilators and, possibly, epinephrine.

Anaphylaxis warrants immediate administration of epinephrine and airway maintenance, along with steroids, antihistamines, and H_2-receptor antagonists.

Meds to manage emergencies

Teach the patient how to use medications such as diphenhydramine (Benadryl) to manage allergic reactions. Provide instruction in using autoinjectable epinephrine (EpiPen) in case a severe reaction occurs. Tell the patient to keep these medications with him at all times, and advise him to keep nonlatex (vinyl or neoprene) gloves on hand for emergencies.

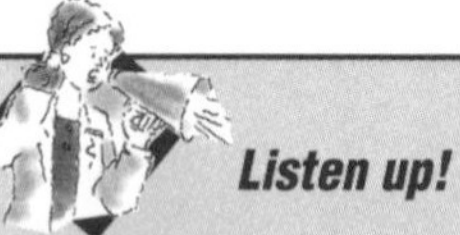

Listen up!

Additional teaching points for latex allergy patients

If your patient has a documented latex allergy, pass along the following pointers for when he enters health care facilities.

Policy
Advise him to enter only those facilities with a latex-free policy, including a latex allergy cart.

Timing
If the patient needs surgery, tell him to request the first operating room available for that day to avoid airborne latex exposure that may occur later in the day.

Premedication
Explain that, before a medical or surgical procedure, the patient is premedicated with diphenhydramine, methylprednisolone (Prednisone), and ranitidine (Zantac) to reduce the severity of any reaction that develops.

Sickle cell anemia

Sickle cell anemia (SCA) is a chronic and incurable inherited blood disease, which occurs mostly in blacks and sometimes in persons from Mediterranean cultures. (See *Working it out.*)

What causes it?

SCA is caused by an inherited mutation in hemoglobin, the part of blood that carries oxygen to other tissues.

Who gets it?

Tell the patient that SCA runs in families, passed on by a recessive gene. Explain that a person with sickle cell trait can pass on the trait, and possibly the disease, to his offspring if his mate also carries the trait. For this reason, encourage testing as part of family planning.

What happens?

In SCA, red blood cells (RBCs) contain hemoglobin S. RBCs with this form of hemoglobin have normal oxygen capacity but are abnormally rigid, rough, and elongated (sickle-shaped). In contrast, normal RBCs, which carry normal hemoglobin A, are disklike and pliable.

When does sickling occur?

Sickling typically occurs with activities or conditions that increase the body's need for oxygen. (See *Sickling situations,* page 174.) Heavy concentrations of sickled cells can thicken the blood and slow circulation, depriving tissues of oxygen. Warn the patient that, without intervention, tiny obstructions can become large infarctions.

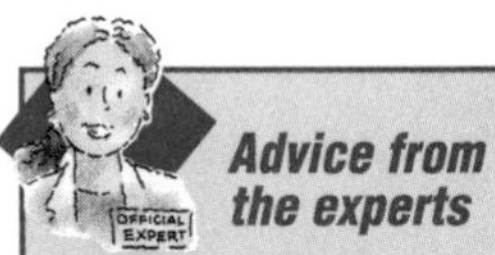

Advice from the experts

Working it out

Because sickle cell anemia (SCA) is a chronic disease, determine how much the patient already knows before you start teaching. SCA usually includes periodic crises, which can leave the patient discouraged and depressed and delay learning. Encourage the patient to express his feelings. If he's been hospitalized before, point out that there's always more to learn about his condition, and the more he learns, the better prepared he'll be to guard against complications.

What's at risk?

Vaso-occlusive crisis is the most common complication of SCA. This painful condition can result from:

- infection
- dehydration
- excessive fatigue.

In addition, the SCA patient is susceptible to serious infection, especially meningitis and pneumonia. An infection can start suddenly and quickly worsen. Although young children are at greater risk, a patient of any age can develop a serious infection.

Teaching about tests

Tell the patient and his family that blood tests — especially hemoglobin electrophoresis — can confirm the SCA diagnosis.

Describe other tests used to detect early organ damage, including routine blood counts, blood chemistry profiles, and urinalysis. (See *Teaching patients about blood and immune system tests,* page 155.)

More tests

Complications may call for additional blood tests and possibly X-rays. A lateral chest X-ray may be ordered to detect the "Lincoln log deformity," a spinal abnormality. This deformity develops in many adults and some adolescents with SCA, leaving the vertebrae resembling logs that form the corner of a cabin.

An eye examination is performed to detect corkscrew- or comma-shaped vessels in the conjunctivae, another possible sign of SCA.

Teaching about activity and lifestyle

Although SCA can't be cured, treatments can alleviate symptoms and prevent painful crises. Physical activities that promote health and fitness are fine, as long as the patient exercises the following precautions as well:

- rest frequently
- increase fluid intake

• don't overdo it (because fatigue can contribute to vaso-occlusive crisis). (See *Other care measures.*)

Explaining spleen care

One reason SCA patients are susceptible to serious infection is the spleen's inability to function properly, which limits the body's defenses. Patients should be careful when exercising, in order to prevent spleen damage. The patient with splenomegaly should avoid contact sports to minimize the risk of a ruptured spleen.

Sickling situations

• Running at high altitudes
• Infection
• Stress
• Strenuous exercise
• Flying in aircraft without adequate air pressure
• Cold

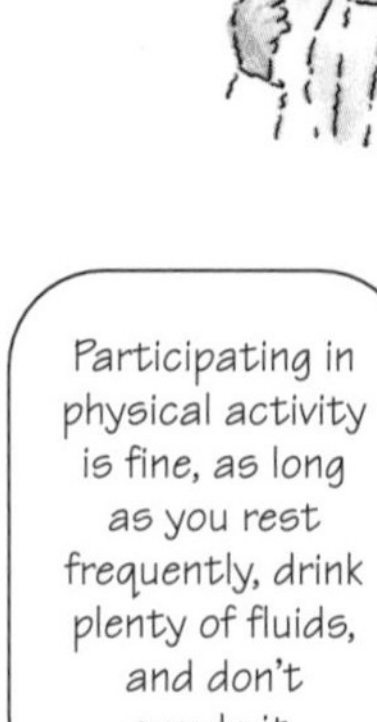

Teaching about diet

Adequate nutrition is essential for patients with SCA. For example, folic acid deficiency exacerbates anemia and may lead to bone marrow depression from increased demands to replace RBCs. Urge patients to add folic acid–rich foods to their diets. These foods include:

• leafy green vegetables
• beef
• liver
• red beans
• wheat germ.

Folic acid supplements are usually given. Also, remind the patient to avoid consuming alcohol and smoking cigarettes because they deplete folic acid in the body.

Let me offer you a drink

In your teaching, don't water down the need for fluids. To maintain adequate hydration and minimize RBC sickling, suggest that parents offer a child with SCA more fluids, such as eggnog, ice pops, and milkshakes.

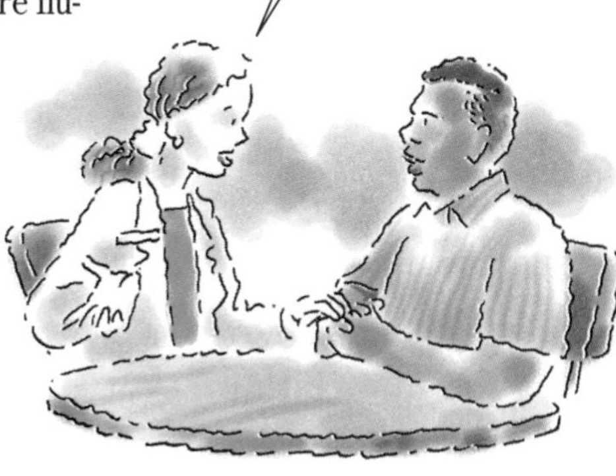
Participating in physical activity is fine, as long as you rest frequently, drink plenty of fluids, and don't overdo it.

Teaching about medication

Although drugs can't cure SCA, certain vaccines, anti-infectives, and chelating agents can minimize complications resulting from SCA or transfusion therapy. Other medications, such as narcotics, may help relieve the pain of vaso-occlusive crisis.

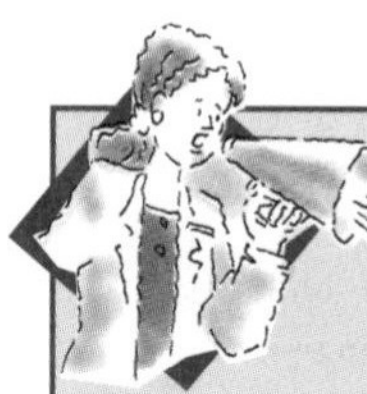

Listen up!

Other care measures

Because sickle cell disorders affect not only the patient, but also those closest to him, provide guidelines for:
- giving crisis care
- maintaining emotional and physical support
- obtaining genetic and psychological counseling as needed.

Crisis care

Review the signs and symptoms of vaso-occlusive crisis so that the patient or his parents can recognize and treat it early. As appropriate, explain how to care for this condition at home.

Tell parents that an infant's first vaso-occlusive crisis may be called the "hand-foot crisis" because the infant's hands or feet, or both, swell and become painful. Advise them to begin home treatment measures but to call the doctor if symptoms persist or worsen.

If the patient must be hospitalized for a vaso-occlusive crisis, explain that I.V. fluids and parenteral analgesics may be given. He may also receive oxygen and blood transfusions.

Call the doctor

Review signs and symptoms that warrant immediate medical attention. For example, instruct parents of young children (ages 8 to 24 months) to report signs of acute sequestration crisis. Stress that this crisis, though rare, is a medical emergency. Other symptoms requiring urgent care include:
- temperature over 101° F (38.3° C)
- stiff neck
- difficulty speaking
- difficulty walking
- numbness
- weakness
- priapism (persistent abnormal erection of the penis) in infants.

Promote parental participation

Include the following points in your teaching sessions with parents of SCA patients:
- Because delayed growth and late puberty are common among SCA patients, reassure adolescent patients that they will grow and mature. They should catch up with their friends by age 17 or 18.
- Urinary frequency and bedwetting may begin around age 6. Explain that this results, not from disobedience or behavior problems, but from the SCA patient's inability to concentrate urine.
- Encourage parents to schedule their child for a yearly eye examination to detect and treat retinal damage resulting from SCA.
- Stress the importance of meticulous leg and foot care because leg ulcers commonly develop during the late teens.
- Promote normal intellectual and social development by cautioning parents against overprotectiveness. Although the SCA patient must avoid strenuous exercise, he can safely enjoy most everyday activities.

Suggest counseling

Refer parents of children with SCA for genetic counseling to answer their questions about SCA in future children. Recommend screening for other family members to determine whether they're SCA carriers.

Besides genetic counseling, parents may benefit from psychological counseling to help them cope with possible feelings of guilt. Recommend an appropriate support group.

Potential pregnancy problems

Tell women that SCA makes pregnancy hazardous. Oral contraceptive use is also hazardous. If appropriate, refer female patients to a gynecologist for counseling. However, if the patient *does* become pregnant, offer guidelines for maintaining a balanced diet and advise her to ask her doctor about taking a folic acid supplement.

Potential priapism problems

Recognize that, in men with SCA, sudden, painful bouts of priapism may develop. Reassure the patient that these common episodes have no permanent, harmful effects.

Vaccine scene

Discuss the need for polyvalent pneumococcal vaccines, which the child may receive at age 6 months and again at age 2 years, with booster vaccines every 4 years. The child usually also receives *Haemophilus influenzae* B vaccine at age 15 months.

Infection prevention

Review prophylactic anti-infective therapy. Low-dose oral penicillin given twice daily until the child reaches age 6 may reduce the risk of pneumococcal infections. After age 6, this preventive measure may not be needed.

Help parents understand the importance of complying with these measures. They should also realize that prophylaxis isn't foolproof; they still have to watch for early signs and symptoms of infection. Warn parents that a child may need to be hospitalized for antibiotic therapy.

Add an antineoplastic agent

Hydroxyurea is an antineoplastic agent that has been found to reduce the frequency of painful crises and need for blood transfusion.

Chalk it up to a chelating agent

A patient who receives regular transfusions may need a chelating agent to remove dangerous iron deposits. The patient can take deferoxamine mesylate (Desferal) at home after receiving detailed instructions on how to mix and administer it. Explain that the drug may color urine orange red.

Instruct the patient or his parents to contact the doctor as soon as possible if any of the following occurs:

- difficulty breathing
- hearing impairment
- visual impairment
- pain at the injection site
- rash.

Armed with analgesics

If a narcotic analgesic is prescribed for vaso-occlusive crisis, tell the patient to follow the doctor's instructions and to report persistent pain.

Break it up

If the patient has a short attention span or the material you're teaching is complicated (such as dressing changes), explain it one step at a time.

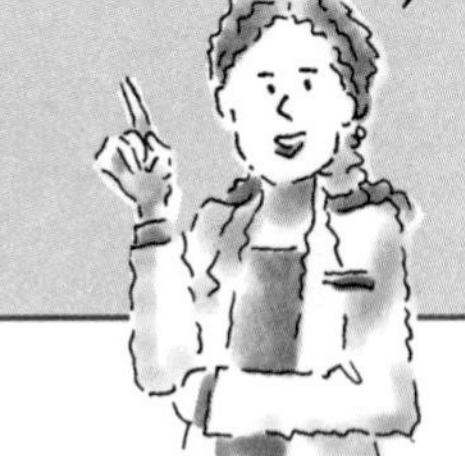

Warm only

Instruct the patient to apply only warm compresses to painful areas. Stress that cold compresses should never be used because this encourages vasoconstriction.

Apply warm compresses to painful areas. Cold compresses should never be used because chilling encourages vasoconstriction.

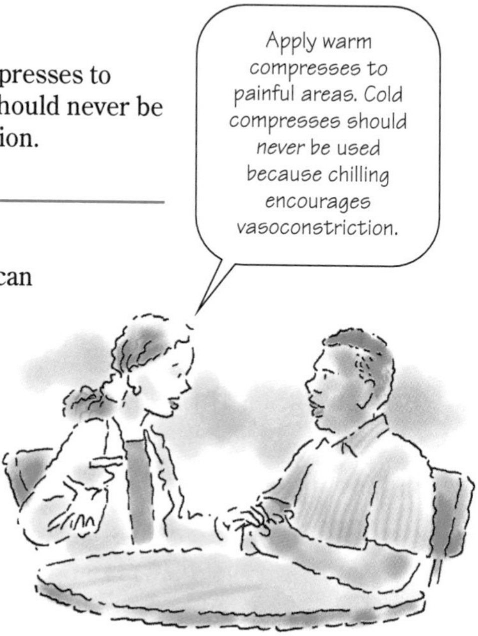

Teaching about surgery

The only currently available treatment that can cure SCA is bone marrow transplant. This treatment isn't commonly done because of the risks and complications associated with it; the mortality rate is 5% to 10%.

Spread the word

Urge the patient to tell all health care providers that he has SCA before he undergoes any treatment, especially major surgery. During any procedure that requires general anesthesia, the patient with SCA needs adequate ventilation to prevent hypoxic crisis. Also urge the patient to wear a medical identification bracelet stating that he has SCA.

Systemic lupus erythematosus

Systemic lupus erythematosus (SLE) is a chronic inflammatory disorder. SLE causes structural changes in connective tissue, the fibers that support many other body tissues. Its unpredictable course includes exacerbations with long periods of complete or near-complete remission. (See *Monitor motivation,* page 178.)

Who's at greatest risk?

SLE strikes women eight times as often as men and is more common among nonwhites, especially among blacks and Asians.

What happens?

The cause of SLE is uncertain, but researchers believe antibodies develop against the body's own tissues. SLE causes various signs and symptoms. The most common are:

- facial erythema (butterfly-shaped rash on the face)
- hair loss

- stiff and aching joints
- musculoskeletal deformity
- photosensitivity.

What else?

The patient may also experience fatigue, weight loss, chills, fever, sensitivity to heat and cold, and musculoskeletal pain. SLE may produce only mild effects, or it may produce potentially life-threatening effects on the heart, blood vessels, kidneys, lungs, and central nervous system.

What triggers flare-ups?

Heredity may predispose some patients to SLE, which has been found in certain families for several generations. Certain factors may trigger a patient's periodic flare-ups. These may include:

- physical or emotional stress
- streptococcal or viral infection
- inadequate rest
- exposure to direct or indirect sunlight, ultraviolet light, or X-rays
- vaccines.

Certain drugs, including sulfonamides, hydralazine, procainamide, penicillin, sulfa drugs and other antibiotics, and some oral contraceptives, may also cause acute exacerbations.

Because SLE is a systemic disease, complications depend largely on the organs affected. (See *Complications of SLE.*)

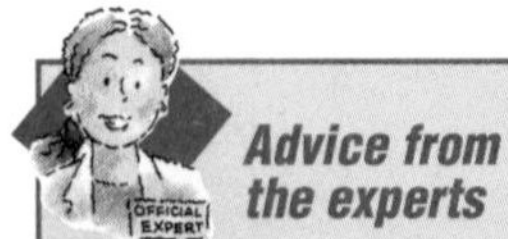

Advice from the experts

Monitor motivation

Pay careful attention to your patient's level of motivation. Systemic lupus erythematosus exhibits three characteristics that can interfere with learning and hinder compliance:

- its chronic nature
- periodic flare-ups
- unpredictable remissions.

Accepting the reality

When the patient experiences a long remission, for instance, she may lose her motivation to comply with therapy. Alternatively, she may meticulously comply with therapy but become discouraged when flare-ups persist. Focus your teaching on helping the patient accept the reality of lifelong treatment and periodic flare-ups.

Teaching about tests

A precise history of the patient's symptoms aids diagnosis. A definitive diagnosis may require months of observation, many laboratory tests, and measurement of the patient's response to different medications.

Draw blood

Blood tests are used to evaluate the immune system and detect certain antibodies. Tests include the antinuclear antibody test (which yields positive results in about 95% of SLE patients), a lupus erythematosus factor test (a positive result strongly suggests SLE), and the anti-DNA antibody test (the most specific test for SLE). Tests may be repeated periodically to monitor the effectiveness of therapy.

Testing effects

Tests used to evaluate the effects of SLE include CBC, ESR, urinalysis, chest X-ray, electrocardiogram, renal function tests, and renal biopsy.

Teaching about activity and lifestyle

If the patient suffers from joint stiffness and inflammation, explain that moderate exercise — such as range-of-motion exercises — promotes optimal health and joint mobility. Using moist or dry heat before exercising can decrease discomfort. Warn the patient against exercising to the point of fatigue. She should also stop during a flare-up and resume exercise slowly thereafter.

Pleasant dreams

Because fatigue is common in SLE, recommend 10 to 12 hours of sleep each night and periodic rests during the day. Make sure the patient understands the need to curtail activities before she tires. Encourage her to maintain a calm, stable environment, if possible, and to practice relaxation exercises and other stress-reduction techniques.

Last words

Explain other treatment measures such as infection control, mouth care, and birth control. (See *More SLE care measures,* page 180.)

Teaching about diet

Foods high in protein, vitamins, and iron can help the patient maintain optimum nutrition and prevent anemia. If the patient loses weight, suggest increasing caloric intake by consuming between-meal snacks or high-protein, high-calorie supplements. Kidney involvement may call for a low-sodium, low-protein diet.

Teaching about medication

The doctor tailors drug therapy to the patient's symptoms and severity of illness.

Complications of SLE

Circulatory disorders

- Raynaud's disease
- Vasculitis, possibly leading to infarctive ulcers, necrotic leg ulcers, or digital gangrene

Cardiopulmonary abnormalities

- Myocarditis
- Endocarditis
- Tachycardia
- Parenchymal infiltrates
- Pneumonitis

Renal abnormalities

- Hematuria
- Urinary tract infections
- Kidney failure

Central nervous system complications

- Emotional instability
- Psychosis
- Organic brain syndrome
- Headache

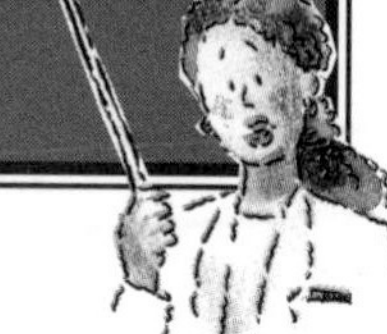

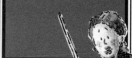

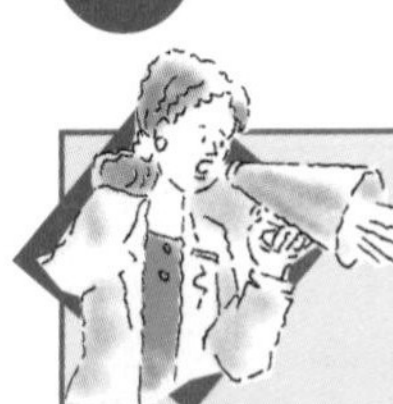

Listen up!

More SLE care measures

Here are additional treatments to discuss with your patient who has systemic lupus erythematosus (SLE).

Therapeutic apheresis

If the patient has life-threatening complications or an acute flare-up that resists corticosteroids, she may undergo therapeutic apheresis. A needle is inserted in each arm and her blood is then pumped through a machine to remove circulating immune complexes. The patient's pulse and blood pressure are monitored during the procedure. Tell her to report any tingling sensations around or in her mouth.

Avoiding infection

Minimizing exposure to infection is important, especially if the patient takes corticosteroids, which suppress the immune response. Advise her to avoid crowds and people with known infections and to consult her doctor about influenza and pneumococcal vaccines.

Caution against excessive bathing because it can dry or break down the skin, leaving it vulnerable to infection. However, each day she should clean and pat dry areas where two skin surfaces touch, such as the underarm or genital area. Tell her to regularly inspect these areas for signs of infection or skin breakdown.

Mouth care

Emphasize meticulous mouth care for preventing and treating oral lesions. Advise the patient to use a soft toothbrush and avoid commercial mouthwashes because of their high sugar content and the irritating and drying effect of the alcohol base. Instruct her to have regular dental checkups and to call her doctor if white plaques appear in her mouth; they may be signs of fungal infection. Suggest eating soft, bland foods if she has open sores.

Sunlight exposure

Tell the patient that sunlight exposure may cause severe hives and blisters. Even brief exposure (20 minutes or less) can produce a rash. Caution the patient to avoid sunlight, even when it's reflected from sand or snow.

Raynaud's disease

If the patient has Raynaud's disease, tell her to protect her hands and feet from cold temperatures to prevent vasospasm. Instruct her to avoid cold water and to wear gloves when handling cold items such as frozen foods.

Family planning

If the patient is in her childbearing years, provide counseling about pregnancy and family planning, as needed. Explain that she may experience menstrual irregularities during flare-ups but her normal cycle will resume during remissions. If she wishes to become pregnant, tell her that keeping her disorder under control and obtaining good prenatal care increase her chances of having a healthy baby. Advise choosing an obstetrician who specializes in high-risk pregnancies, ideally one with experience in caring for pregnant SLE patients.

If the patient wishes to avoid pregnancy, discuss birth control options. Explain that oral contraceptives may aggravate the disorder and that many doctors recommend a diaphragm; explain how to obtain and use one. Warn her against becoming pregnant and possibly exposing a fetus to medications that may produce birth defects.

Other advice

Tell the patient to call the doctor if fever, cough, or skin rash occurs or if chest, abdominal, muscle, or joint pain worsens. Finally, provide the names of organizations that can offer further information and support.

Aspirin and anti-inflammatories

Aspirin and other nonsteroidal anti-inflammatory drugs (NSAIDs) can relieve pain and fever and fight inflammation. Warn about common adverse effects, such as gastric upset and ulcers.

Advise the patient to report unintended weight gain and such GI symptoms as loss of appetite, nausea, vomiting, diarrhea, and abdominal cramps. Tell her to call her doctor immediately if she has black, tarry stools or if her vomit contains blood or resembles coffee grounds.

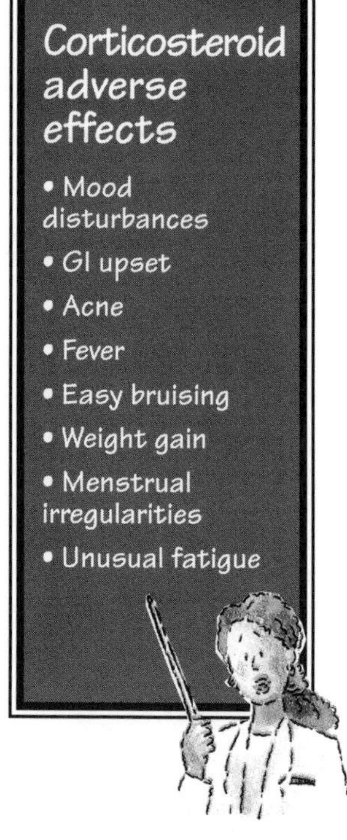

Corticosteroid adverse effects
• Mood disturbances
• GI upset
• Acne
• Fever
• Easy bruising
• Weight gain
• Menstrual irregularities
• Unusual fatigue

Corticosteroids

For severe SLE or acute exacerbations, systemic corticosteroids are the treatment of choice. Initial high dosages often bring noticeable improvement within 48 hours. When symptoms come under control, the dosage is tapered slowly. (See *Corticosteroid adverse effects.*)

Lessening lesions

Topical corticosteroids may also be used to treat skin or mucosal lesions. Demonstrate how to apply the cream and warn her not to use nonprescription preparations without her doctor's approval. Adverse effects may include burning, itching, irritation, dryness, acne, hypopigmentation, hypertrichosis, allergic contact dermatitis, secondary infection, and atrophy.

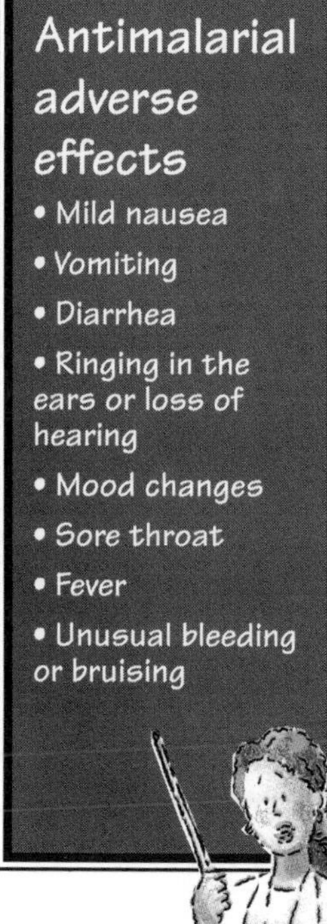

Antimalarial adverse effects
• Mild nausea
• Vomiting
• Diarrhea
• Ringing in the ears or loss of hearing
• Mood changes
• Sore throat
• Fever
• Unusual bleeding or bruising

Antimalarials

Antimalarial drugs also may be used to treat skin and mucosal lesions. The patient must take the antimalarial regularly and may not achieve full benefits for up to 6 months. (See *Antimalarial adverse effects.*)

Watch the eyes

Because antimalarials can cause retinopathy, recommend that an ophthalmologist examine the patient every 3 to 4 months to detect early signs of retinal damage. If the patient notices any changes in her vision, such as blurring or blind spots, tell her to contact her doctor immediately.

Immunosuppressants

If the patient fails to respond to NSAIDs, corticosteroids, or antimalarials, the doctor may prescribe an immunosuppressant drug. (See *Immunosuppressant adverse effects.*)

Immunosuppressant adverse effects

- Unusual bleeding or bruising
- Chills
- Fever
- Sore throat
- Partial hair loss (hair grows back when drug usage stops)
- Interference with blood cell production

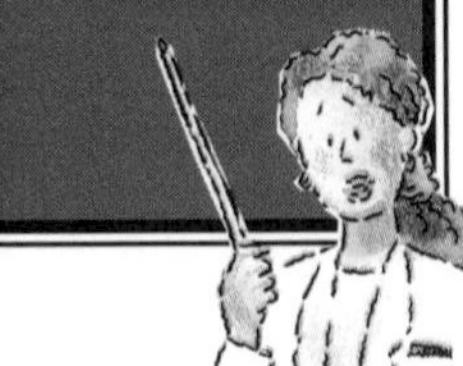

Thrombocytopenia

Thrombocytopenia is a congenital or acquired bleeding disorder. It's marked by a shortage of platelets (thrombocytes), cells that are needed for normal blood clotting.

What causes it?

This disorder has several causes, including:

- decreased or defective platelet production in the bone marrow
- sequestration (abnormal platelet collection) in the spleen
- increased platelet destruction in the bloodstream
- conditions related to infection
- use of some drugs
- primary immune disorder or other disease
- vitamin deficiency.

What happens?

In thrombocytopenia, decreased platelet function impairs blood clotting. Bruising and bleeding commonly accompany this disorder. The severity of these signs varies with the degree of thrombocytopenia.

Beyond bruising

Severe thrombocytopenia can cause acute hemorrhage, which may be fatal without immediate treatment. The most common sites of severe bleeding include the brain and the GI tract. Pulmonary bleeding or cardiac tamponade also can occur.

Describe the symptoms of intracranial bleeding. Tell the patient to report symptoms immediately, even if he hasn't suffered a head injury. (See *Symptoms of intracranial bleeding.*)

Anything else?

Capillary or mucosal bleeding may lead to GI bleeding, epistaxis, menorrhagia, or gingival or urinary tract bleeding. Explain the significance of black, tarry stools or "coffee-ground" emesis and bloody urine. By reporting bleeding signs promptly, the patient may prevent serious blood loss from a tiny ulcer or other internal lesion.

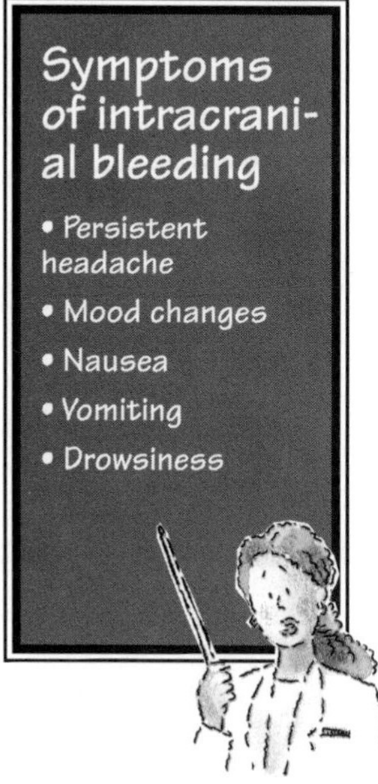

Teaching about tests

Frequent, small blood samples may be needed for platelet counts, especially after repeated platelet infusions. Test results reveal whether the condition is responding to infusion therapy or platelets are being destroyed.

Other tests include platelet antibody studies, platelet survival studies, and bone marrow studies.

Teaching about activity and lifestyle

The lower the patient's platelet count falls, the more cautious he must be in activities. If the patient has severe thrombocytopenia, instruct him to avoid sports and other strenuous physical activities in which he might twist a joint, strain a muscle, sustain hard blows or kicks, or traumatize vital organs. (See *Living with thrombocytopenia,* page 184.)

Even minor bumps

Even minor bumps or scrapes can cause bleeding. In extreme situations, spontaneous hemorrhage can occur. Suggest that a family member or other caregiver provide supervision and assistance to prevent injury and monitor for bleeding. (See *Avoiding excessive bleeding,* page 185.)

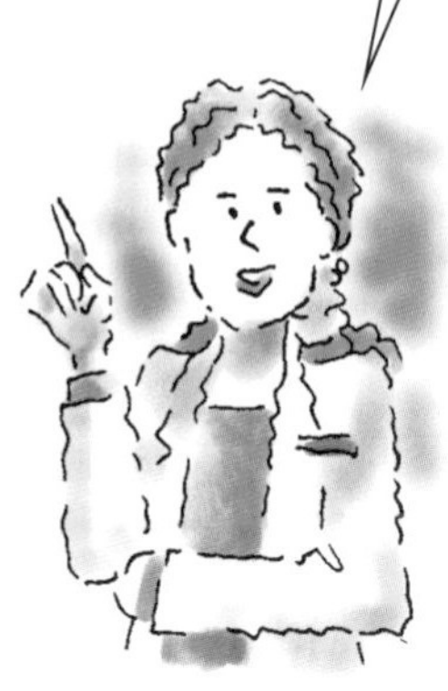
The lower your platelet count falls, the more cautious you must be in activities.

Teaching about medication

Corticosteroids may be prescribed to suppress the patient's immune response if the disorder doesn't resolve spontaneously. Therapy may be brief or long-term.

Patients with HIV-induced thrombocytopenia can improve platelet counts by taking zidovudine (AZT).

These don't help

Some medications can cause thrombocytopenia. Advise your patient not to take any over-the-counter drugs. Evaluate all the medications your patient takes to ensure they aren't contributing to the reduced platelet count.

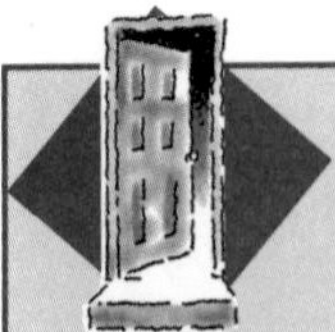

No place like home

Living with thrombocytopenia

Here are some pointers to give your patient for dealing with thrombocytopenia in daily life.

The tooth of the matter
Practice good dental hygiene to avoid bleeding and to prevent the need for tooth extractions or restorations. Be sure to use a soft toothbrush and proper tooth flossing technique. Avoid using a sawing motion that cuts the gums. (If his platelet count drops below 30,000/μl, he may have to stop flossing altogether.) Also avoid using toothpicks.

Nose knowledge
If experiencing frequent nosebleeds, use a humidifier at night. Moisten inner nostrils twice a day with an anti-infective ointment, such as Neosporin Ointment.

No strain
Avoid straining while having a bowel movement or while coughing.

Self-monitoring
Examine skin for ecchymoses and petechiae. Ideally, have someone else check skin areas that are difficult to see. Report any bleeding from the mucous membranes or GI tract as well as any new petechiae or ecchymoses.

Test stools for occult blood. A female patient should report increased menstrual flow to her doctor. Carry medical identification to alert others about thrombocytopenia.

Teaching about procedures

The patient may need an I.V. infusion of platelets to stop abnormal bleeding caused by a low platelet count (typically under 20,000/μl). If platelet destruction results from an immune disorder, however, platelet infusions may have only minimal effect and may be reserved for life-threatening bleeding.

Getting the chills

The patient receiving repeated platelet infusions may develop antibodies to WBCs in the platelets, producing fever and chills. Acetaminophen (Tylenol) may be used to decrease or prevent discomfort.

The patient also may develop antibodies to plasma proteins, which typically causes hives. Explain that he may be given an antihistamine before a platelet infusion to prevent this reaction.

Immune globulin treatment

If appropriate, discuss immune globulin treatment. Mention that it's moderately successful in some patients who have immune thrombocytopenia.

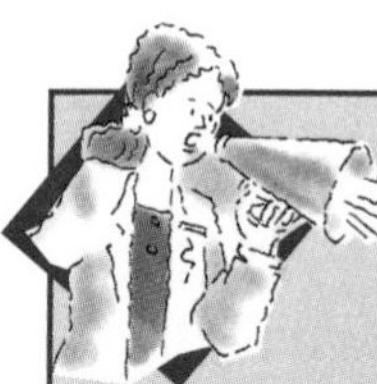

Listen up!

Avoiding excessive bleeding

Because your patient has a tendency to bleed easily and for a longer time than normal, he may need to change his daily activities and modify his living habits. Provide the following list of do's and don'ts to help him function safely and avoid excessive bleeding.

Do's

- Use an electric razor.
- Wear gloves when washing dishes, raking, or gardening.
- Take your temperature only by mouth.
- Wear socks and shoes that fit properly. Footwear that's too large can cause abrasions. Footwear that's too small can pinch the blood vessels in your feet.
- Regularly check your urine, stools, and sputum for blood.
- Use a thimble while hand sewing.
- Inform all health care workers of your condition before undergoing any procedure, including routine dental care.
- Use a nasal spray containing normal saline solution or run a vaporizer to moisten your breathing passages and prevent nosebleeds.
- Use a soft toothbrush and floss gently unless your doctor advises otherwise.
- Keep your head elevated when lying down.

Don'ts

- Avoid shaving, cutting paper, or removing paint with a straightedged razor blade.
- Never go barefoot. Always protect your feet with shoes.
- Avoid leaving knives, scissors, thumbtacks, or other sharp objects on countertops or tables where they could accidentally cut you. Store them in protective containers instead.
- Refrain from contact sports and roughhousing.
- If possible, avoid intramuscular or subcutaneous injections.
- Avoid plucking your eyebrows.
- Reject substances that increase your risk for bleeding, such as alcohol, nicotine, caffeine, and products containing aspirin or ibuprofen.

Teaching about surgery

Splenectomy may be necessary to correct thrombocytopenia caused by platelet destruction. Because the spleen is the primary site of platelet removal and antibody production, a splenectomy usually significantly reduces platelet destruction. Signs of hypersplenism include abdominal pain, nausea, vomiting, and an enlarged, tender spleen.

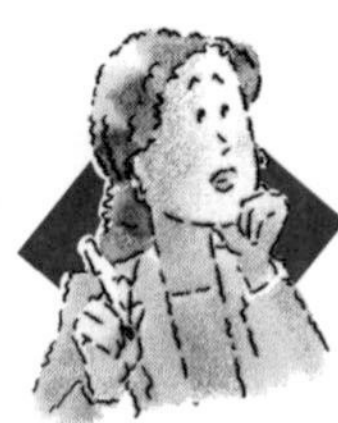

Quick quiz

1. Tell a patient diagnosed with AIDS to prevent an infection by:

A. eating plenty of raw fruits and vegetables.
B. exercising frequently and at regular intervals, even if he's tired.
C. practicing thorough hand-washing technique.

Answer: C. Thorough hand washing is the most effective way to prevent an opportunistic infection.

2. When teaching a patient with hemophilia, explain that the most common treatment for excessive bleeding is:

A. direct pressure on the bleeding site.
B. a clotting factor replacement product.
C. transfusion of whole blood.

Answer: B. The primary treatment for hemophilia is I.V. administration of the missing clotting factor.

3. The goal of an exercise regimen for a patient with rheumatoid arthritis is:

A. to reduce pain and stiffness in the affected joint.
B. to reduce the amount of synovium in the joint.
C. to feel pain-free.

Answer: A. The proper exercise regimen can make it easier to flex and extend the joints, and may also help prevent some loss of joint function.

Scoring

☆☆☆ If you answered all three questions correctly, jump for joy. You must be immune to failure.

☆☆ If you answered two questions correctly, that's okay. You're definitely not allergic to hard work.

☆ If you answered fewer than two questions correctly, don't worry. Reviewing the material should improve your knowledge count.

Getting connected

Sickle cell site

For more information about sickle cell anemia, direct the patient to the following Web site:

- Sickle Cell Information Center (www.emory.edu/PEDS/SICKLE).

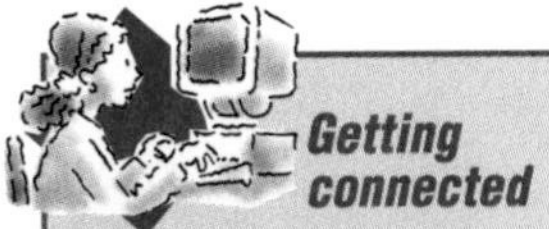

Asking about arthritis

For more information about arthritis, direct the patient to the Arthritis Foundation Web site (www.arthritis.org).

6

Musculoskeletal disorders

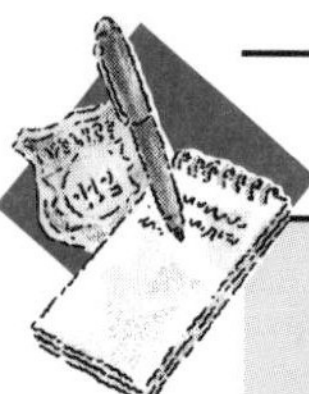

Just the facts

In this chapter, you'll learn how to teach patients with the following musculoskeletal disorders:

- carpal tunnel syndrome
- chronic low back pain
- fractures
- osteoarthritis
- osteoporosis
- strains and sprains.

Carpal tunnel syndrome

Carpal tunnel syndrome is a serious occupational health problem. It affects people who use their hands repetitively and strenuously; examples include homemakers, computer operators, cashiers, assembly line workers, meat cutters, machinists, mechanics, and carpenters.

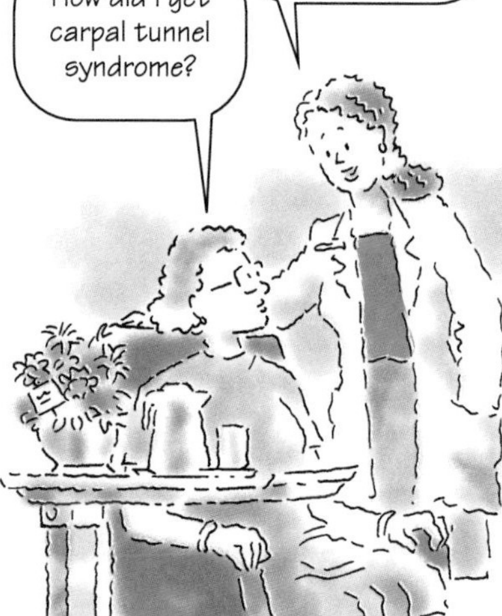

How did I get carpal tunnel syndrome?
Probably from repeated, strenuous use of your hands.

How did it happen?

Carpal tunnel syndrome occurs when the median nerve is compressed between the inelastic carpal ligament and other parts of the carpal tunnel.

The median nerve controls many movements on the forearm, wrist, and hand, such as turning the wrist toward the body and flexing the index, middle, and ring fingers. Compression of this nerve causes loss of movement and sensation in the wrist and fingers.

Why did it happen?

The exact cause of carpal tunnel syndrome is unknown. However, occupations that require rapid, repetitive wrist motions involving excessive wrist flexion or extension predispose a person to this condition. Other suspected risk factors include vitamin B_6 deficiency and conditions that cause edema, such as:
- diabetes
- heart failure
- pregnancy
- premenstrual fluid retention
- renal failure
- rheumatoid arthritis.

The patient may also have underlying conditions that can aggravate carpal tunnel syndrome. (See *What makes carpal tunnel syndrome worse.*)

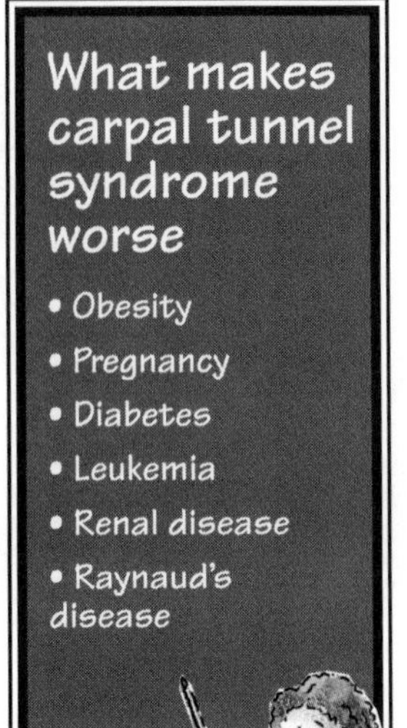

What makes carpal tunnel syndrome worse

- Obesity
- Pregnancy
- Diabetes
- Leukemia
- Renal disease
- Raynaud's disease

What are the consequences?

Review possible symptoms — which can affect one or both hands — including:
- weakness
- burning
- pain
- numbness
- tingling.

The patient may be able to relieve discomfort by vigorously shaking or dangling his arms at his sides. Vasodilation and venous stasis (blood pooling) may cause some signs and symptoms to intensify at night and in the morning. In severe cases, the patient may experience more serious signs and symptoms. (See *It's severe carpal tunnel syndrome.*)

Teaching about tests

The physical examination may include Phalen's test and a check for Tinel's sign to help gauge the severity of signs and symptoms. To confirm the condition, the doctor may order electrophysiologic tests. (See *Teaching about electrophysiologic tests,* page 190.)

Teaching about activity and lifestyle

Resting the affected wrist can relieve symptoms but not cure the underlying problem. Help the patient identify activities that aggravate or trigger symptoms. Advise him to eliminate or modify these activities, or at least slow the pace and decrease the activity.

Don't ignore the risks

Emphasize that continued overuse of the affected wrist increases the problem. Wrist function continues to decline and, if left untreated, the patient may experience permanent nerve damage with loss of movement and sensation.

Don't move

An immobilization device, such as a glove or lock-up splint, can relieve pressure and reduce wrist movement. Remind the patient to wear the device continuously (even during sleep, if necessary) and to keep the wrist elevated to reduce swelling.

Move

Review exercises to maintain joint motion, prevent wrist stiffness, and preserve the function and strength of muscles. (See *Carpal tunnel workout,* page 191.)

It's severe carpal tunnel syndrome

- Paresthesia of the thumb, index, and middle fingers and half of the ring finger
- Inability to make a fist
- Inability to grasp or hold small objects
- Atrophy of the fingernails
- Dry, shiny skin on the hands
- Atrophy of the thenar eminence (the padded area of the palm below the base of the thumb)

Teaching about medication

The drugs most commonly prescribed to treat carpal tunnel syndrome are nonsteroidal anti-inflammatory drugs (NSAIDs), taken orally, and corticosteroids, given by injection into the carpal tunnel tendons. For a vitamin B_6 deficiency, pyridoxine may be prescribed.

NSAIDs

NSAIDs help control pain and reduce inflammation when taken as prescribed. It may take 2 to 4 weeks to reach maximum effectiveness. Pregnant patients should avoid NSAIDs.

Help the medicine go down

Advise the patient to take the following drugs with food or antacids to avoid stomach upset:
- indomethacin (Indocin)

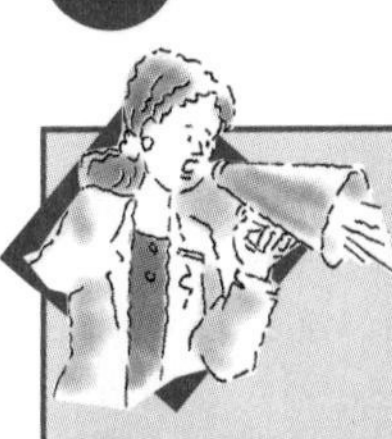

Listen up!

Teaching about electrophysiologic tests

Electrophysiologic tests are nerve stimulation procedures that use electrical current in amounts that are too small to be harmful. Reassure the patient that these tests aren't painful, although they may feel uncomfortable or strange. Explain that before testing begins, a technician may ask about the patient's signs and symptoms.

Finger to wrist

A digital electrical stimulation test is used to confirm carpal tunnel syndrome. The technician places electrodes around the index and middle fingers to stimulate the fingers electrically, and attaches an electrode over the median nerve in the wrist to record nerve stimulation. If the median nerve is compressed, the stimulating current takes longer than usual to travel from the fingers to the wrist, or the stimulation may be weak, depending on the degree of compression.

Did the thumb move?

In the motor function test of the median nerve, the technician places stimulating electrodes over the median nerve at the wrist and recording electrodes over the thumb and directly below the thumb on the inside of the hand. The technician then watches for thumb movements. Delayed movement usually signals median nerve compression and carpal tunnel syndrome.

Needles and nerves

In electromyography, the technician inserts very fine needles into the wrist and thumb to check for irritability (spontaneous electrical activity) of the hand muscles innervated by the median nerve.

- mefenamic acid (Ponstel)
- phenylbutazone (Butazolidin)
- piroxicam (Feldene).

Corticosteroids

To reduce inflammation, a steroid preparation may be injected following administration of a local anesthetic. This brings almost immediate—but temporary—pain relief.

Pyridoxine

Pyridoxine is taken daily for at least 3 weeks to treat vitamin B_6 deficiency. Tell the patient to store the drug in a dark bottle protected from light. Also, suggest a nutritious diet that includes sources of vitamin B_6. (See *Sources of B_6*, page 192.)

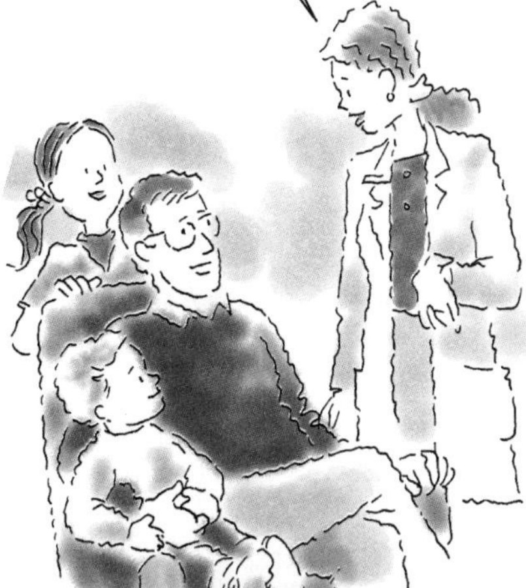
As part of your therapy, corticosteroids may be injected into the carpal tunnel tendons. Expect immediate — but temporary — pain relief.

Teaching about surgery

Treatment for carpal tunnel syndrome usually begins with conservative measures if the disorder is mild or symptoms are expected to subside on their own (such as after

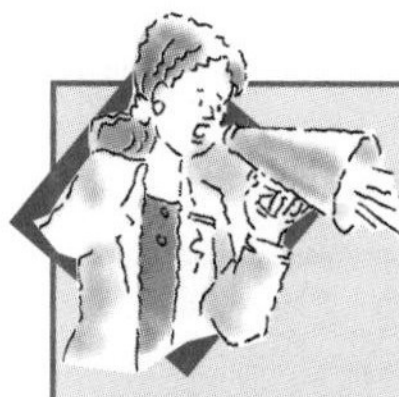

Listen up!

Carpal tunnel workout

If the patient must limit hand motions to relieve carpal tunnel syndrome, he needs to exercise the wrist, hand, fingers, and thumb daily to maintain muscle tone. The doctor, nurse, or physical therapist shows him how to support, control, and move his hand correctly. Urge the patient to do the recommended exercises with the affected hand and, if needed, the other hand. Provide the instructions below.

Wrist and hand exercises

1. Extend the arm—palm down, fingers straight—keeping the palm flat. Then slowly raise the fingers as far as they'll comfortably go without flexing the wrist. Next, slowly lower the fingers as far downward as they'll comfortably go.

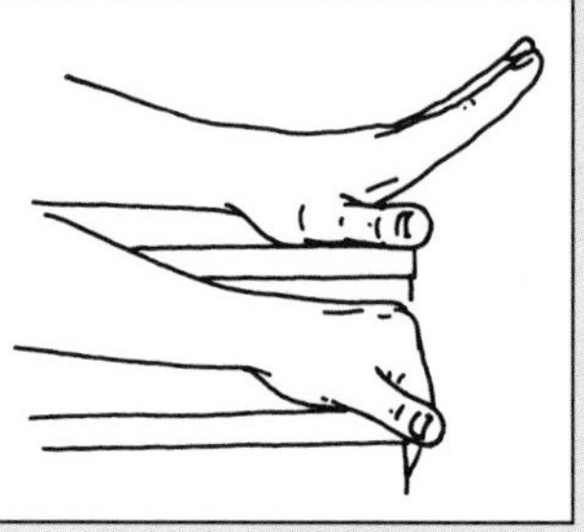

2. With the arm still in the extended position, wave or rock the hand from side to side and then gently twist the hand from side to side. Next, move the hand in small circles, first in one direction and then in the opposite direction.

Finger and thumb exercises

1. With a rubber band around the fingers for mild resistance, spread the fingers as far apart as possible. Then bring them back together and make a fist.

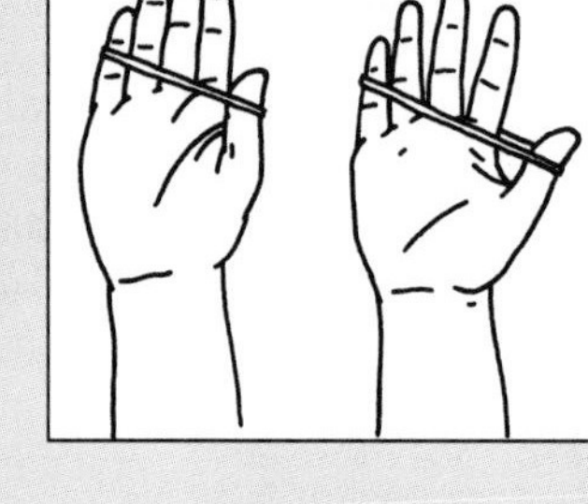

2. Hold up the hand and touch the little finger and thumb together. Repeat this movement, touching the other three fingers to the thumb.

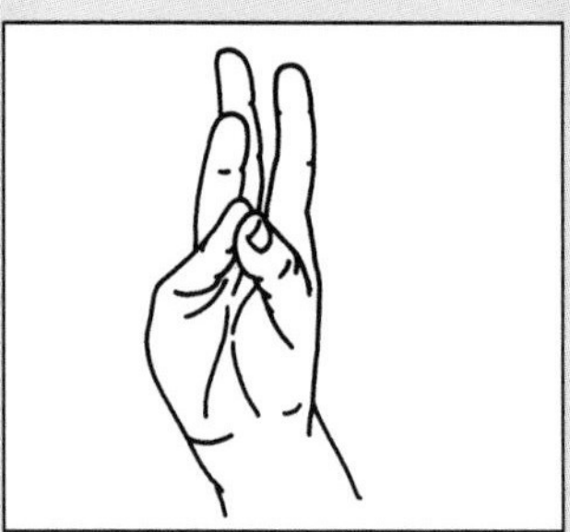

3. Finally, bend all the fingers up and down, as though waving goodbye.

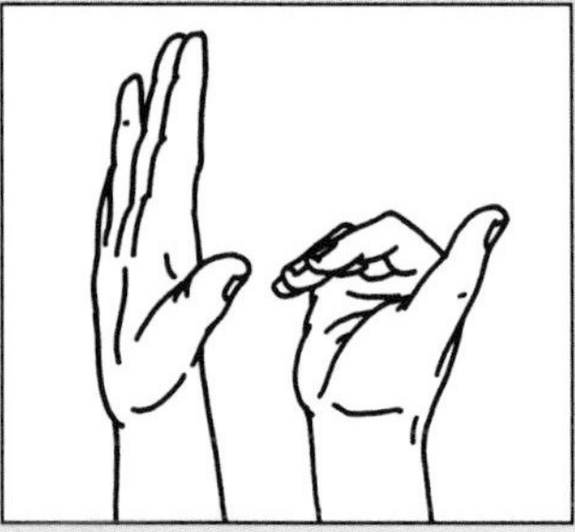

pregnancy). Surgery to decompress the median nerve may be recommended if symptoms are severe or muscle atrophy occurs.

What to expect after surgery

Review measures taken after surgery, such as pain management, dressing care, and elevation of the hand.

Explain that the patient's fingers will be checked for circulation, sensation, and movement every 1 to 2 hours for 24 hours after surgery. Teach the patient to watch for signs and symptoms of infection: redness, warmth, swelling, or pus at the incision site and temperature elevation. Tell him to call the doctor immediately if these occur.

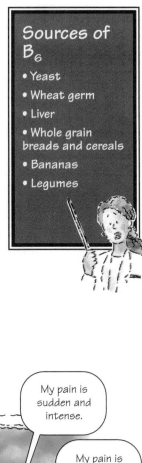

Sources of B_6

- Yeast
- Wheat germ
- Liver
- Whole grain breads and cereals
- Bananas
- Legumes

Chronic low back pain

Chronic low back pain is pain that lasts for more than 6 months or that recurs every 3 months to 3 years. Experts say that 70% to 80% of the world's population suffer from disabling low back pain at some time in their lives. It often forces difficult career and lifestyle changes.

How does it feel?

Pain from a back condition varies. It may be:

- sudden and intense
- dull and diffuse
- deep and aching.

Back pain may affect one or both sides of the body (unilateral or bilateral). It may be exacerbated by anything that puts pressure on the spine, such as sneezing, coughing, and straining. Lying down may relieve the pain.

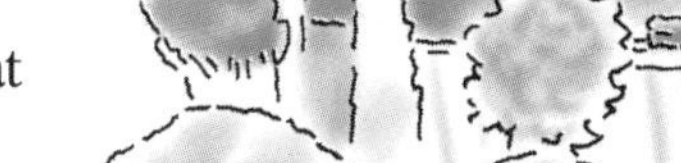
All of these symptoms may be associated with low back pain.
My pain is sudden and intense.
My pain is dull and diffuse.
My pain is deep and aching.

What causes it?

Low back pain is generally caused by stress on the vertebrae or a herniated disk, also called a ruptured or slipped disk. Certain physical factors can put the patient at risk for low back pain. (See *Risk factors for low back pain.*)

What should I do?

Begin teaching by helping the patient identify what triggers his low back pain. Then, together, develop strategies to help him avoid recurrent pain or live productively with it.

Is stress an important factor?

Stress may trigger a cycle of pain. For example, if the patient feels pressure from his job or personal life, the back muscles may tighten, causing pain and pressure. Then a cycle begins: Stress causes tension, which causes pain, which causes more stress, and so on. If it's not broken, this cycle can immobilize the patient.

Teaching about tests

Tests for chronic low back pain include a thorough history and physical assessment to reveal decreased reflexes, muscle wasting, paresthesia, and numbness.

Testing, testing

Imaging tests, such as computed tomography (CT) and magnetic resonance imaging (MRI) scans, myelography, or diskography may help determine the cause of chronic low back pain.

Laboratory tests may include a complete blood count (CBC), calcium level (increased in metastatic bone tumor), uric acid level, erythrocyte sedimentation rate (ESR), and rheumatoid factor tests. These tests are used to determine if gout or a rheumatoid disease, such as arthritis, is causing the patient's back pain.

To check for lumbar disk disease and sciatic nerve involvement, the doctor may perform a straight leg test, a sciatic nerve test, and sitting root tests.

Spinal X-rays are ordered if the level and extent of the suspected injury warrants them. (See *Teaching patients about musculoskeletal tests,* pages 194 to 196.)

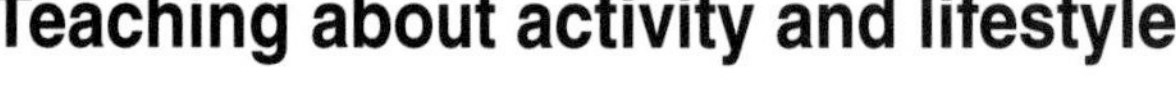

Teaching about activity and lifestyle

The primary treatments for chronic low back pain are conservative. (See *Primary treatment for chronic low back pain,* page 197.) If these measures fail, the doctor may

(Text continues on page 197.)

Risk factors for low back pain

- Poor posture
- Poor body mechanics
- Obesity
- Poor physical fitness
- Jobs that require intense physical labor or awkward positioning for prolonged periods (such as truck driving and nursing)
- Sprained or strained ligament
- Torn muscle
- Pinched nerve
- Arthritis
- Degenerative disorders such as lumbar disk disease

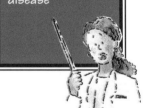

Teaching patients about musculoskeletal tests

Test and purpose	What to teach the patient
Arthrography • To detect abnormalities of the menisci, cartilage, and ligaments of the knee • To detect shoulder abnormalities, such as a torn rotator cuff and anterior capsule derangement • To evaluate the need for surgery	• This radiographic test involves injecting air or a radiopaque contrast medium into the joint space. It's performed by a doctor in the X-ray department and takes about 1 hour. • After the patient's joint is anesthetized, the doctor injects a contrast medium. The patient may experience a tingling sensation or pressure in the joint. X-rays are then taken as the contrast medium fills the joint space. The patient is asked to quickly assume various positions for these X-rays, then to remain as still as possible. If the knee is being studied, the patient may have to take a few steps. • After the test, the patient may experience some swelling or discomfort or may hear noises in the joint. He should apply ice to the joint to reduce swelling and take a mild analgesic for pain. If symptoms persist for more than 2 days, the patient should contact the doctor. • The patient should rest the joint for at least 12 hours after the test. If the doctor applies an elastic bandage after a knee arthrogram, the patient must keep the bandage in place for several days. He must also learn how to rewrap it.
Arthroscopy • To detect and diagnose meniscal, patellar, condylar, extrasynovial, and synovial diseases • To monitor disease progression • To perform joint surgery or biopsy • To monitor the effectiveness of therapy	• This test allows direct examination of the inside of a joint. It's a safe, convenient approach for surgery, if necessary. Arthroscopy is usually done in the operating room under general or local anesthesia by an orthopedic surgeon, and it takes 30 to 60 minutes. • The patient must not eat or drink after midnight before the test. Immediately before the test, he receives a sedative and the area around the joint is shaved. • During the test, the patient may feel transient discomfort as the local anesthetic is injected (if applicable). The doctor makes a small incision and inserts the arthroscope into the joint cavity. • After the test, the patient is allowed to walk as soon as he's fully awake. He'll experience mild soreness and a slight grinding sensation in his knee for a day or two. He should notify the doctor of severe or persistent pain or fever with signs of local inflammation, and avoid excessive use of the joint for a few days after the test.
Bone biopsy • To distinguish between benign and malignant bone tumors • To detect metastatic bone diseases and infection	• This test allows direct examination of a small sample of bone and takes 15 to 30 minutes (for needle biopsy) or 30 to 60 minutes (for open biopsy). • The patient may receive a local or general anesthetic. For a general anesthetic, he must not eat or drink for 12 hours before the test. • If the patient is undergoing needle biopsy with a local anesthetic, he'll feel a sharp, sticking sensation as the local anesthetic is injected into the skin. The doctor makes a small incision, then inserts the needle into the bone. The patient will feel pressure as the needle is advanced into the bone. • After the test, the patient will experience some pain and tenderness for 1 to 3 days after a needle biopsy or for 2 to 6 days after an open biopsy. He should call the doctor if pain or tenderness worsens, if drainage from the biopsy site increases, or if fever develops. He can resume his normal activities after the test as soon as he's comfortable doing so. If he has undergone open biopsy, the doctor will remove the stitches or sutures in 5 to 10 days.

Teaching patients about musculoskeletal tests *(continued)*

Test and purpose	What to teach the patient
Bone scan (bone scintigraphy) • To detect or rule out malignant bone lesions when radiographic findings are normal but cancer is confirmed or suspected • To detect occult bone trauma due to pathologic fractures • To monitor degenerative bone disorders • To detect infection	• This painless test can often detect bone abnormalities before conventional X-rays can. • Fasting before the test isn't necessary. However, the patient should avoid eating a meal or drinking large amounts of fluids right before the test. • After applying a tourniquet on the patient's arm, the doctor injects a small dose of a radioactive isotope. The isotope emits less radiation than a standard X-ray machine. A 2- to 3-hour waiting period follows injection of the isotope. Then the patient is asked to lie in a supine position on a table within the scanner. The scanner moves slowly back and forth, recording images for about 1 hour. He must lie as still as possible during the test. He may be asked to assume various positions on the table. • Encourage the patient to drink plenty of fluids after the test.
Computed tomography scan • To aid diagnosis of bone tumors and other abnormalities	• This test helps detect bone abnormalities and takes 30 to 90 minutes. • If the patient is scheduled to receive a contrast medium, he mustn't eat for 4 hours before the test. • The patient is asked to put on a hospital gown and remove all jewelry before the test. He must empty his bladder just before the test. • The patient is asked to lie on a table within the large tunnel-like scanner. Then he may be given a contrast medium by mouth or by injection. During the test, the table he's lying on moves a small distance every few seconds. The scanner will rotate around him and may make a clicking or buzzing noise. He must remain still during the test. Although he'll be alone in the room, he can communicate with the technician through an intercom system. • If the patient received a contrast medium, he should drink plenty of fluids after the test.
Diskography • To identify a degenerated or extruding intervertebral disk	• During this X-ray study of the spine, which uses fluoroscopy, a contrast medium is injected into the disk space to identify a degenerated or extruding intervertebral disk.
Joint aspiration (arthrocentesis) • To aid in differential diagnosis of arthritis • To identify the cause of joint effusion • To relieve pain and distention resulting from accumulation of fluid within the joint • To administer local drug therapy (usually corticosteroids)	• This test removes a fluid sample from within the joint space for analysis. It takes about 10 minutes. • The patient is asked to assume a position and then remain still. After cleaning the skin over the joint, the doctor inserts the needle. After withdrawing the fluid, he applies a small bandage to the puncture site. • After the test, medical staff may apply ice or cold packs to the joint to reduce pain and swelling. If the doctor removed a large amount of fluid, the patient may need to wear an elastic bandage. He should avoid using the joint excessively after the test, in order to avoid joint pain, swelling, and stiffness. He should report any increased pain, tenderness, swelling, warmth, or redness as well as fever; these may signal infection.

(continued)

Teaching patients about musculoskeletal tests

Test and purpose	What to teach the patient
Myelography • To detect spinal abnormalities, such as tumors, herniated intervertebral disks, fractures, and inflammation	• This test reveals obstructions in the spinal canal. It takes about 1 hour. • The patient lies in a prone position on a tilting X-ray table. After cleaning the skin on the patient's lower back with an antiseptic, the doctor injects an anesthetic. The patient may experience a stinging sensation. Next, the doctor inserts a needle between two vertebrae of the spinal cord and injects an oil- or water-based contrast medium. The patient may feel a transient burning sensation during injection. He may also feel flushed and warm and may experience a headache, a salty taste, or nausea and vomiting. X-rays are taken as the table is tilted vertically and then horizontally to allow the contrast medium to flow through the spinal canal. After completing the test, the doctor withdraws the oil-based contrast medium or allows the water-based medium to be absorbed. He then applies a small dressing to the puncture site. • If an oil-based medium is used, the patient must remain flat in bed for 6 to 8 hours after the test and avoid abrupt movement. He must drink plenty of fluids and can resume his normal diet. If nausea prevents this, he may receive I.V. fluids and an antiemetic. • If a water-based medium is used, the patient must sit in a chair or lie with the head of the bed elevated for 6 to 8 hours after the test, and then remain on bed rest for an additional 6 to 8 hours. He must drink plenty of fluids and can resume his normal diet, as tolerated. If the patient is on phenothiazine therapy, he must temporarily discontinue the drug, as ordered by the doctor. The patient must notify the doctor if he has a headache for more than 24 hours after the test or if he develops weakness, numbness, or tingling in his legs.
Photodensitometry • To measure cortical bone density as an aid in early diagnosis of osteoporosis	• This test can reveal osteoporosis before it's apparent on conventional X-rays. It takes about 20 minutes. • The patient's hand is positioned next to a small piece of aluminum alloy. As X-rays are taken, a computer compares the density of the bone to that of the aluminum.
Photon absorptiometry (single) • To measure cortical bone density as an aid in early diagnosis of osteoporosis	• This painless test can reveal even slight bone loss. It takes about 20 minutes. • The patient's arm is positioned in a cradle as X-rays are taken.
Photon absorptiometry (dual) • To measure trabecular bone density as an aid in early diagnosis of osteoporosis	• This painless test can detect osteoporosis before most other tests. It takes about 20 minutes and causes no discomfort. • The patient lies on his back in a tunnel-like machine that takes X-rays of his lumbar spine.
Transiliac bone biopsy • To allow direct examination of osteoporotic changes in bone cells	• This procedure reveals characteristic osteoporotic changes in bone cells. • Before the procedure, the skin over the iliac crest is cleaned and anesthetic is applied. • During the procedure, the doctor makes a small incision, introduces a hollow needle, and aspirates a tiny core of bone marrow. The patient can expect brief discomfort. • After the needle is removed, pressure is applied to the puncture site for 10 to 15 minutes.

recommend more aggressive therapies, such as epidural steroid injection, chemonucleolysis, or surgery.

Take it lying down

If bed rest is prescribed, explain the benefits:

1. It limits motion of the vertebral column.
2. It relieves nerve root compression.
3. It reduces disk swelling.

Teach the patient to lie in a position that reduces tension on the spine, such as semi-Fowler's or a side-lying position. For added support, recommend placing a bed board under the mattress.

Primary treatment for chronic low back pain

- Bed rest
- Medication
- Back strengthening exercises
- Heat application
- Traction
- Physical therapy
- Weight reduction, if necessary

Walk this way

Demonstrate the correct way to perform routine activities, such as walking, standing, sitting, lifting, and carrying. Have the patient repeat the demonstration so you can evaluate his understanding. (See *Posture power,* page 198.)

Follow the program

Emphasize the importance of following an exercise program prescribed by a doctor or physical therapist. The patient should check with the doctor before participating in sports.

Strengthened, stretched, and well-curved

Explain that, by performing regular back exercises, the patient can accomplish the following:
- increase blood flow to the tissues
- strengthen the back and abdominal muscles
- stretch the ligaments that attach muscles to bones
- maintain a normal curve of the spine. (See *More ways to combat back pain,* page 199.)

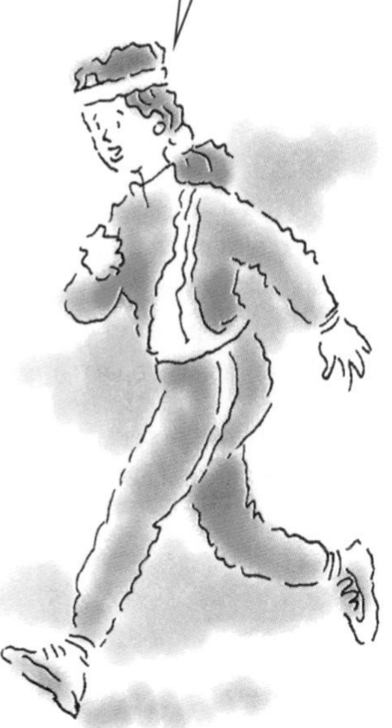
Back exercises can improve blood flow, strengthen muscles, stretch ligaments, and help maintain a normal curve of the spine.

Teaching about diet

Explain to overweight patients that excess weight strains the spine. If the doctor prescribes a weight-loss diet, make sure the patient has a written copy of it. When teaching about meal planning, include other family members — especially the one who does most of the cooking.

Teaching about medication

The doctor may prescribe drug therapy for acute pain, commonly beginning with muscle relaxants, analgesics

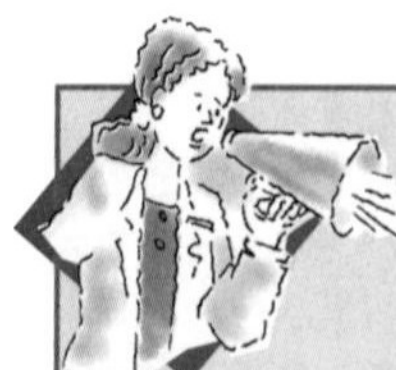

Listen up!

Posture power

If your patient has chronic back pain, emphasize that good posture is a must — whether he's standing, sitting, or lying down. Point out that good posture strengthens the abdominal and buttock muscles that support the hard-working back.

Standing and walking

When the patient stands correctly, he should be able to draw an imaginary line from his ear through the tip of his shoulder, middle of his hip, back of his knee, and front of his ankle. He won't be able to do this if he stands with his lower back arched, his upper back stooped, or his abdomen sagging forward.

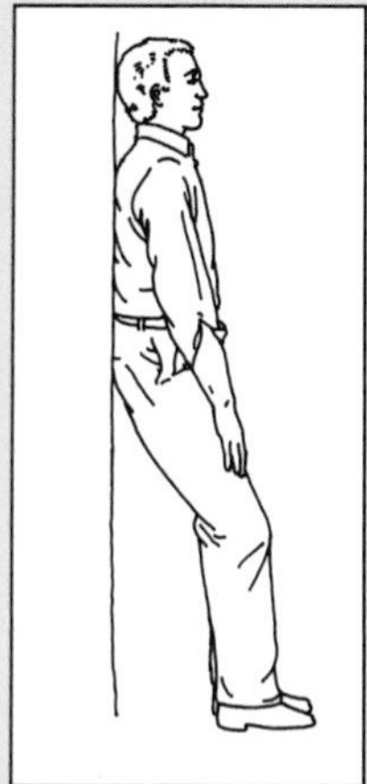

To correct his posture, instruct the patient to stand 1′ (0.3 m) away from a wall. Then have him lean back against the wall with his knees slightly bent. Tell him to tighten his stomach and buttock muscles to tilt his pelvis back and flatten his lower back.

As he holds this position, have him inch up the wall until he's standing. His lower back should still be pressed against the wall. Inform him that this is the posture he should assume when walking.

Sitting

If possible, the patient should choose a hard, straight-backed chair to sit on. Tell him to place a rolled towel or a small pillow behind his lower back. To keep his back from tiring when sitting for a long time, instruct him to raise one leg higher than the other by propping it on a footrest.

Lying down

Advise the patient to sleep on a firm mattress. If he must sleep on a soft mattress, recommend supporting it with a bed board or a piece of plywood placed underneath it.

The best position for sleeping is lying on the side with the knees bent and a pillow between them. Explain that this position prevents the spine from twisting when he drops his upper leg. Tell the patient not to curl up excessively, though, because this can put too much pressure on his back bones.

Caution the patient not to sleep on his stomach or on high pillows. These positions can strain his back, neck, and shoulders. Sleeping on the back is okay if he keeps a pillow under the knees or places a small pillow or rolled towel under the small of his back.

Lifting and carrying

Instruct the patient to maintain the natural low back curve with his pelvis tucked in while lifting and carrying. Tell him to turn and face the object he wants to lift. As he keeps his feet flat and shoulder-width apart, have him bend his knees, lower himself to the object, and place his hands around it. Then with his knees bent and back straight, tell him to use his arm and leg muscles (instead of his back muscles) to lift the object. Warn him to avoid lifting heavy objects above his waist.

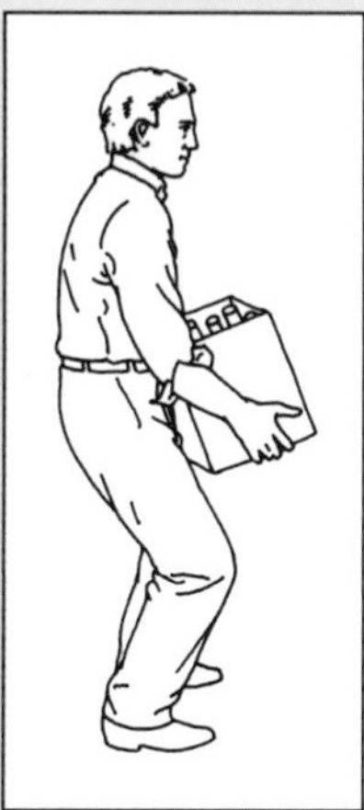

Advise him to carry the object by holding it close to his body. Tell him to avoid carrying unbalanced loads or anything heavier than he can easily manage. Advise him to get help for large or bulky items.

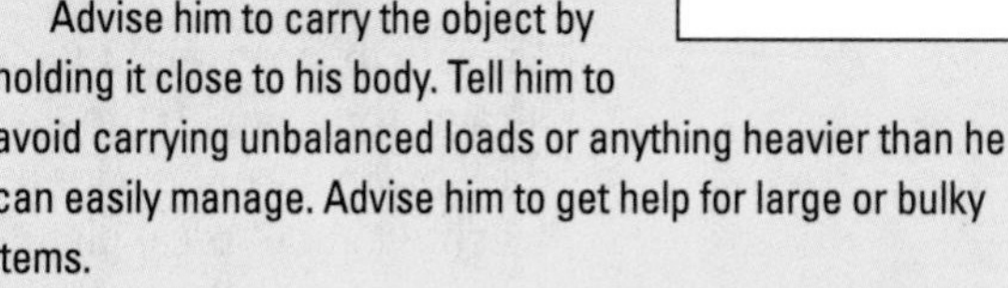

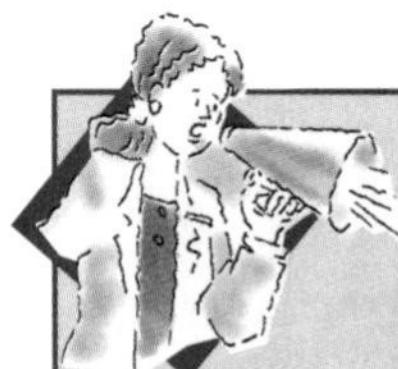

Listen up!

More ways to combat back pain

Other items to teach may include home care measures and alternatives to surgery.

Pain relief plus

Suggest that the patient use pillows, a bed board, or a firm mattress to ensure comfortable positioning. Applying local heat or cold may reduce muscle spasms. If the patient has decreased sensation, advise frequent skin checks to ensure safety during heat or cold therapy.

Traction

Traction may enhance the benefits of bed rest. Traction holds the spine in position, reduces muscle spasms, and widens the intervertebral space. This reduces bulging or rupture of the disk. Explain that traction is discontinued if it doesn't bring satisfactory results.

If traction is to be used at home, teach the patient and members of his family about:

- devices used in traction
- how traction works
- duration of traction therapy.

Chemonucleolysis

Chemonucleolysis is an alternative to surgery if other measures don't relieve pain from a herniated disk but is used only for conditions without nerve involvement. Pain is eased by the injection of enzymes (chymopapain or collagenase) into the disk to dissolve the nucleus pulposus.

More info

Refer the patient to appropriate organizations for further information and support, as necessary.

(narcotics or NSAIDs), and steroids to reduce pain and inflammation. The patient should never suddenly stop taking steroids. Rather, the dosage should be reduced gradually. Review the adverse effects of muscle relaxants, such as drowsiness and vertigo.

Getting to the root of the matter

If the patient's pain involves the nerve root and isn't relieved by conservative measures, an epidural injection of a steroid or anesthetic (or both) may be ordered.

Explain that if this injection doesn't provide adequate pain relief, more injections may be required. However, the injection can be repeated only a limited number of times.

Teaching about surgery

When conservative measures fail to relieve pain, surgery may be recommended. If the patient has signs or symptoms of spinal cord compression, such as incontinence, surgery is performed without delay. (See *Surgical procedures for chronic low back pain,* page 200.)

Laminae relief

In a laminectomy, the surgeon removes one or more bony laminae (the flattened portion on either side of the vertebra's arch). This is most commonly done to relieve pressure on the spinal cord or spinal nerve roots resulting from a herniated disk.

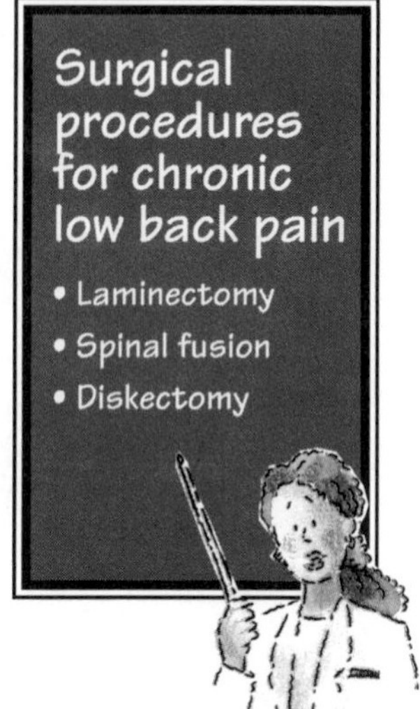

Surgical procedures for chronic low back pain
• Laminectomy
• Spinal fusion
• Diskectomy

No confusion about fusion

After laminae removal, bone chips from the hip, lower leg, or a bone bank may be grafted between vertebral spaces. This procedure — known as spinal fusion — stabilizes the spine. Spinal fusion alone may be done when trauma or disease weakens the vertebrae.

Disk dismissed

Alternative treatment may include removal of a herniated disk. In some cases, the procedure can be done on an outpatient basis using local anesthesia.

Fractures

Fractures are the most common orthopedic injury. In teaching about fractures, emphasize the importance of complying with therapy to avoid permanent deformity or disability. Inadequate or improper care of a fracture can lead to life-threatening complications, such as fat embolism (with pelvic and long-bone fractures) and compartment syndrome (with elbow, wrist, knee, and ankle fractures).

How did it happen?

A fracture results from excessive stress on a bone, typically from major trauma. There are exceptions, however, such as the following:
• A stress fracture can occur when a normal bone is subjected to repeated stress (such as prolonged standing, walking, or running).
• If the patient has a bone-weakening disease, such as osteoporosis or a bone tumor, minor trauma or even normal activities may lead to a pathologic or spontaneous fracture.

There are several signs that may indicate that a fracture has occurred. (See *It could be a fracture.*)

How long before it heals?

Healing begins almost immediately after a fracture occurs. However, the rate of healing depends on the type of fracture. A displaced fracture in which the fragments must be realigned may take months or even years to fully heal.

What's at risk?

Mention that complications can arise shortly after the injury or may develop later. Also discuss compartment syndrome — a serious complication caused by tissue swelling within muscle groups. The swelling compresses nerves and arteries, causing muscle ischemia (reduced blood supply to the muscle). This condition makes its entrance in one of two ways:

 suddenly, right after injury

 gradually, over several days.

If untreated, this condition can cause permanent dysfunction and deformity. Irreversible muscle damage can occur within 6 hours. Examples of such damage are:
- paralysis
- sensory loss
- permanent disability. (See *Signs of compartment syndrome,* page 202.)

Anything else?

If the patient has a long-bone fracture, explain the need to be monitored for another complication—fat embolism. This potentially life-threatening complication can occur as the bone marrow releases fat into the pulmonary capillaries, obstructing breathing. Alternatively, the fat may pass into the arteries, eventually affecting the central nervous system.

> **It could be a fracture**
> - Pain and tenderness of the injured part
> - Loss of normal limb contours
> - Limb shortening
> - Swelling
> - Bruising
> - Decreased range of motion
> - Abnormal movement
> - Crepitus (a crackling sound)

Teaching about tests

X-rays reveal most fractures. X-rays are typically taken from two angles; they're also taken of the joints above and below the fracture. The doctor may also order a CT scan. (See *Teaching patients about musculoskeletal tests,* pages 194 to 196.)

Teaching about activity and lifestyle

Activity restrictions are needed for proper healing. Explain that a doctor or physical therapist will decide:

- when he can begin a program of passive and active range-of-motion (ROM) exercises
- when he can start to use the injured body part.

Back up the doctor's recommendations for restricting weight-bearing use of the injured limb. Review instructions for using crutches or other assistive devices for ambulation.

Let's talk safety

For all patients with fractures, review safety measures. (See *Playing it safe.*) If appropriate, discuss the patient's rehabilitation program, which may include physical and occupational therapy.

> **Signs of compartment syndrome**
>
> - Worsening pain that's unrelieved by analgesics
> - Increased swelling
> - Numbness and tingling in the affected limb
>
> **Warning**
>
> Tell the patient not to elevate the limb or apply ice. It may further reduce blood supply to the affected area.

Teaching about diet

Stress the importance of consuming a nutritious diet that includes foods rich in:
- calcium (dairy products, salmon, and broccoli)
- vitamin A (carrots, sweet potatoes, and other yellow or orange fruit or vegetables)
- vitamin C (citrus fruits and tomatoes)
- vitamin D (found in fortified milk and produced by sun-exposed skin).

These foods promote healing, calcium absorption, and bone remodeling. Vitamin and mineral supplements are sometimes prescribed to hasten healing, but their benefits are controversial.

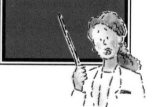

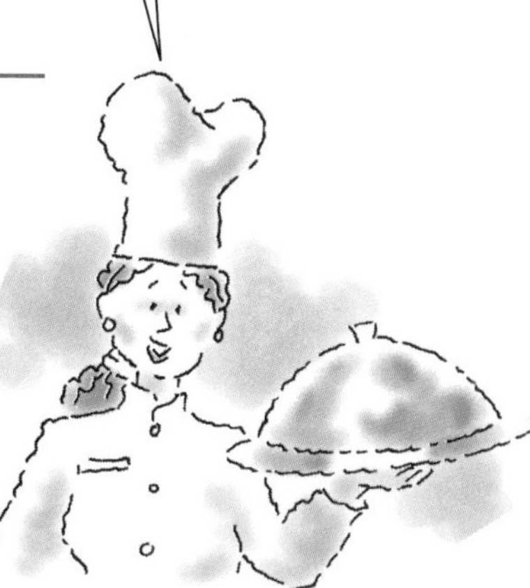
Allow me to recommend a nutritious diet that includes foods rich in calcium and vitamins A, C, and D.

Teaching about medication

A narcotic or nonnarcotic analgesic may be prescribed to reduce pain. The most frequently prescribed nonnarcotic analgesics are acetaminophen and NSAIDs such as ibuprofen.

If the patient has an open fracture, antibiotics are prescribed. Tell the patient to take the drug exactly as directed and complete the entire course of prescribed therapy.

Look out

Warn the patient about these possible adverse effects of drugs:

- NSAIDs may cause stomach upset and GI bleeding. Tell the patient to call the doctor immediately if he has any signs of bleeding, such as black, tarry stools or bloody vomitus.
- If the patient is taking a narcotic such as codeine, caution him to avoid driving and other activities that require alertness until the effects of the drug are known. This medication may cause constipation; advise consulting the doctor about using a stool softener.

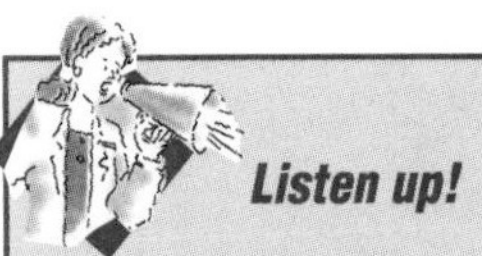

Playing it safe

Because most fractures result from trauma, teach the patient measures to prevent fractures from recurring, such as:

- installing safety rails around the shower or bath
- wearing nonskid, flat-soled, supportive shoes
- removing throw rugs from the environment
- avoiding slippery, wet, or irregular flooring.

Equipment quiz
If the patient needs crutches or other ambulatory devices, make sure he can use this equipment safely.

Teaching about procedures

The first step in healing the fracture is to realign bone fragments — a procedure called reduction. The next step is to immobilize the injured area.

Case closed

Closed reduction is a method of fracture realignment. In closed reduction, the doctor manipulates and realigns the bone fragments. In some patients, traction may be used to achieve closed reduction.

Immobilize and stabilize

After the fracture is reduced, external support devices, such as a sling, cast, brace, and splint, may be used to immobilize and stabilize the healing bone.

Teaching about surgery

If closed reduction isn't possible or advisable, surgery to perform open reduction may be needed to realign bone fragments.

Open reduction with internal fixation

In this procedure, an incision is made and the fracture is aligned during surgery. Internal fixation devices are used to maintain the bone's position. (See *Internal fixation devices,* page 204.)

Open reduction with external fixation

The patient with a severe open fracture and extensive soft-tissue injuries may require an external fixation device. Explain that metal pins are surgically inserted above and below the fracture to hold the bones together. The pins are then attached firmly to the device's frame.

Watching for wobbly pins

Teach the patient to clean the external pin sites daily using a mixture of normal saline solution and peroxide. Tell him to watch for and report loose pins as well as signs or symptoms of infection, such as redness, swelling, warmth, fever, or drainage.

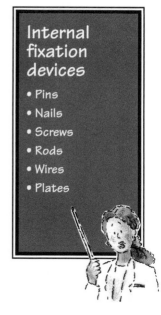

Internal fixation devices

- Pins
- Nails
- Screws
- Rods
- Wires
- Plates

Osteoarthritis

Osteoarthritis (also called degenerative joint disease) is a chronic, degenerative disorder affecting about 20 million Americans in all age groups. This noninflammatory disorder may follow trauma or be a complication of congenital malformations.

What happens?

As osteoarthritis develops, the following occurs:

- The smooth, elastic cartilage of a joint gradually wears down or erodes.
- The bones underneath the worn cartilage stiffen, and bony spurs develop around the joint. This narrows the space between the joints.
- During movement, the bones rub together, causing pain and loss of joint function.

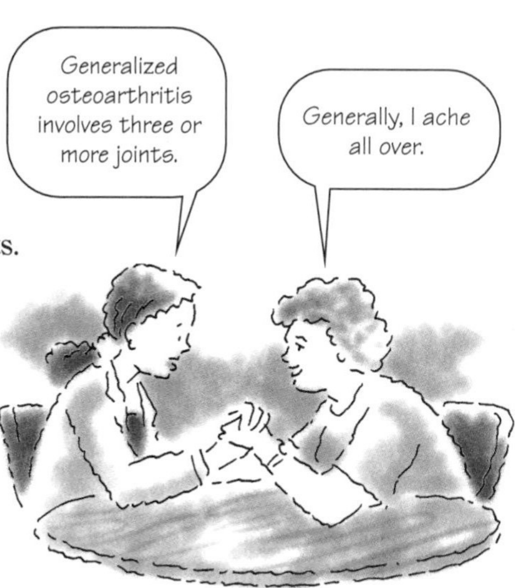

Generally, I ache all over.

What's primary osteoarthritis?

Primary osteoarthritis may affect joints of the thumb, hip, knee, and spine. It seems to be related to aging. In some cases, it appears to be hereditary.

Is it local or general?

Mention that primary osteoarthritis may be localized or generalized. Generalized osteoarthritis involves three or more joints.

What's secondary osteoarthritis?

Secondary osteoarthritis results from a predisposing factor. (See *Predisposing factors for secondary osteoarthritis.*) It can affect any joint.

Why so stiff?

Reassure the patient that osteoarthritis doesn't cause systemic signs or symptoms; its effects are limited to joints. These effects are usually gradual, beginning with joint stiffness lasting less than 15 minutes. Soreness progresses to joint pain, which worsens with activity and is relieved with rest.

Predisposing factors for secondary osteoarthritis

- Traumatic injury
- Infection
- Congenital abnormalities such as hip dysplasia
- Endocrine disorders such as diabetes mellitus
- Developmental disorders such as scoliosis
- Calcium deposition disease

Teaching about tests

To confirm osteoarthritis, the doctor may order X-rays, arthroscopy, MRI, and a bone scan. (See *Teaching patients about musculoskeletal tests,* pages 194 to 196.)

Rule it out

Routine laboratory tests may be used to rule out other conditions (such as rheumatoid arthritis or infection) or to reveal an underlying metabolic disorder. Tests may include CBC, blood chemistry profile, ESR, joint aspiration, and urinalysis.

Teaching about activity and lifestyle

Osteoarthritis has no cure, but treatment may be used to manage pain, restore or maintain joint mobility, and preserve independence.

A balanced exercise program is the key to treatment. The patient and health care team work together to plan a program to meet the patient's needs.

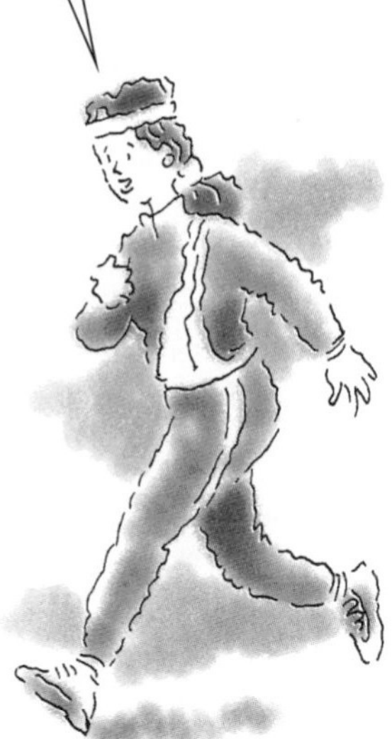

Stop and go

A good exercise program alternates between:

- activity (to maintain joint mobility and muscle strength)
-  rest (to prevent undue joint fatigue).

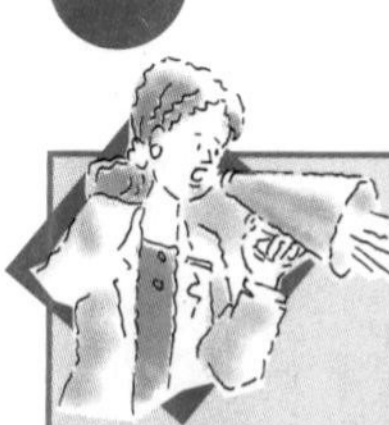

Listen up!

Range-of-motion exercises

Here are guidelines and specific active range-of-motion exercises to provide to your patient.

Day by day
The patient should perform exercises daily to get the most benefit from them. She should repeat each exercise three to five times or as often as her doctor recommends. (As the patient gets stronger, she may be told to increase her activity level.)

Organize it
Advise the patient to organize her routine. For example, if she's exercising all her major joints, advise her to begin at her neck, and then work toward her toes.

Slowly and gently
The patient should move slowly and gently so she doesn't injure herself. If an exercise hurts, she should stop doing it. Then she should consult with her doctor regarding whether to keep doing that particular exercise.

Take a break
The patient should take a break and rest after an exercise that's especially tiring. Also suggest that she space her exercises over the course of a day if she doesn't want to do them in a single session.

First the neck
The patient should slowly tilt her head as far back as possible. Next, have her move it to the right, toward her shoulder.

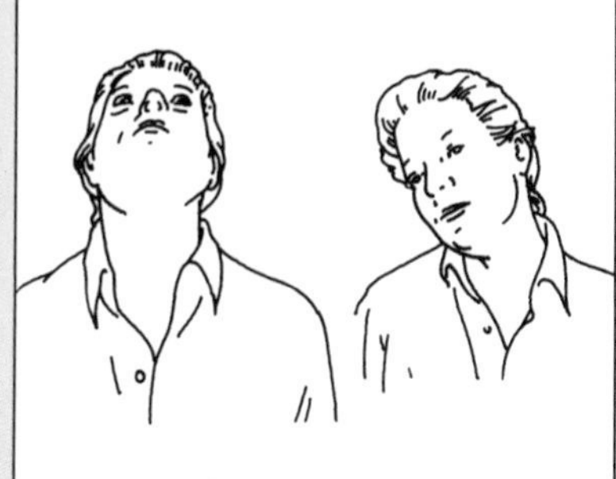

Next, she should keep her head to the right and lower her chin as far as it will go toward her chest. Next, she should move her head toward her left shoulder. To complete a full circle, she should move her head back to its usual upright position.

After the patient performs the recommended number of counterclockwise circles, she should reverse the exercise, and perform an equal number of clockwise circles.

Now the shoulders
The patient should raise her shoulders as if she were about to shrug. Next, have her move her shoulders forward, down, back, then up in a single circular motion. Next, she should move her shoulders backward, down, forward, then up again in a single circular motion.

The patient should continue to alternate forward and backward shoulder circles throughout the exercise.

Work those elbows
The patient should extend her arm straight out to the side. She should then open her hand, palm up, as if to catch a raindrop. Next, she should slowly reach back with her forearm so that she touches her shoulder with her fingers. She should then slowly return her arm to its straight position. Have the patient repeat with her other arm.

Instruct the patient to continue to alternate arms throughout the exercise.

Don't forget the fingers
The patient should spread the fingers and thumb on each hand as wide apart as possible without causing discomfort. Then she should bring her fingers back together in a fist.

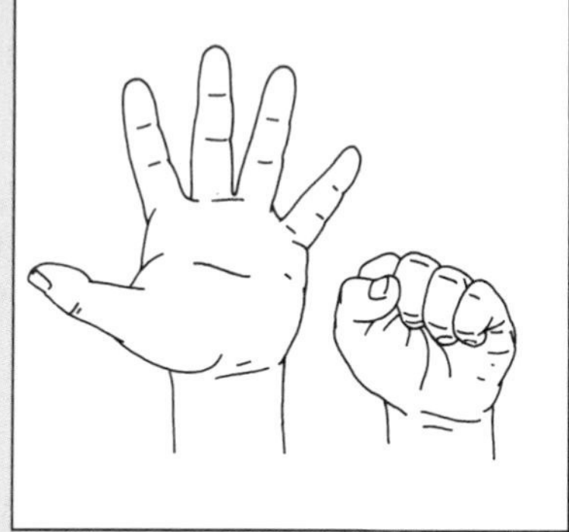

Range-of-motion exercises *(continued)*

Next, the wrist and hands

The patient should extend her arms, palms down and fingers straight. Keeping her palms flat, she should slowly raise her fingers and "point" them back toward herself. Next, she should slowly lower her fingers and "point" them as far downward as she comfortably can.

Work the legs and knees

The patient should lie on her bed or on the floor. She should bend one leg so the knee is straight up and the foot is flat on the bed or floor.

Next, she should bend the other leg, raise her foot, and slowly bring her knee as far toward her chest as she can without discomfort. Then the patient should straighten this leg slowly while she lowers it. Tell the patient to repeat this exercise with the other leg.

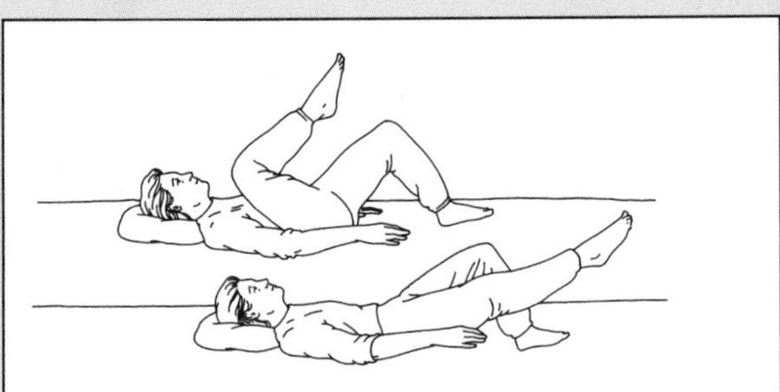

Focus on the ankle and foot

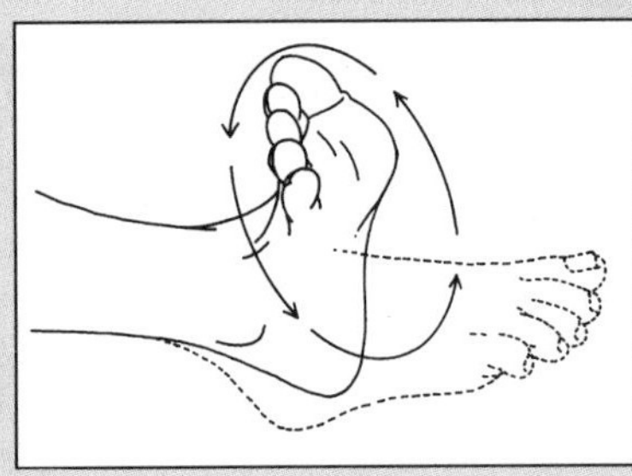

The patient should raise one foot, pointing her toes away from herself. Next she should move this foot in a circular motion — first to the right, then to the left.

Next, she should point her toes back toward herself. With her foot in this position, she should make a circle — first right, then left.

Next, she should perform the same exercise with her other foot.

Last but not least, the toe

The patient can perform this exercise sitting in a chair or lying on her bed. First, she should stretch her legs out in front, with her heels resting on the floor or the bed. Then she should slowly bend her toes down and away from herself. Next, she should bend her toes up and back toward herself. Finally, she should spread out her toes so that they're totally separated. Then she should squeeze her toes together.

Urge the patient to alternate exercise and rest in daily activities, too. The amount and type of activity and rest depend on the severity of the disease, which joints are affected, and the patient's lifestyle.

Improving flexibility

Demonstrate how to perform full, active ROM exercises. Emphasize that these exercises improve flexibility. (See *Range-of-motion exercises.*)

Feeling stronger

Show the patient how to perform isometric exercises to maintain muscle strength. (See *Isometric exercises,* page 208.)

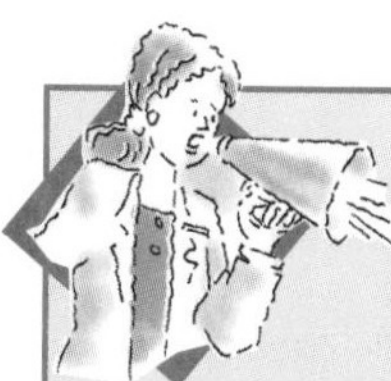

Listen up!

Isometric exercises

To perform isometric exercises, the patient exercises against a resistive force. This force increases the muscle-strengthening effect of the exercise. Remind him to repeat each exercise as many times as the doctor directs (typically three).

In general

Emphasize that, when doing isometric exercise, the joints aren't moved. Instead, the patient contracts his muscles against the resistance of a stationary object, such as a bed, a wall, or another body part. Explain that pressing the palms together (pushing with one, resisting with the other) until he feels tightness in his chest and upper-arm muscles is a basic isometric exercise.

The patient doesn't have to be in any special position for most isometric exercises, so he can do them anytime and anywhere. Tell him to hold each contraction from 3 to 5 seconds, and to repeat the entire series at least five times a day.

For the first week, tell him not to contract his muscles fully; this will give them a chance to get used to the exercises. After that, he should contract them fully.

First the neck

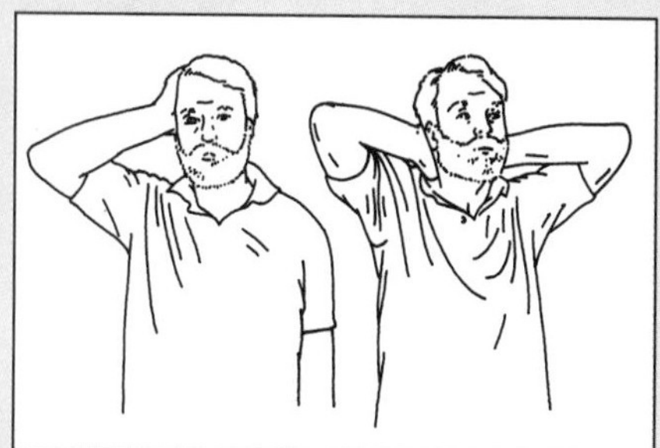

The patient places the heel of his right hand above his right ear. Without moving his head, neck, or arm, have him push his head toward his hand. Tell him to repeat this exercise with his left hand above his left ear.

Next, have him clasp his fingers behind his head and push his head against his hands without moving his neck or hands

Now the shoulder and chest

First, the patient should hold his right arm straight down at his side. Then have him grasp his right wrist with his left hand. Instruct him to try to shrug his right shoulder — but to prevent this by keeping a firm grip on his right wrist. Next, tell him to do a reverse version of this exercise with his left arm and shoulder.

Ready for the arm

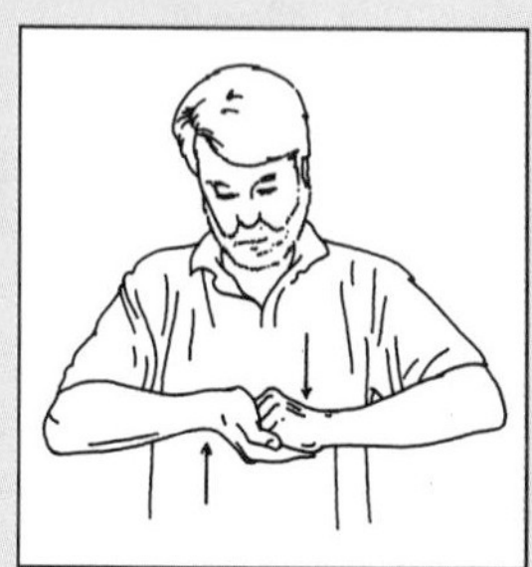

The patient should hold his right arm straight down at his side and then bend his elbow at a 90-degree angle. Tell him to turn his right palm up and place his left fist in it, and then try to bend his right arm upward while resisting this force with his left fist. Tell him to then do this exercise with his left arm and right fist.

Do those abdominals

The patient sits on the floor or bed with his legs out in front of him. Tell him to bend forward and place his hands palms down on the midfront of his thighs. He then tries to bend farther forward while pressing his palms against his thighs for resistance.

Now the buttocks

The patient should stand and squeeze his inner thighs and buttocks together as tightly as possible. When doing this exercise in bed, a pillow between the knees makes it more effective.

Don't forget the thigh

For leg support, the patient should sit on the floor or on a bed. With his legs completely straight, have him vigorously tighten the muscles above his knees so his kneecaps move upward.

At last, the calf

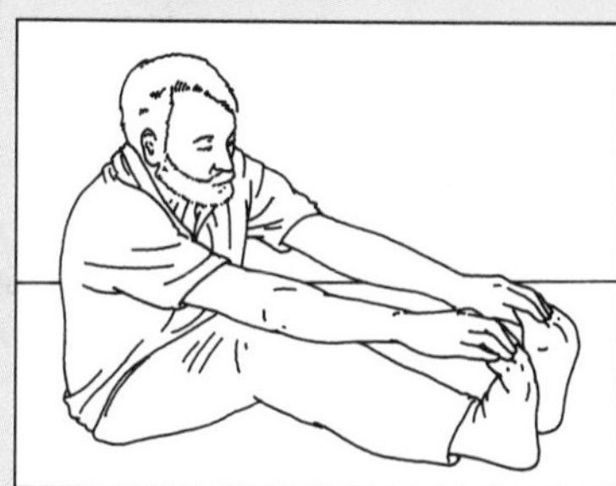

The patient sits up and grasps his toes, then pulls back gently and holds this position briefly. Then, have him push his toes forward and down as far as possible, holding this position briefly.

Reducing pain

To reduce pain and swelling, advise cutting down the number of repetitions the patient does. To improve ROM, recommend increasing repetitions. If exercises don't help or if new joints become involved, tell the patient to check with the doctor. Generally, pain that lasts until the next exercise period (or several hours) indicates that the exercise was too strenuous.

I'm home!

Don't forget to review home care measures. (See *Living with osteoarthritis.*)

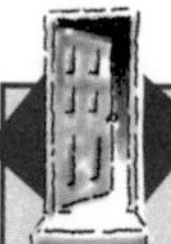

No place like home

Living with osteoarthritis

Discuss these self-care measures that the patient may take at home:

- To decrease stiffness and promote comfort, the doctor may recommend massage and the application of moist heat and cold.
- To compensate for decreased mobility, the patient may need to use assistive devices and splints to support painful joints.
- Emphasize the importance of employing safety measures in the patient's home. Suggest adapting the home, if necessary.
- Tell the patient where he can obtain aids for personal care, such as for eating, driving, and walking.
- Refer the patient to appropriate organizations for additional information and support.

Teaching about diet

Because excess weight adds stress to already painful joints, advise the patient to follow a prescribed weight-reduction program.

Teaching about medication

Drugs used to treat osteoarthritis include aspirin and other salicylates and NSAIDs. Teach the patient the name, purpose, and dosage of each drug. Tell him to report adverse effects. (See *Adverse effects of salicylates and NSAIDs,* page 210.)

Teaching about surgery

Occasionally, surgery is needed to correct deformity or improve function. The doctor may recommend orthopedic surgery to correct underlying congenital anomalies or defects caused by trauma.

Teach the patient about his specific surgical procedure, such as debridement, osteotomy, arthrodesis, and partial or total joint replacement. After surgery, show him how to care for his brace, cast, or other device, as appropriate, and how to resume safe exercise.

Debridement

When the patient is scheduled for joint debridement, explain that the goals of this procedure are:

 to smooth irregular joint surfaces

to remove loose bone or cartilage particles and inflamed synovium.

Tell the patient that, after surgery, the affected joint is immobilized for a few days.

Osteotomy

The doctor may recommend an osteotomy to correct joint misalignment. Usually performed on the knee, this procedure involves removing a section of the bone to realign the joint. Reassure the patient that osteotomy usually relieves joint pain and improves joint mobility and stability.

Arthrodesis

Also called fusion, arthrodesis involves fusing a joint to relieve pain or provide support. Although typically performed on the spine, other joints may be eligible for this surgery.

Joint replacement

Severe joint pain and disability may warrant partial or total joint replacement. Hip and knee replacements are the most common. Joint replacement usually relieves pain and greatly improves joint function.

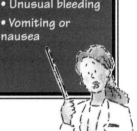

Adverse effects of salicylates and NSAIDs

- Abdominal pain
- Bloody or tarry stools
- Bloody urine
- Headache
- Hearing loss
- Rash
- Severe diarrhea
- Tinnitus
- Unusual bleeding
- Vomiting or nausea

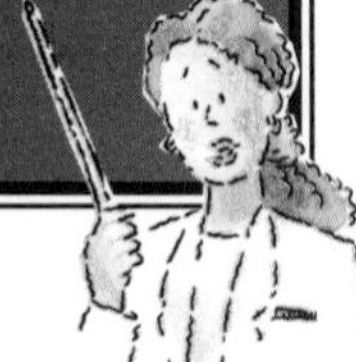

Passive but continuous

Review postoperative care, such as continuous passive motion for a total knee replacement and hip abduction after a total hip replacement.

Osteoporosis

Osteoporosis causes a gradual loss of bone mass while the size of the bones remains constant. This leaves bones porous and brittle. Osteoporosis affects up to 15 to 20 million Americans, causing more than 1 million fractures each year. Sometimes called the "silent disease," osteoporosis often goes undetected until the patient sustains a fracture.

What causes it?

There are several risk factors that predispose patients to osteoporosis. (See *Risk factors for osteoporosis.*)

What is type I osteoporosis?

Osteoporosis is classified as either type I or type II. Also called postmenopausal osteoporosis, type I osteoporosis is related to estrogen loss and affects older women between ages 55 and 75 with no secondary underlying condition. Fractures of the vertebrae and wrist are the most common with this form.

What is type II osteoporosis?

Type II osteoporosis most commonly occurs secondary to an underlying condition, such as hyperparathyroidism, or from an iatrogenic cause such as long-term corticosteroid use. It affects both men and women but is seen in twice as many women as men. Fractures of the vertebrae, hip,

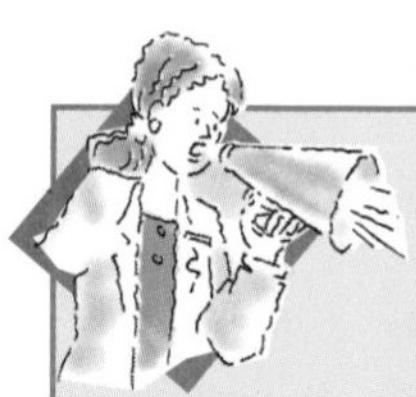

Listen up!

Risk factors for osteoporosis

Everyone loses some bone tissue with age. However, some are more likely to experience extensive bone loss. The following list describes factors that increase a person's risk for osteoporosis.

Can't do anything about it

The risk factors listed below are unalterable:

- sex. Osteoporosis affects four times as many women as men.
- age. After age 50, the osteoporosis risk increases.
- race. Whites and Asians are at greater risk than Blacks.
- body frame. Osteoporosis affects more petite, small-framed persons than average-sized, large-framed persons.
- onset of menopause in women. Earlier onset of menopause (whether natural or surgically induced) increases the risk of osteoporosis.

Adjustments may be possible

For some patients, alterations in lifestyle may eliminate these risk factors:

- a calcium-deficient diet
- a sedentary lifestyle
- regular alcohol and tobacco use or excessive caffeine consumption
- long-term corticosteroid, heparin, or certain antibiotic and anticonvulsant drug use
- multiparity or breast-feeding more than one nontwin infant.

Medical conditions

Osteoporosis may also be associated with the following medical conditions:

- chronic renal failure
- Cushing's syndrome
- eating disorders such as anorexia
- hyperparathyroidism
- hyperthyroidism
- intestinal absorption disorders requiring special therapy (such as intestinal bypass or gastrectomy)
- liver disease
- rheumatoid arthritis.

hands, wrists, and long bones are the most common complication. A calcium-poor diet may contribute to type II osteoporosis.

With type II osteoporosis, a fracture may result even from a simple activity, such as rising from a chair, raising a window, and bending over. Urge the patient to report even minor injuries to the doctor, particularly if pain or swelling persists.

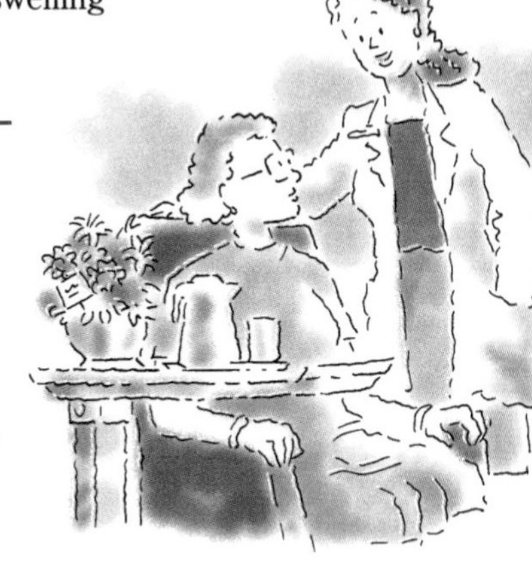
Because you have osteoporosis, you should report even minor injuries to the doctor.

Teaching about tests

To confirm osteoporosis and differentiate type I and type II, the doctor may order blood and urine studies, X-rays, a bone biopsy, and a CT scan. (See *Teaching patients about musculoskeletal tests,* pages 194 to 196.)

X-rays can reveal fractures and advanced bone loss. Special X-ray studies are used to measure the mineral content and mass (density) of long bones.

Teaching about activity and lifestyle

Urge the patient to follow a weight-bearing exercise program to prevent further bone loss. Moderate weight-bearing exercise activates osteoblastic bone formation, improves muscle strength, promotes circulation, and enhances intestinal absorption of calcium. (See *Recommended weight-bearing exercises.*)

Let's go for a swim instead

For an elderly patient, the doctor may recommend swimming if weight-bearing exercise isn't feasible.

Safety first

Make sure the patient understands the importance of adding safety practices and proper body mechanics to everyday activities. (See *Exercise carefully.*)

Home sweet home

For all patients with osteoporosis, discuss additional care measures they can perform at home. (See *Living with osteoporosis,* page 214.)

Recommended weight-bearing exercises

- Walking
- Jogging
- Bicycling
- Low-impact aerobics

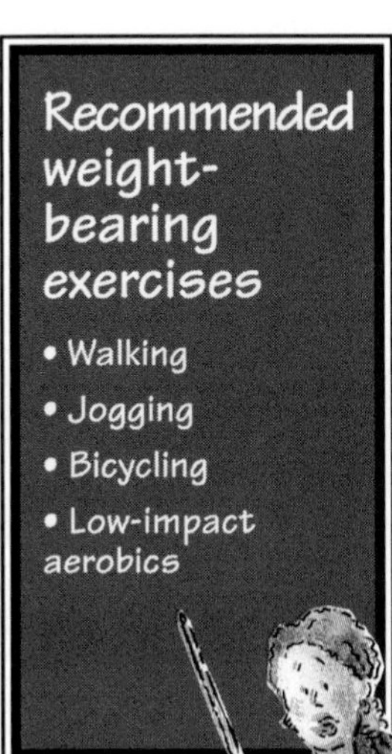

Teaching about diet

Although daily dietary calcium can't replace lost bone, it may slow or prevent further bone loss. Help the patient plan her menu selections to boost her calcium intake.

Keeping calcium convenient

Advise the patient to keep a supply of calcium-rich foods on hand. (See *Calcium-rich foods.*)

Living without lactose

A patient who is lactose-intolerant or can't consume dairy products may need calcium supplements or calcium-containing antacids such as Tums. She should avoid foods and beverages that contain caffeine because they also contain phosphorus, which contributes to bone loss.

Advice for smokers and meat eaters

A patient who smokes or consumes a lot of sugar and meat should follow her doctor's recommendations for getting more calcium.

Listen up!

Exercise carefully

Instruct the patient with osteoporosis to be cautious while exercising. Advise her to avoid activities that involve twisting, jumping, or straining the back (such as golf, tennis, and bowling) because these may cause fractures.

Calcium-rich foods

- Milk
- Cheese
- Yogurt
- Ice cream
- Collard greens
- Turnip greens
- Broccoli
- Oysters
- Salmon
- Sardines
- Egg yolk
- Beans
- Nuts
- Lettuce
- Tofu

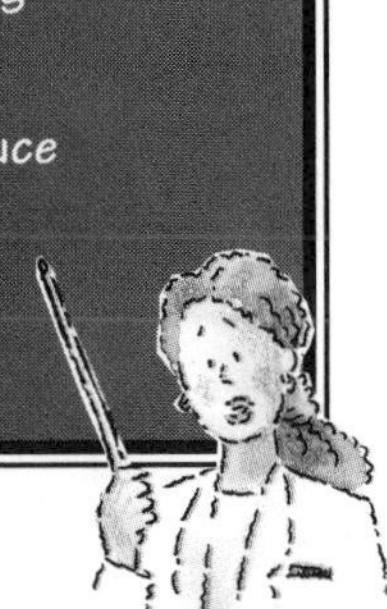

Teaching about medication

Tell the patient about drugs that may be prescribed to prevent or slow bone loss:
- calcium and vitamin D supplements
- calcitonin
- estrogen (for menopausal women)
- thiazide diuretics.

Review how to take these medications, and discuss possible adverse effects. If appropriate, mention that certain new drugs may improve the long-term prospects for successful osteoporosis treatment. For example, a new antiresorptive drug, such as Fosamax, may reduce the risk of fractures.

Calcium supplement

If the patient isn't getting enough calcium in her diet, the doctor may recommend an over-the-counter calcium supplement.

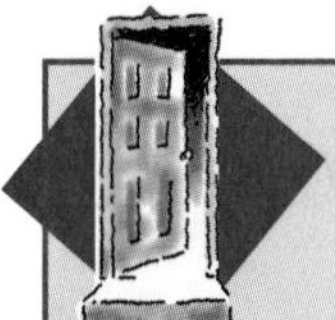

No place like home

Living with osteoporosis

Make sure your patient understands the importance of diligent self-care to deal with osteoporosis. Safety practices and proper body mechanics go hand in hand in preventing fractures.

If the shoe fits
Advise the patient to wear comfortable, well-fitting shoes with rubber heels to help cushion and protect the spine during walking. Discourage high heels.

Careful!
To prevent falls, suggest the following:
- Remove throw rugs.
- Place a nonskid mat in the bathtub.
- Install handrails on stairs.
- Don't walk about in dimly lit rooms.
- Don't lift heavy objects.
- Don't twist suddenly.
- Don't bend from the waist.

A nice device
If appropriate, suggest a cane or walker to help the patient maintain balance and decrease lower back pain. Tell the patient about other devices that can make daily activities easier, such as:
- a shoe horn
- a long-handled sponge
- a reacher-grabber.

More info
Finally, refer the patient to appropriate resources for further information and support, such as the National Osteoporosis Foundation.

Extra! Extra! How to get extra calcium!

Instruct the patient to take the calcium supplement 1 hour before meals to ensure maximum absorption. Recommend that she avoid laxatives and multivitamins containing zinc, which decrease calcium absorption.

The doctor may recommend taking a vitamin D supplement along with the calcium to maximize intestinal absorption.

Between not during

To ease adverse effects of calcium supplements — gas and constipation — suggest increasing fluid intake and increasing fiber between meals.

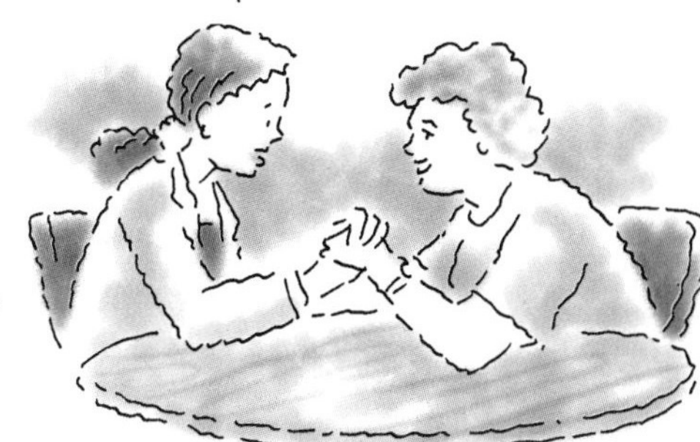
To get the most out of your calcium supplement, take it 1 hour before meals.

Calcitonin

Calcitonin is a hormone normally produced by the body. It prevents bone loss by inhibiting bone resorption. Calcitonin (from salmon) slows the progression of osteoporosis and is used to treat postmenopausal osteoporosis.

Breathe in

Calcitonin is usually given intranasally, although it's also available as an I.M. or a subcutaneous injection. Teach the patient to take the nasal spray through alternating nostrils daily. Also instruct her to keep calcitonin refrigerated and to use it in combination with calcium and vitamin D supplements as prescribed to prevent further bone loss.

Estrogen

Estrogen replacement therapy may be recommended for a postmenopausal patient or for a menopausal patient at high risk for osteoporosis. Because estrogen replacement therapy may increase the risk of endometrial and breast cancer, advise the patient to discuss the pros and cons of this treatment option with her doctor before beginning therapy.

Etidronate

Etidronate disodium (Didronel) is the first drug proven to restore lost bone and increase bone mass. However, as a treatment for osteoporosis, the drug is still experimental.

Sign on the dotted line

Negotiate learning with your patient. If the patient is noncompliant, suggest a contract that spells out learning goals, a timetable, and your obligation as well as the patient's.

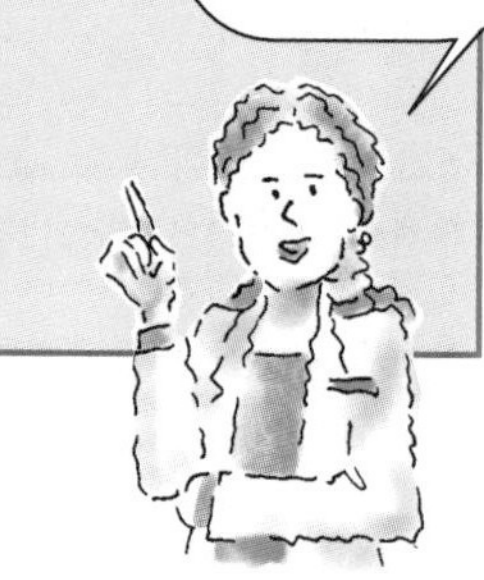

Strains and sprains

A sprain or a strain may seem like a minor injury to many patients. However, left untreated, such injuries may seriously compromise the patient's ability to regain normal strength and function. Failure to rehabilitate the injured extremity may lead to more serious re-injury.

What is a sprain?

A sprain results from stretching or tearing the capsule or ligament surrounding a joint, resulting in acute pain and swelling. An ankle sprain, for instance, may occur from twisting the ankle during a fall or stepping on an uneven surface.

What is a strain?

A strain is a partial, microscopic tear in a muscle or tendon or both. An acute strain results from a sudden forced movement that overstretches the muscle or tendon. The patient may not feel pain until sometime after the initial injury, such as during continued activity.

A chronic strain results from repeated muscle overuse, commonly during sports, such as tennis, golf, and basketball. A strain can also occur when a person uses poor body mechanics in lifting or carrying.

Teaching about tests

A physical examination of the injured area is used to evaluate joint stability. An X-ray or a CT scan may be used to evaluate the severity and determine the location of the injury. Sprains and strains are classified by the extent of tissue damage, from grade I (mild damage) to grade III (severe damage). (See *Teaching patients about musculoskeletal tests,* pages 194 to 196.)

Teaching about activity and lifestyle

Instruct the patient to rest the injured part for 24 hours or longer as the doctor directs. After that, he may resume some activities using a sling, wrap, cast, splint, or crutches.

Home sweet home

The doctor may recommend an appropriate rehabilitation program as well as home care measures. (See *Living with a strain or sprain.*)

Teaching about medication

Analgesics may be prescribed to relieve pain. NSAIDs decrease inflammation. Review the prescribed dosages and possible adverse effects of these drugs. Advise the patient with a history of ulcers or sensitivity to salicylates to take NSAIDs with meals to help prevent stomach upset.

Stop if...

Instruct the patient to stop taking pain medication and tell the doctor if nausea, vomiting, abdominal pain, or dark stools occur.

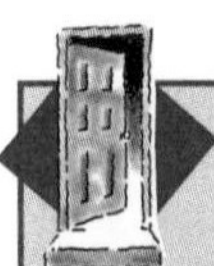

No place like home

Living with a strain or sprain

Here is some advice you can offer your patient to speed recovery from a sprain or strain.

Get with the program
If the patient has a sprain, tell him his rehabilitation program may begin with range-of-motion exercises, followed by isometric exercises for the injured limb. As healing progresses, conditioning and strengthening exercises may be added. Stress the importance of exercising uninjured extremities as well as the injured one because this helps prevent loss of muscle tone and vascular problems. Exercise also helps to prevent thrombus formation.

Check it out
Instruct the patient to check pulses, warmth, mobility, and sensory function around the injury site and to report any changes to the doctor right away.

Express yourself
Finally, encourage the patient to express his concerns about his condition.

Teaching about procedures

An immobilization device helps relieve pain and promote healing. The type of device used depends on the severity of the patient's injury and his degree of disability.

For example, a moderate sprain may require an air cast—an inflatable device with an adjustable, rigid, lightweight shell. For a severe sprain, a plaster or Fiberglas cast may be used for more rigid support. (See *Make sure it's dry.*)

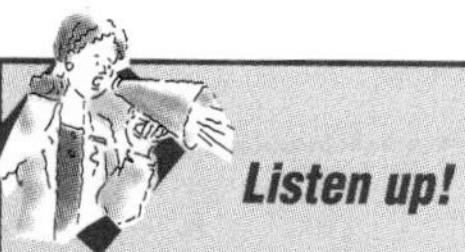

Make sure it's dry

Caution the patient not to bear weight on the injured limb until a plaster or Fiberglas cast is completely dry. Otherwise, he may reshape the cast and produce pressure points.

Ice advice

Emphasize that rest and ice reduce pain and swelling. Tell the patient to place an ice pack over the injury for 24 to 36 hours, applying it at 30-minute intervals and moving it every 5 minutes to avoid frostbite.

The first 24 hours and after

To reduce swelling, the patient should elevate the injured extremity above heart level for the first 24 hours after the injury. To further ease swelling, recommend wrapping the injured part in an elastic bandage to compress the tissue. After 24 hours, mild heat is applied to promote absorption of blood and fluid from the area.

Teaching about surgery

Surgical intervention—usually arthroscopy—may be necessary for a sprain that causes joint instability or doesn't respond adequately to conventional measures. Tell the patient that, after surgery, he'll wear an immobilization device for several weeks, depending on the location and severity of the injury.

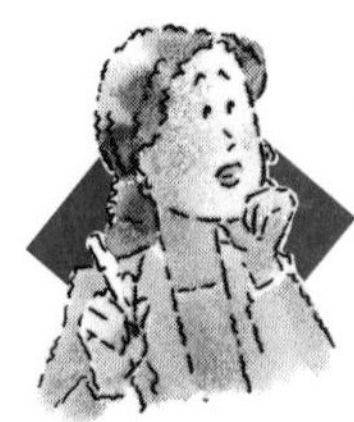

Quick quiz

1. When discussing symptoms with a patient with carpal tunnel syndrome, you're most likely to discuss:

A. itching in the hands.
B. weakness, burning, pain, numbness, or tingling in one or both hands.
C. muscle bulging in the hands.

Answer: B. Other symptoms include inability to make a fist, and paresthesia in parts of the hand.

2. You should teach the patient with chronic low back pain that pain may be exacerbated by:

A. lying down.
B. regular back exercises.
C. any activity that increases pressure on the spine.

Answer: C. This activity includes sneezing, coughing, and straining. Lying down may relieve the pain. A prescribed exercise program will help improve the condition.

3. When teaching a patient with osteoporosis, activities you should encourage are:

A. moderate weight-bearing activities.
B. bed rest.
C. sports, such as tennis and golf.

Answer: A. These activities promote bone formation, improve muscle strength, promote circulation, and enhance intestinal absorption of calcium.

Scoring

☆☆☆ If you answered all three questions correctly, take a bow. Your skills are well-aligned.

☆☆ If you answered two questions correctly, nice work. With practice, you could muscle your way to the top of the class.

☆ If you answered fewer than two questions correctly, don't get weak in the knees. There's still time to bone up on the topic.

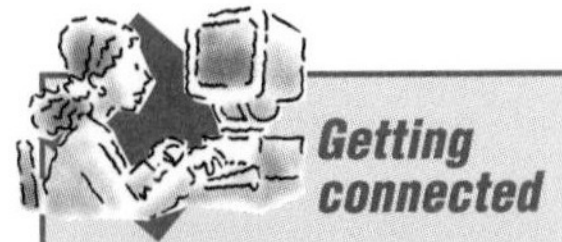

Osteoporosis on-line

For more information about osteoporosis, direct the patient to the following Web sites:

- National Osteoporosis Foundation (www.nof.org)
- Osteoporosis and Related Bone Diseases National Resource Center (www.osteo.org).

7

Renal and urologic disorders

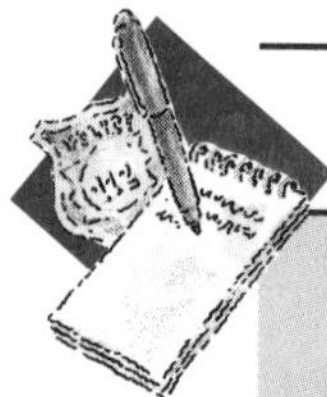

Just the facts

In this chapter, you'll learn how to teach patients with the following renal and urologic disorders:

- acute renal failure
- chronic renal failure
- glomerulonephritis
- neurogenic bladder
- renal calculi
- urinary tract infection.

Acute renal failure

Acute renal failure is the sudden inability of the kidneys to remove waste materials from the blood and maintain proper fluid and electrolyte balance. The first sign of acute renal failure is oliguria (a sudden decrease in urination) or, rarely, anuria (total absence of urination). (See *Classifying acute renal failure*.)

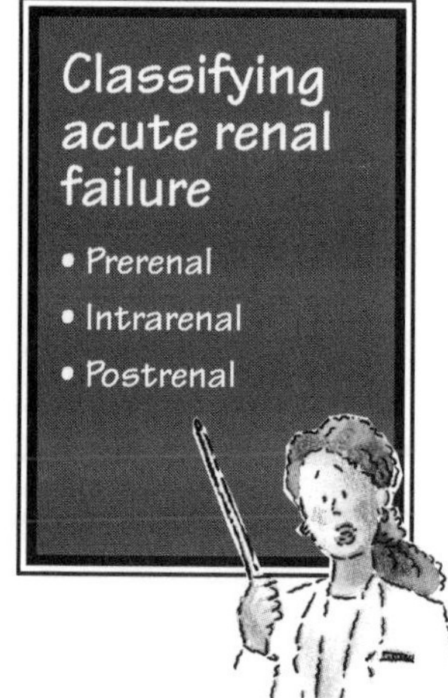
Classifying acute renal failure
• Prerenal
• Intrarenal
• Postrenal

What's prerenal failure?

Prerenal failure results when factors outside the kidneys impair renal perfusion, including heart failure and other cardiovascular disorders, hypovolemia, and renovascular obstruction.

What's intrarenal failure?

Intrarenal failure results from disorders that damage the kidneys themselves, such as acute tubular necrosis. Parenchymal changes from disease and nephrotoxic substances can also contribute to intrarenal failure.

What's postrenal failure?

Postrenal failure results from an obstruction in the urinary tract anywhere from the tubules to the urethral meatus. This obstruction may be caused by renal calculi or ureteral constriction, for example.

What's at risk?

Although early detection and aggressive therapy usually reverse acute renal failure, compliance is a key factor. Less than full compliance can lead to fluid and electrolyte imbalance, acidosis, infection, and uremia. In addition, compliance is necessary to prevent or delay chronic renal failure. (See *It gets complicated!*)

Teaching about tests

Tell the patient that he'll undergo careful screening to reveal preexisting risk factors that can affect kidney function, such as exposure to nephrotoxic substances.

Blood tests

Blood tests may include a complete blood count (CBC) and blood urea nitrogen (BUN), electrolyte, protein, creatinine, and uric acid levels. The patient undergoes follow-up blood tests regularly during treatment to ensure proper management of the disorder. (See *The other arm, please.*)

Urine tests

Urine tests are used to evaluate the kidneys' ability to dilute and concentrate urine, determine the extent of kidney failure, and check for infection. Tests for urine osmolality, sodium levels, and creatinine clearance require a urine specimen.

Other tests

Diagnostic studies may include computed tomography (CT) scan, kidney-ureter-bladder (KUB) radiography, magnetic resonance imaging (MRI), renal angiography, renal ultrasonography, and retrograde ureteropyelography. These tests reveal abnormal kidney size or shape, fluid accumulation, and obstructed urinary outflow. Renal

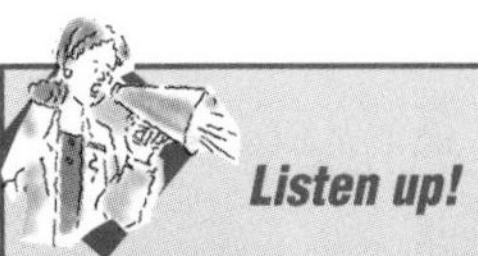

Listen up!

The other arm, please

If the patient has an arteriovenous access device for dialysis, instruct him to tell the technician not to use the affected arm when drawing blood, inserting I.V. lines, or taking blood pressure.

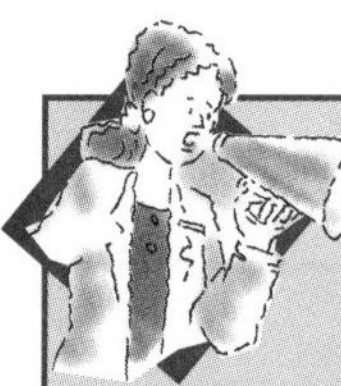

Listen up!

It gets complicated!

Help your patient understand the following possible complications of acute renal failure and signs and symptoms he should watch for and report.

Uremia

Explain that uremia is an accumulation of protein waste products in the blood. When these waste products reach toxic levels, such complications as uremic pericarditis and uremic pneumonitis may result.

The signs and symptoms of uremia include:

- nausea
- vomiting
- headache
- decreased level of consciousness
- dizziness
- decreased visual acuity
- breath with urine odor
- elevated blood pressure.

Hypervolemia

Tell the patient that hypervolemia is an abnormal increase in the volume of fluid circulating in the body. This excess fluid may accumulate in the vessels or tissues. Unchecked, hypervolemia can result in such serious complications as hypertension, heart failure, and pulmonary edema.

Teach the patient to report signs of hypervolemia:

- sudden weight gain
- swollen hands and feet
- increased blood pressure.

Hypovolemia

Explain that hypovolemia is an abnormal decrease in the volume of fluid circulating in the body. Untreated, it can progress to shock.

Teach the patient to report signs and symptoms of hypovolemia:

- weight loss
- dry skin and mucous membranes
- decreased urine output
- muscle cramps
- fatigue
- dizziness
- decreased blood pressure.

Hyperkalemia

Point out that hyperkalemia occurs when too much potassium accumulates in the blood. Hyperkalemia can cause an irregular heart rate, possibly leading to cardiac arrest and death. Instruct the patient to notify the doctor if he experiences signs and symptoms of hyperkalemia, including:

- weakness
- malaise
- nausea
- diarrhea
- abdominal cramps.

biopsy may be ordered if the results are inconclusive. (See *Teaching patients about renal and urologic tests,* pages 223 to 225.)

Teaching about activity and lifestyle

The patient with severe acute renal failure must limit activity to conserve energy. Later, if his condition improves, the doctor may suggest increasing the activity level. If bed rest is ordered, teach the patient early, progressive ambulation, as approved by the doctor.

Following up

Before your patient goes home, make sure he understands the importance of follow-up monitoring and care measures. (See *At home with acute renal failure.*)

Teaching about diet

Diet alone can't reverse acute renal failure, but it does play an important role in therapy.

Have some carbohydrates!

Collaborate with the doctor and dietitian to teach the patient how to adjust his diet. A diet high in carbohydrates and low in protein, sodium, potassium, and phosphorus can prevent further kidney damage while maintaining nutritional balance. Be sure to include family members in your dietary teaching, especially those who prepare the patient's meals.

(Text continues on page 226.)

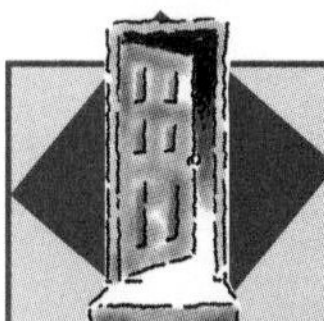

No place like home

At home with acute renal failure

Review the following teaching topics to ensure the acute renal failure patient's understanding of follow-up care.

Balancing act
Make sure the patient knows how to monitor his fluid balance. Show him how to measure and record his daily weight, blood pressure, and fluid intake and output.

Pressure points
Show the patient the proper technique for taking accurate blood pressure readings, and instruct him to compare each blood pressure reading with his baseline reading. Tell him to notify the doctor if his blood pressure exceeds the desired reading the doctor has specified for him.

Infection prevention
Also encourage the patient to monitor his temperature and to stay alert for signs and symptoms of possible urinary tract infection, such as a change in the odor, color, or consistency of his urine.

Be sure to acknowledge the patient's fear of losing kidney function or becoming dependent on dialysis. To allay his fears, stress that early detection and aggressive therapy can usually reverse acute renal failure and prevent its progression to chronic renal failure.

Support
Finally, refer both the patient and his family to a local group or national organization for information and support.

Teaching patients about renal and urologic tests

Test and purpose	What to teach the patient
Antegrade pyelography • To evaluate obstruction of the upper collecting system by stricture, calculus, clot, or tumor • To evaluate hydronephrosis revealed during excretory urography or ultrasonography and to enable placement of a percutaneous nephrostomy tube • To evaluate the function of the upper collecting system after ureteral surgery or urinary diversion • To assess renal functional reserve before surgery	• This test allows radiographic examination of the kidney and takes about 1 hour. • The patient lies in a prone position on an X-ray table and takes a sedative to help him relax. Medical staff clean the skin over the kidney with an antiseptic solution and numb it with a local anesthetic. Then the doctor inserts a needle into the kidney to inject contrast medium. Urine may also be collected from the kidney for testing and a tube is left in the kidney for drainage, if necessary. The patient may feel mild discomfort as the local anesthetic is injected and transient burning and flushing from the contrast medium. The X-ray machine will make loud, clacking sounds as it exposes films of the kidney. • After the test, the patient's blood pressure, heart rate, and respiration are monitored every 15 minutes for the first hour, every 30 minutes for the second hour, and every 2 hours for the next 24 hours. Also, his dressing is checked for blood or urine leakage, and his fluid intake and urine output are monitored for 24 hours. If a nephrostomy tube is inserted, it is checked to ensure that it's patent and draining well. • The patient should report posttest chills, fever, and rapid pulse or respiration to the doctor immediately. He should also report pain in the abdomen or flank or sudden onset of chest pain or dyspnea.
Cystometry • To evaluate detrusor muscle function and tonicity • To help determine the cause of bladder dysfunction	• This test evaluates bladder function, especially as it relates to the urgency to void and the ability to suppress voiding. It takes about 40 minutes. The patient must urinate just before the test. • The patient lies in a supine position on an examining table while medical staff pass a catheter into the bladder. As saline solution or carbon dioxide enters the bladder, the patient is asked to report his sensations, such as when he first feels the urge to void, when his bladder feels full, and when he has a strong urge to void. • The patient may experience transient urinary burning or frequency after the test.
Cystoscopy • To visualize internal bladder structures • To help confirm hydronephrosis • To locate an obstruction associated with hydronephrosis	• This 20-minute test is usually performed in the doctor's office. The patient may receive a general anesthetic; if so, he shouldn't eat for 8 hours before the test. If he'll have a local anesthetic, he may receive a sedative to help him relax before the test. (If the patient is a woman, she won't receive any anesthetic.) If the doctor plans to take bladder X-rays, the patient may receive a bowel preparation to clean his bowels and ensure sharper, clearer X-ray images. • The patient lies in a supine position (with his hips and knees flexed) on an X-ray table. The genitalia are cleaned with an antiseptic solution, and he's covered with a sterile drape. Next, the doctor administers a local anesthetic, if appropriate, and introduces the cystoscope through the urethra and into the bladder. The patient's bladder is filled with irrigating solution, and the cystoscope is rotated to inspect the bladder wall surface. If a local anesthetic is used, the patient may feel a burning sensation as the cystoscope advances through the urethra. He may also feel an urgent need to void as the bladder fills with the irrigating solution.

(continued)

Teaching patients about renal and urologic tests *(continued)*

Test and purpose	What to teach the patient
Cystourethroscopy • To directly visualize the bladder wall, ureteral orifices, and urethra • To provide a channel for invasive procedures, such as biopsy, lesion resection, removal of calculi, or passage of a ureteral catheter to the renal pelvis	• This test permits visualization of the bladder and urethra, and takes about 20 minutes. • If a general anesthetic has been ordered, the patient must fast for 8 hours before the test. If a local anesthetic has been ordered, the patient may receive a sedative before the test to help him relax. • The patient lies in a supine position on an X-ray table, with his hips and knees flexed. His genitalia are cleaned with an antiseptic solution, and he's draped. Then the doctor administers a local anesthetic, if appropriate, and introduces the cystourethroscope through the urethra into the bladder. Next, the doctor fills the bladder with irrigating solution and rotates the scope to inspect the entire surface of the bladder wall. If a local anesthetic is used, the patient may feel a burning sensation when the cystourethroscope is passed through the urethra. He may also feel an urgent need to urinate as the bladder is filled with irrigating solution. • The patient's blood pressure, heart rate, and respiration are monitored every 15 minutes for the first hour after the test, then every hour until stable. He should drink plenty of fluids and take the prescribed analgesics. However, he should avoid alcohol for 48 hours after the test. Urinary burning and frequency will soon subside. He must take antibiotics, as ordered, to prevent bacterial infection. • The patient should report flank or abdominal pain, chills, fever, or decreased urine output to the doctor immediately. In addition, he should notify the doctor if he doesn't void within 8 hours after the test or if bright red blood continues to appear after three voidings.
Kidney-ureter-bladder radiography • To evaluate the size, structure, and position of the kidneys • To screen for abnormalities (such as calcification) in the region of the kidneys, ureters, and bladder	• This test shows the position of the urinary system organs and helps detect abnormalities in them. The test takes only a few minutes, and the patient isn't required to restrict food or fluids. • The patient lies in a supine position in correct body alignment on a radiographic table. He extends his arms overhead while medical staff check the iliac crests for symmetrical positioning. If the patient can't extend his arms or stand, he may lie on his left side with his right arm up. The male patient's gonads are shielded to prevent irradiation of the testes. (The female patient's ovaries can't be shielded because they're too close to the kidneys, ureters, and bladder.) Then a technician takes a single X-ray.
Nephrotomography and renal computed tomography scan • To differentiate between a renal cyst and a solid tumor • To detect and evaluate renal pathologic conditions, such as tumor, obstruction, calculi, polycystic kidney disease, congenital anomalies, and abnormal fluid accumulation around the kidneys	• This test helps detect renal abnormalities by providing cross-sectional images of the kidney. In renal computed tomography, a computer translates these images for display on an oscilloscope screen. The test takes about 1 hour. • The patient must fast for 8 hours before the test if he's scheduled to receive a contrast medium. If he has a history of hypersensitivity to iodine or iodine-containing foods, the doctor may forgo administration of the contrast medium or may prescribe antiallergenic prophylaxis. • The patient lies on an X-ray table as the scanner rotates around his body. He should be aware that the machine will make loud, clacking sounds. He should lie still to avoid distorting the X-ray films. After the technician takes a series of films, the patient may receive an injection of contrast medium. He may experience transient flushing, headache, and metallic taste as well as a burning or stinging sensation at the injection site. • If the patient received a contrast medium, he should report any posttest flushing, nausea, itching, or sneezing to the doctor.

Teaching patients about renal and urologic tests *(continued)*

Test and purpose	What to teach the patient
Renal biopsy • To aid diagnosis of renal parenchymal disease • To monitor progressive renal disease and to assess effectiveness of treatment	• This test helps diagnose kidney disorders and takes about 15 minutes. The biopsy needle is in the kidney for only a few seconds. • The patient should restrict food and fluids for 8 hours before the test. He'll receive a mild sedative before the test to help him relax. • The patient lies in a prone position with a sandbag under his abdomen. After the biopsy site is numbed with a local anesthetic, the patient is asked to hold his breath as the doctor inserts a biopsy needle through his back into the kidney. The patient may experience a pinching pain as the needle is inserted. • After the test, pressure is applied to the biopsy site to stop superficial bleeding, followed by the application of a pressure dressing. The patient must lie flat on his back without moving for at least 12 hours to prevent bleeding. His blood pressure, heart rate, and respiration are closely monitored.
Renal ultrasonography • To determine the size, shape, and position of the kidneys, their internal structures, and perirenal tissues • To evaluate and localize urinary obstruction and abnormal accumulation of fluid • To assess and diagnose complications following kidney transplantation	• This test helps detect abnormalities in the kidneys and takes about 30 minutes. The test is safe and painless; in fact, it may feel like a back rub. • The patient lies in a prone position, exposing the area to be scanned. The technician then applies ultrasound jelly and guides a transducer over this area. During the test, the patient may be asked to breathe deeply to assess kidney movement during respiration.
Retrograde cystography, ureteropyelography, or urethrography • To diagnose bladder rupture without urethral involvement, neurogenic bladder, recurrent urinary tract infections (UTIs), reflux, diverticula, and tumors • To diagnose urethral strictures, laceration, diverticula, and congenital abnormalities • To examine the renal collecting system	• These tests evaluate the structure and integrity of the bladder, renal collecting system, and urethra. Each takes about 30 minutes to 1 hour. • If a general anesthetic is ordered, the patient must fast for 8 hours before the test. However, before retrograde ureteropyelography, he must drink plenty of fluids to ensure adequate urine flow. • For *retrograde urethrography* and *retrograde cystography,* the patient is placed in a supine position on an X-ray table. A catheter is inserted into the urethra (for urethrography) or the bladder (for cystography); then a contrast medium is instilled through the catheter. The patient is asked to assume various positions while X-ray films are taken. • For *retrograde ureteropyelography,* the patient is positioned on an X-ray table with his legs in stirrups and a contrast medium is injected through a urethral catheter. X-ray films are taken while the catheter is in place and again after it's withdrawn. The patient may experience some discomfort when the catheter is inserted and when the contrast medium is instilled. The X-ray machine will make loud, clacking sounds as it exposes the films. • After *retrograde urethrography,* the patient should report flushing, nausea, itching, or sneezing to the doctor immediately. • After *retrograde cystography* or *ureteropyelography,* the patient's blood pressure, heart rate, and respiration are monitored frequently until stable. His urine volume and color are also monitored. The patient should notify the doctor if blood continues to appear in his urine after the third voiding or if he develops chills, fever, or increased pulse or respiratory rate.

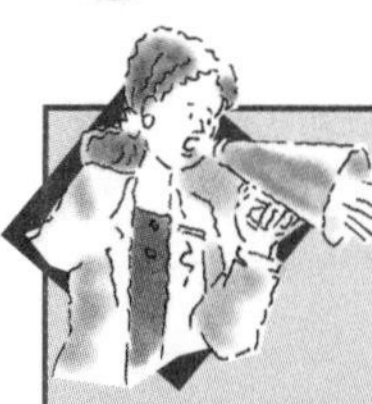

Listen up!

Measuring fluid intake and output

The doctor will probably want your patient to keep a daily record of his fluid intake and output. Explain to the patient that this record can help the doctor judge his progress and response to treatment.

What are intake and output anyway?
Inform the patient that fluid *intake* includes everything he drinks, such as water, fruit juice, and soda. It also includes foods that become liquid at room temperature, such as gelatin, custard, and ice cream. Intake even includes liquid medicines and solutions delivered through tubing into one of the veins (I.V.) or into his stomach.

Explain that *output* includes everything that leaves his body as a fluid — urine, drainage from a wound, diarrhea, and vomitus.

Don't guess
Because the patient's intake should balance his output, urge him to keep very accurate records. Tell him to measure fluids whenever possible instead of guessing the amount.

Measuring intake
Instruct the patient to measure and record the amount of fluid he has with each meal, with medicine, and between meals. Tell him to pour any liquid into a measuring cup or other graduated container before putting it in a glass or cup. Tell him to subtract any amount he doesn't drink from the measurement. Remind him that labels on cans and bottles indicate exact amounts. If the patient is receiving medicine or nutrition I.V. or through a stomach tube, instruct him to record the amount of fluid that's infused.

Measuring output
Before throwing away any urine from a bedpan, urinal, or portable toilet, the patient (or his caregiver) should measure and record the amount. Advise him to keep a measuring container handy just for this purpose.

If the patient has a drainage bag in place, instruct him or his caregiver to measure and record the amount of fluid in the bag before discarding it. Finally, advise the patient to measure and record any vomitus or liquid bowel movements as output.

Making it metric
The doctor may want the patient to measure his fluid intake and output metrically. To convert fluid ounces (oz) to the metric equivalent of milliliters (ml), instruct the patient to multiply by 30. To convert milliliters to ounces, tell him to divide by 30.

APPROXIMATE EQUIVALENTS

Household	Metric
1 quart (32 oz)	960 ml
1 pint (16 oz)	480 ml
1 measuring cup (8 oz)	240 ml
2 tbs (1 oz)	30 ml

Fluids: More or less

Depending on the cause and stage of acute renal failure, the patient may need to either restrict or increase fluid intake. Pass on the following pointers:

- If the patient must restrict fluids, he should suck on ice chips when thirsty. He should include the ice chips as part of his daily fluid intake.

• Divide fluid intake over the course of the day. To avoid overload, measure fluid intake and urine output precisely.
• The patient should weigh himself at the same time each day, using the same scale and wearing the same type of clothing. He should notify the doctor if his weight increases or decreases by more than 5% from one day to the next. (See *Measuring fluid intake and output.*)

Teaching about medication

The doctor may discontinue medications that are concentrated in the kidneys and excreted in the urine. Explain that, because acute renal failure delays urine excretion, it increases the risk of toxic drug reactions. Tell the patient not to discontinue or adjust the dosage of any medication without the doctor's approval.

Teaching about procedures

Postrenal failure usually requires catheterization to drain urine from the bladder. A procedure (surgical or nonsurgi-

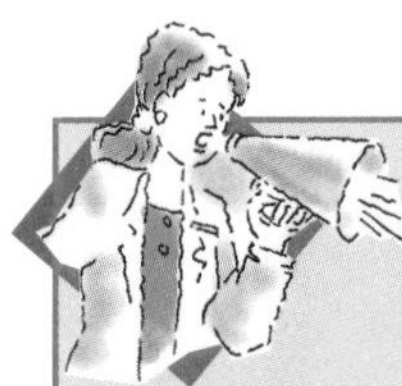

Listen up!

Describing dialysis

The patient may receive hemodialysis or peritoneal dialysis.

Hemodialysis
To perform hemodialysis, a surgeon catheterizes the subclavian or femoral veins. Explain the three basic steps that follow:
• The patient's blood exits the body through the catheter or fistula.
• The blood then circulates through a dialyzer that removes waste products.
• The patient's blood is returned to his body.

The process takes 3 to 5 hours and is repeated three or four times a week until the patient's own kidney function improves. After hemodialysis, the patient may feel tired for several hours as his body adjusts to the treatment.

Peritoneal dialysis
This procedure may be performed manually, by an automatic or semiautomatic cycler machine, or as continuous ambulatory peritoneal dialysis.

Explain the basic procedure of all three methods:
• A catheter is inserted into the peritoneal cavity through a small incision in the patient's abdomen.
• A dialysate solution is instilled through the catheter into the peritoneal cavity, where it remains long enough to allow excess fluid, electrolytes, and accumulated wastes to move through the peritoneal membrane into the dialysate.
• After the prescribed dwelling time, the dialysate is drained from the patient's peritoneal cavity, taking toxins with it.

cal) may be needed to free the obstruction. If the patient requires surgery, explain the procedure, including who will perform it, where it's performed, and how long it will take.

In the final analysis, dialysis

If acute renal failure doesn't respond promptly to other treatment measures, the patient commonly undergoes dialysis. (See *Describing dialysis,* page 227.)

Chronic renal failure

Chronic renal failure is the progressive failure of normal kidney function. In your teaching, emphasize that patients today survive longer than ever before, thanks to dialysis and kidney transplantation.

Why?

Explain that chronic renal failure results from progressive, irreversible damage to the nephrons, the kidneys' structural and functional units.

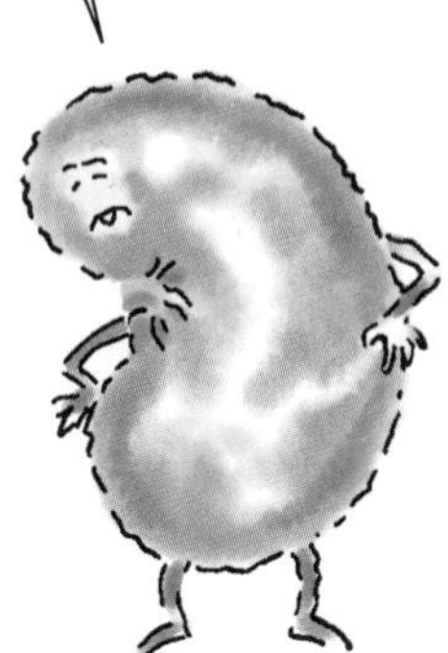
Oy vey! Progressive, irreversible damage to my nephrons leads to chronic renal failure.

Teaching about tests

Describe routine blood and urine tests used to evaluate kidney function, radiologic tests used to visualize abnormalities, and renal biopsy used to examine tissue. (See *Teaching patients about renal and urologic tests,* pages 223 to 225.)

Blood tests

Blood studies include CBC, coagulation studies (such as activated partial thromboplastin time and prothrombin time), electrolyte levels, creatinine, BUN, cholesterol, magnesium, iron and, periodically, calcium and phosphorus analyses.

Urine tests

Urine studies include urinalysis with microscopic study, creatinine clearance and protein loss determinations, and cultures (if infection is suspected). Teach the patient how to collect a clean-catch midstream specimen or 24-hour urine specimen as needed.

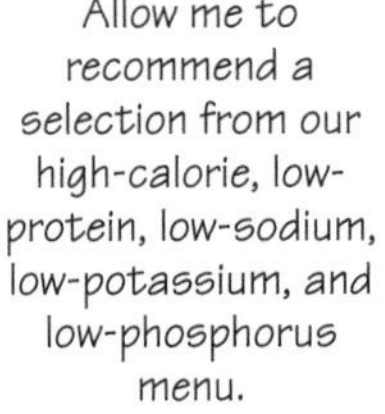

Allow me to recommend a selection from our high-calorie, low-protein, low-sodium, low-potassium, and low-phosphorus menu.

Teaching about activity and lifestyle

Through regular exercise, the patient can maintain muscle strength and mobility and prevent bone demineralization. Urge the patient to avoid excessive fatigue and to conserve energy by alternating activity with rest. As needed, explain how to protect a dialysis access site during exercise.

Help with self-help

Discuss ways the patient can help manage other difficulties of renal failure. (See *Getting by,* page 230.)

Teaching about diet

A diet high in calories but low in protein, sodium, potassium (including salt substitutes), and phosphorus is easy on the kidneys and may slow the progression of renal disease. Encourage the patient to take prescribed vitamin supplements.

Keeping up with change

Explain that dietary needs change as renal disease progresses. Emphasize the need to carefully regulate fluid intake based on urine output.

Teaching about medication

The doctor may prescribe drugs, such as diuretics, to help control the systemic effects of renal failure and to relieve symptoms.

Teaching about procedures

If the patient requires dialysis, explain its purpose, and discuss the two types: hemodialysis and peritoneal dialysis. Point out that dialysis doesn't cure or reverse renal disease and won't compensate for loss of the kidney's endocrine or metabolic function. (See *Describing dialysis,* page 227.)

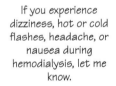

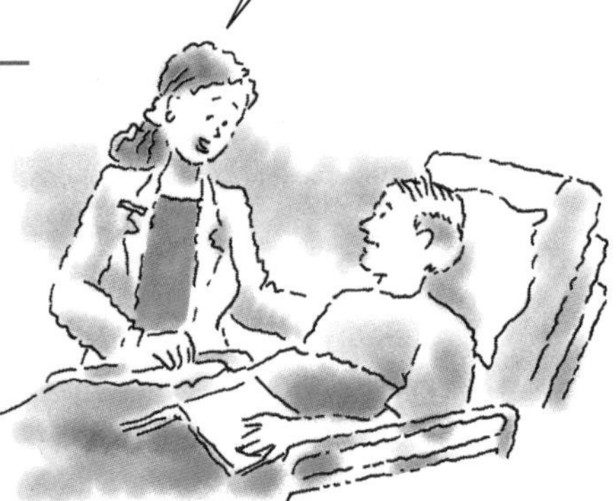
If you experience dizziness, hot or cold flashes, headache, or nausea during hemodialysis, let me know.

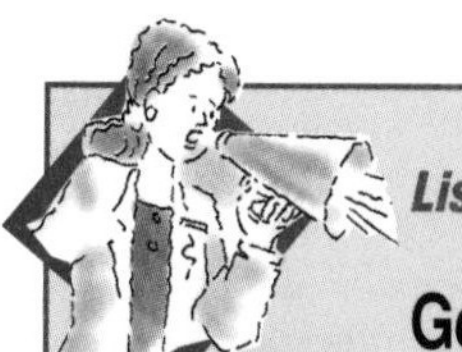

Listen up!

Getting by

Teach your patient how to manage these signs and symptoms of chronic renal failure.

Itching

Itching, which results from dry skin, calcium and phosphorus imbalances, and uremic toxins, can be relieved by antipruritic drugs and by using moisturizing soaps and lotions. Tell the patient to avoid using deodorant soaps and bathing daily in hot water.

Cramps

Tell the patient to promptly report muscle cramps to the doctor so that he can treat their cause.

Mouth odor

To minimize uremic mouth odor, encourage good oral hygiene and regular dental visits. Good oral hygiene also helps prevent infections.

Depression

Lifelong kidney disease disrupts the patient's normal activities, lifestyle, and relationships and may trigger serious depression. To help the patient manage depression, encourage him to express his feelings and formulate ways to empower him, such as joining support groups.

Sexual dysfunction

In any patient with chronic renal failure, anemia may cause fatigue and weakness while medications, especially antihypertensives, can cause impotence. Altered body image, resulting from pallor, discolored skin, uremic mouth odor, or the presence of a vascular access device or peritoneal catheter, may contribute to sexual difficulties.

Stick with the regimen

To help the patient deal with his sexual concerns, encourage him to follow his treatment regimen closely; this should improve his feelings of well-being. If antihypertensive drugs cause impotence, the patient should discuss with the doctor the option of changing drugs.

Talk about it

Give the patient an opportunity to talk openly about psychological obstacles. Ask for a sexual history and encourage him to share his feelings. Advise him to pursue sexual activity when he's most energetic—perhaps in the morning or after a rest. Explain that time pressures and stress inhibit sexual pleasure. Because role reversal may affect his relationship with his partner, be sure to include his spouse in your discussion. Reassure them that sexual activity won't damage the patient's health.

Touch, stroke, caress

If intercourse isn't possible, discuss other forms of sexual expression, such as touching, stroking, and caressing. Advise the patient that a close, supportive relationship with his partner is crucial in managing his disorder.

Hypotension during hemodialysis

Tell the patient to notify the nurse if he experiences any of the following symptoms of hypotension during hemodialysis:
- dizziness
- hot or cold flashes
- headache or nausea.

A lifelong commitment (unless...)

Emphasize that the patient needs to continue hemodialysis for life unless he receives a successful transplant or changes to peritoneal dialysis.

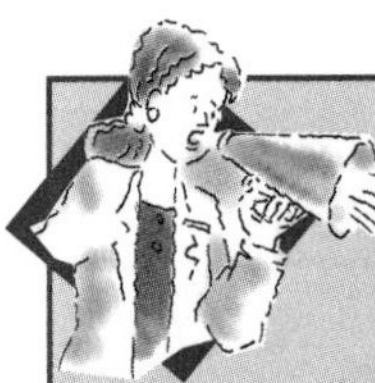

Listen up!

Transplant talk

Tell the transplant candidate that successful transplantation restores renal function. Stress that he'll need medical follow-up for the rest of his life. Inform him that the donor kidney can come from a healthy family member or from a donor. Tell him that before transplantation, he'll have a comprehensive examination and tests to identify and treat any disorders that might complicate recovery.

Quick! We're ready

Review what to expect before surgery. If a donor kidney is to be used, the patient is notified when a kidney is available; then surgery is performed immediately. Stress the importance of staying healthy during the waiting period so the surgery can be performed safely on short notice.

How long?

Tell the patient that surgery usually takes 3 to 4 hours.

A close watch

After surgery, the patient is monitored closely in an intensive care or transplant unit. A catheter is inserted in his bladder to monitor urine output.

Protection against rejection

Immunosuppressive drugs are given to prevent rejection. Explain that immunosuppressive therapy, with such drugs as cyclosporine, continues for as long as the transplanted kidney remains in place.

Just in case

If a donor kidney doesn't function immediately (possibly from damage related to removal or transplantation), dialysis can sustain the patient until treatment restores renal function.

It gets complicated

Discuss possible longer-term complications of transplantation, including recurrent glomerulonephritis in the new kidney, drug-induced diabetes mellitus, aseptic necrosis of the hip joints, cancer, muscle wasting, and coronary artery disease.

Teaching about surgery

Nephrectomy (the removal of part or all of a kidney) is indicated if the kidneys are severely infected, greatly enlarged from cystic disease, or causing renin-induced hypertension. Show the patient the incision site in the flank over the affected kidney.

Better quality of life at one-third the cost

For patients with end-stage renal disease, especially for those who want to avoid dialysis or improve their quality of life, kidney transplantation is the treatment of choice. Also, the cost of maintaining a successful kidney transplant is one-third that of dialysis. (See *Transplant talk.*)

Glomerulonephritis

Glomerulonephritis encompasses a variety of kidney disorders that cause inflammation in the glomeruli (the filtering structures of the kidney). The major types of glomerulonephritis include acute (poststreptococcal glomerulonephritis and infectious glomerulonephritis), chronic, and rapidly progressive forms.

What's poststreptococcal glomerulonephritis?

Poststreptococcal glomerulonephritis is the more common form of acute glomerulonephritis. This form follows a streptococcal infection of the respiratory tract or, less commonly, a skin infection such as impetigo. Symptoms usually develop about 1 to 4 weeks after the original infection. (See *Signs of poststreptococcal glomerulonephritis*.)

This form of glomerulonephritis may resolve spontaneously in about 2 weeks. Usually, the disorder strikes children, most of whom recover fully. It tends to be more serious in adults; about 30% progress to chronic renal failure within months.

Tell the patient with poststreptococcal glomerulonephritis to expect an initial phase of oliguria (decreased urine output), lasting 10 to 14 days, followed by a phase of copious urine output.

Signs of poststreptococcal glomerulonephritis

- Fatigue
- Fluid retention
- Hematuria
- Oliguria (less than 400 ml [13.5 oz] of urine daily)
- Proteinuria
- Mild to severe hypertension
- Dyspnea
- Cough
- Smoky or coffee-colored urine (indicating blood in the urine)

What's infectious glomerulonephritis?

Infectious glomerulonephritis is usually associated with a bacterial, viral, or parasitic infection elsewhere in the body. It differs from poststreptococcal glomerulonephritis in that its symptoms occur during or within a few days of the original infection.

What's chronic glomerulonephritis?

Chronic glomerulonephritis is a diverse group of disorders that cause progressive kidney damage. It destroys the glomeruli and renal tubules, causing kidney shrinkage and loss of function.

This form of glomerulonephritis usually develops insidiously and asymptomatically, typically over many years. Kidney inflammation and scarring occur imperceptibly.

By the time signs and symptoms emerge, chronic glomerulonephritis may be irreversible, eventually resulting in renal failure. The course of the disorder may vary. (See *Signs of chronic glomerulonephritis*.)

Explain that chronic glomerulonephritis may occur as a primary kidney disorder or follow a systemic disorder. Acute glomerulonephritis also may progress to the chronic form.

What's rapidly progressive glomerulonephritis?

Rapidly progressive glomerulonephritis swiftly destroys the glomeruli, resulting in irreversible renal failure within days or months. Acute glomerulonephritis or other factors may trigger this rare disorder.

What's at risk?

Emphasize that untreated glomerulonephritis can lead to complications that may result in end-stage renal disease, an irreversible condition that requires dialysis or kidney transplantation.

Mention also that glomerulonephritis increases the risk for nephrotic syndrome, a group of signs and symptoms that result from glomerular damage. Nephrotic syndrome can lead to chronic renal failure. (See *Signs of nephrotic syndrome,* page 234.)

Teaching about tests

Diagnosis of glomerulonephritis requires a detailed medical history, an assessment of signs and symptoms, and laboratory tests. Encourage the patient to report even seemingly trivial signs and symptoms — for example, unexplained weight gain, a change in urinary frequency, or a waistband that suddenly feels snug.

If it's acute

If acute glomerulonephritis is indicated, throat or skin cultures may be used to identify the causative bacteria. Imaging studies, such as renal CT scan, MRI, KUB radiography, and renal ultrasonography, may be ordered to evaluate the kidneys' structure and function. Additional tests may include renal angiography, renal biopsy, and retrograde ureteropyelography. (See *Teaching patients about renal and urologic tests,* pages 223 to 225.)

Signs of chronic glomerulonephritis

Early
- High blood pressure
- Hematuria
- Proteinuria

Midstage
- Edema in the legs and around the eyes
- Persistent hypertension (indicating kidney damage)
- Mild headaches
- Orthopnea
- Dyspnea during exertion

Late-stage
- Nausea
- Vomiting
- Pruritus (itchy skin)
- Malaise
- Fatigue
- Mild to severe anemia
- Severe hypertension
- Azotemia (abnormal nitrogen in the blood)

In all cases

Blood and urine tests are routinely performed in all types of glomerulonephritis. These may include CBC; hemoglobin and hematocrit evaluations; electrolyte analyses; tests to determine serum protein, creatinine, uric acid, and BUN levels; and analyses, such as antistreptolysin O antibody titer, to detect streptococcal organisms. Follow-up tests may be ordered to monitor the patient's progress and response to therapy.

Signs of nephrotic syndrome

- Swelling around the eyes on waking in the morning (an early sign)
- Frothy urine
- Progressive, generalized edema
- Nausea and vomiting
- Anorexia
- Abdominal pain
- Light-headedness on standing
- Lethargy
- Depression
- Pallor

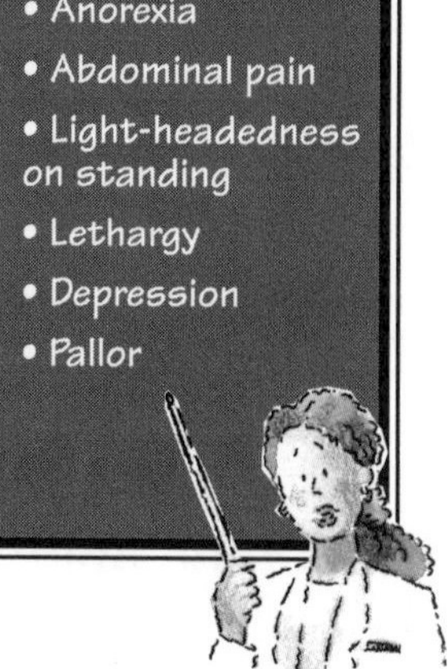

Teaching about activity and lifestyle

Encourage the patient with acute glomerulonephritis to comply with the bed rest plan recommended by his doctor. Stress that rest promotes healing whereas overactivity may cause hematuria and proteinuria.

Pillow talk

Warn the patient with edema that he may become short of breath during exertion. If he has orthopnea, advise him to elevate his head while lying down and to use an extra pillow if necessary. Show him how to turn and reposition himself to prevent skin breakdown.

Making a comeback

After the period of bed rest, encourage the patient to resume daily activities gradually. Because he'll tire easily at first, suggest that he take frequent rest breaks and limit his activities, depending on his degree of renal compromise.

Teaching about diet

A prescribed diet is typically high in calories and low in sodium, potassium, and fluid. (For a list of high-potassium foods to avoid as well as recommended low-potassium foods, see *High or low potassium?* For a list of high-sodium foods, see *Saturated with sodium*, page 236.)

More or less

The doctor may order protein replacement or restriction. Accordingly, help the patient plan dietary changes that incorporate his food preferences.

Advice for the thirsty

Show the patient how to measure his fluid intake and output. Explain how this can help prevent fluid overload and related edema and other complications. If his fluid intake is restricted, suggest that he suck on sugarless hard candy to relieve a dry mouth and use ice chips rather than a glass of water to relieve his thirst.

Teaching about medication

For acute poststreptococcal glomerulonephritis, the doctor may order an antibiotic. For chronic glomerulonephritis, he may prescribe an immunosuppressant, such as azathioprine, cyclosporine, or a corticosteroid, to block the normal antigen-antibody response. Other key medications include antihypertensive drugs, such as hydralazine, to treat hypertension and diuretics, such as furosemide, to control edema.

Riskier now

Explain that the doctor may periodically discontinue or change previously prescribed medications. Because this disorder leaves the kidneys less efficient at removing drugs from the body, the patient is at increased risk for toxic effects from medications.

Teaching about procedures

Explain that procedures, such as dialysis or plasmapheresis, may be recommended, depending on the patient's condition and type of glomerulonephritis.

Discussing dialysis

If the doctor orders dialysis for kidney failure that doesn't respond to other treatments, explain the two types of dialysis: hemodialysis and peritoneal dialysis. They remove toxic wastes from the blood when the kidneys can't perform this function. (See *Describing dialysis,* page 227.)

Planning for plasmapheresis

If the doctor recommends plasmapheresis to remove circulating antibody complexes from the blood, inform the patient that this special blood-filtering technique removes blood from the body, separating its components to allow

High or low potassium?

Avoid foods with high potassium

- Apricots
- Avocados
- Bananas
- Cantaloupe
- Carrots
- Cauliflower
- Chocolate
- Dried beans
- Dried fruit
- Liver
- Oranges
- Peanuts, nuts
- Potatoes
- Prune juice
- Pumpkin
- Spinach
- Sweet potatoes
- Tomatoes

Eat foods with low potassium

- Apples, pears
- Cranberries
- Grapes
- Canned carrots
- Corn
- Green beans
- Summer squash
- Noodles, rice, white bread

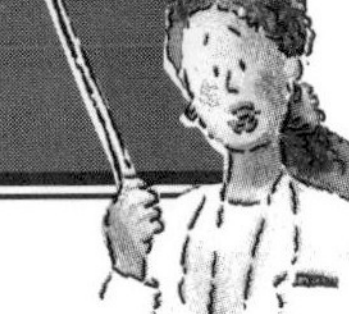

removal of the causative antibody complexes. The purified blood components are then returned to the body.

Suggesting surgery

If conservative treatments fail and kidney failure develops, the patient may need to consider nephrectomy or kidney transplantation. (See *Transplant talk*, page 231.)

Neurogenic bladder

Neurogenic bladder results from altered bladder innervation and may lead to urinary tract infections (UTIs), hydronephrosis, and calculi formation. It affects more than 1 million Americans of all ages.

What is it?

Tell the patient that neurogenic bladder involves a dysfunction caused by a lesion of the central or peripheral nervous system. This leads to inadequate bladder storage capacity and voiding problems, such as incontinence and incomplete emptying.

What causes it?

Many possible underlying causes may lead to neurogenic bladder, including multiple sclerosis, stroke, dementia, diabetes mellitus, and tumors.

What is spastic neurogenic bladder?

Spastic neurogenic bladder results from spinal cord damage above the sacral segments of the spinal cord. (See *Signs of spastic neurogenic bladder.*)

What is flaccid neurogenic bladder?

Flaccid neurogenic bladder results from spinal cord damage at or below the sacral segments of the spinal cord. The bladder becomes flaccid, resulting in overfilling and overdistention, less efficient bladder and detrusor muscle contractions, and lack of bladder sensation, so the patient doesn't realize when his bladder is full. Other effects include urine retention, UTIs, and overflow incontinence.

Saturated with sodium

- Bouillon
- Canned foods
- Celery
- Cheeses
- Chinese food
- Dried fruit
- Frozen foods
- Monosodium glutamate
- Mustard
- Olives
- Pickles
- Preserved meat
- Salad dressing and prepared sauces
- Sauerkraut
- Snack foods (crackers, chips, pretzels)
- Soy sauce

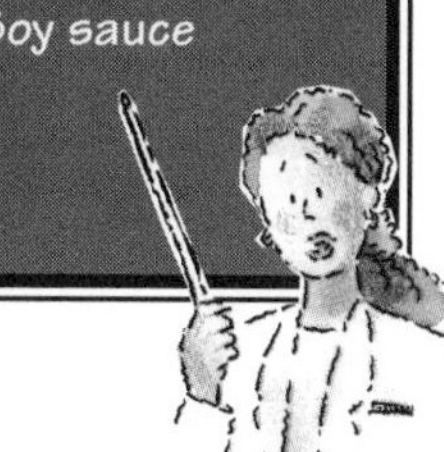

What's at risk?

Warn the patient that untreated neurogenic bladder can lead to recurrent UTIs, calculi formation, hydronephrosis, and renal failure (a life-threatening complication).

Teaching about tests

One of your primary goals when caring for a patient with this disorder is to guide him through a lengthy diagnostic workup to identify his bladder dysfunction.

Tell me everything

Tell the patient he will need to provide a thorough medical history, emphasizing neurologic and urologic problems. Routine laboratory tests, including a urinalysis and urine culture, may be used to screen for renal or urinary tract disease and UTI. Other diagnostic tests may include excretory urography, cystourethroscopy, urodynamic tests (cystometry, external sphincter electromyography, and uroflometry), retrograde cystography, and voiding cystourethrography. (See *Teaching patients about renal and urologic tests,* pages 223 to 225.)

Teaching about activity and lifestyle

Teach the patient to recognize when the bladder is full. (See *It's a full bladder,* page 238.) Instruct him to record what time he voids, the length of time between voidings, fluid intake, and urine output. This record keeping will help avoid bladder distention.

Help the patient help himself

Explain self-care measures that can help the patient empty the bladder and avoid UTIs. (See *Self-care for neurogenic bladder,* page 238.)

Teaching about diet

Advise the patient to drink 8 to 10 glasses (at least 64 oz [2 L]) of fluids each day to flush his urinary system and reduce the risk of UTIs. He should drink 8 oz (237 ml) every 2 hours and try to void 30 minutes later. Remind the pa-

Signs of spastic neurogenic bladder

- Loss of conscious sensation in the bladder
- Decreased bladder capacity
- Hypertrophy of the bladder wall
- Spontaneous detrusor muscle contractions
- Urinary sphincter spasms
- Urinary frequency and retention
- Recurrent urinary tract infections
- Lack of urinary control, including stress incontinence

tient to count as fluids any foods that are liquids at room temperature, such as gelatin, pudding, and ice cream.

Crave cranberry

Recommend drinking cranberry juice daily to help keep the urine acidic and decrease the risk of UTIs. Instruct the patient to avoid foods rich in calcium and phosphorus to reduce the risk of developing kidney stones. Ascorbic acid (vitamin C) may be prescribed to help maintain urine acidity.

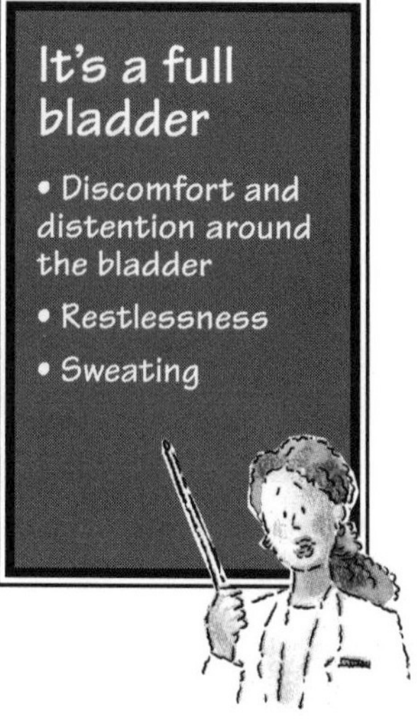

It's a full bladder
• Discomfort and distention around the bladder
• Restlessness
• Sweating

Teaching about medication

Drug therapy — usually the first-line treatment for neurogenic bladder — can correct incontinence by:

- helping the bladder empty more efficiently
- improving coordination between the detrusor muscle and the urethral sphincter.

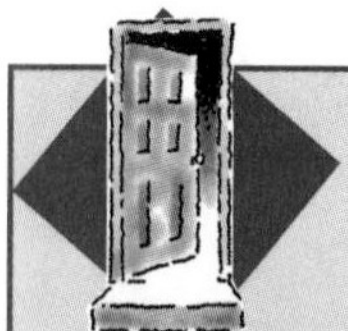

No place like home

Self-care for neurogenic bladder

Discuss with the patient methods to help him empty his bladder at home.

Manual stimulation
If the patient has a spastic neurogenic bladder, teach him to activate urination and relax the urethral sphincter by stimulating "trigger areas." Tell him to sit on the toilet and stroke his abdomen or genitalia, then pull gently on his pubic hair. Or he can digitally stimulate the anal sphincter.

Credé's method
If the patient has a flaccid neurogenic bladder, teach him to manually empty the bladder. Instruct him to sit on the toilet and apply pressure to his abdomen over the bladder, moving his fingers downward in a "milking" motion.

Valsalva's maneuver
This method is also effective for the patient with a flaccid neurogenic bladder. Instruct him to sit on the toilet, then forcibly exhale while keeping his mouth closed. This helps the bladder release urine and promotes complete emptying.

Intermittent self-catheterization
In conjunction with a bladder training program, intermittent self-catheterization is especially useful for a patient with a flaccid neurogenic bladder. Discuss the importance of cleaning the catheter to decrease the chance of infection.

Indwelling catheterization
Usually, indwelling catheterization is reserved for patients who lack the manual dexterity to perform a bladder training program, such as those with multiple sclerosis or other neuromuscular problems.

Drugs used to treat neurogenic bladder may include anticholinergics such as propantheline bromide (Pro-Banthine), antispasmodics such as flavoxate hydrochloride (Urispas), cholinergics such as bethanechol chloride (Urecholine), and external sphincter relaxants such as dantrolene sodium (Dantrium).

Teaching about procedures

If your patient has an indwelling catheter, teach him and his family how to care for it at home and how to cope with any problems. Discuss what to do if the catheter becomes blocked and how to recognize signs and symptoms of infection. Urge the patient to contact the doctor or nurse if these problems arise. (See *Caring for an indwelling catheter.*)

Teaching about surgery

An artificial urinary sphincter or a bladder pacemaker may be implanted if other measures fail to improve the pa-

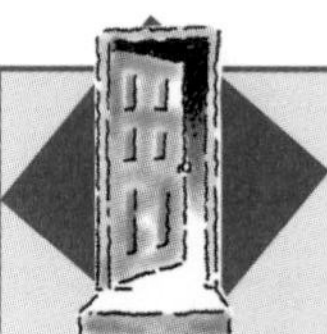

No place like home

Caring for an indwelling catheter

If your patient has an indwelling catheter, teach him ways to prevent or at least control bladder infection.

Catheter care

Tell the patient to wash the catheter area with soap and water twice daily to keep it from becoming irritated or infected. Also instruct him to wash the rectal area whenever he has a bowel movement. He should dry the skin gently but thoroughly.

Instruct the patient to wash the drainage tubing and bag with soap and water once daily, followed by a rinse with a solution made from about 1 part white vinegar to 7 parts water. Tell him to empty his leg drainage bag at least every 4 hours and his bedside drainage bag at least every 8 hours.

Stress the need to always keep the drainage bag below bladder level. Warn the patient never to pull on the catheter. Tell him to disconnect it from the drainage tubing only to clean the bag.

Call now

Advise the patient to call the doctor right away if he has:

- urine leakage or discharge around the catheter
- pain in the bladder area
- abdominal pain and fullness
- scanty urine flow
- blood or particles in his urine
- temperature above 100° F (37.7° C)
- cloudy urine.

tient's bladder function. If necessary, an alternative route for urine excretion may be surgically created.

Cutaneous ureterostomy

In this surgery, one or both ureters are detached from the bladder and brought through the skin to form one or two stomas.

Ileal conduit

In this surgery, the ureters are connected to a small portion of the ileum excised especially for the procedure, followed by creation of a stoma from one end of the ileal segment.

Before and after

Tell the patient to fast for several hours before either surgery because a general anesthetic is used. Point out that, after surgery, his vital signs will be monitored until he's stable, and his dressings will be checked periodically and changed at least once every shift. Also, he will have a nasogastric tube in place after surgery.

How does this work?

Review the doctor's explanation of the urine collection device used after surgery. Encourage the patient to handle the device to help ease his acceptance of it. Reassure him that he'll receive complete training on how to use it after he returns from surgery.

Voice of experience

If possible, arrange for a visit by a well-adjusted ostomy patient who can provide a firsthand account of the surgery and offer insight into the realities of stoma and collection-device care. Include members of the patient's family in the session, especially those who will provide routine care at home.

Not alone

Finally, refer the patient and his family to a support group such as the United Ostomy Association or the American Gastroenterological Association (www.gastro.org).

Renal calculi

Calculi, also called kidney stones, vary in size from minute granular deposits—called sand or gravel—to bladder stones the size of an orange. Small calculi seldom cause problems because they're easily carried through the ureter and out of the body with urine. A larger calculus, however, can cause excruciating pain if it enters the ureter. It may also become lodged there.

Gadzooks! Renal calculi can range in size from minute granular deposits to the size of an orange.

How does it start?

Explain that calculi usually begin when tiny specks of undissolved material remain in the urinary tract. As more material clings to these specks, they gradually develop into calculi. Calculi typically form in the kidneys but can develop anywhere in the urinary tract, including the ureters and bladder.

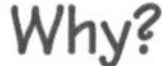

Why?

The kidneys excrete some substances that are insoluble and are normally excreted with minimal crystal formation. Various risk factors may lead to increased crystal formation and stone development. (See *Risk factors for renal calculi.*)

Risk factors for renal calculi

Discuss with your patient the following predisposing factors for renal calculi:

- *metabolic disorders.* These disorders include cystinuria, renal tubular acidosis, hypercalcemia, hyperoxaluria, hyperuricuria, and hypomagnesemia.
- *geography.* The Northwest, Southeast, and Southwest of the United States are known as "calculi belts."
- *climate.* Exposure to sunlight increases vitamin D production (and calcium absorption).
- *diet.* Eating too much animal protein can raise calcium oxalate and uric acid levels by 50% in calculus-forming patients.
- *dehydration.* Diminished water intake and reduced urine production concentrate calculus-forming substances.
- *urinary tract abnormalities.* Narrow tracts can trap and form stones.
- *sedentary jobs.* These jobs are linked to upper urinary tract calculi.
- *obstruction.* Urinary stasis (as in spinal cord injury) allows calculus constituents to accumulate.
- *drug therapy.* Certain medications, vitamins C and D, and calcium supplements can promote calculi development.

Other causes

Chemotherapeutic drugs and external radiation may cause cellular breakdown and acute hyperuricemia. Furosemide may cause hyperuricemia as well.

What's at risk?

Calculi too large for natural passage can obstruct the urinary tract. Unless calculi are removed, urine trapped above the obstruction sets the stage for renal infection. Eventually, the kidneys' collection system may become abnormally dilated—holding up to several liters of urine. This condition, called hydronephrosis, may lead to renal insufficiency if untreated.

Teaching about tests

Explain that the patient will be asked to provide a thorough medical history, focusing on the type, location, and duration of pain and the presence of fever.

Blood tests

Blood is drawn for CBC and to determine calcium, phosphorus, BUN, creatinine, glucose, uric acid, and electrolyte levels. Tests to measure serum calcium and phosphorus may be repeated on 3 different days to determine average levels. (See *Teaching patients about renal and urologic tests,* pages 223 to 225.)

Urine tests

Teach the patient how to collect a clean-catch urine specimen and a 24-hour urine collection for routine urinalysis and special urine testing.

Teaching about activity and lifestyle

As part of any treatment for renal calculi, advise the patient to watch for and report passage of bloody urine and the following signs or symptoms of infection:
- increased pain
- inability to void
- change in the color or odor of his urine
- temperature over 101° F (38.3° C).

Strain, save, analyze

After calculi removal, instruct the patient to strain his urine after voiding and to save any solid material for analysis. Explain that knowing the composition of calculi helps the doctor pinpoint what's causing them to form.

Teaching about diet

Because most renal calculi contain calcium (combined with phosphate and some other substances), the patient should reduce his intake of calcium and phosphorus.

Hold the calcium and phosphorus!

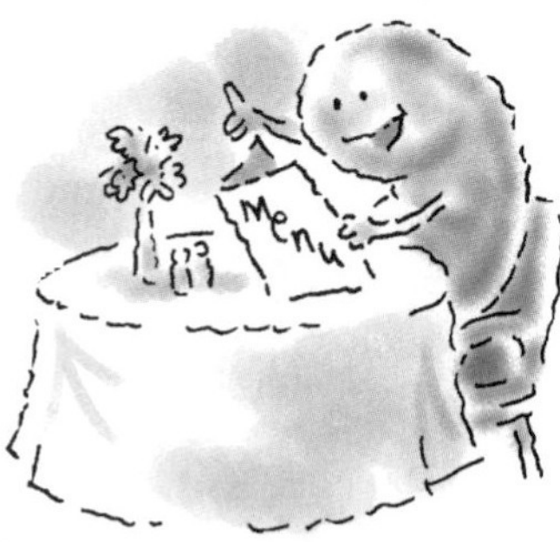

I'll pass

To avoid calculi recurrence, teach the patient which foods to avoid. (See *Eat less or none at all.*)

Drink up

If the patient is on a nonrestricted fluid diet, instruct him to drink at least 12 glasses of fluid each day, to keep urine volume at about 2 quarts (2 L) daily.

Teaching about medication

Drug therapy depends on the composition of the patient's calculi and may continue indefinitely to prevent recurrence. Ammonium chloride or acetohydroxamic acid (Lithostat) may be prescribed to acidify the urine, which helps prevent more calculi from forming.

Teaching about procedures

As appropriate, teach the patient about invasive and noninvasive procedures to remove calculi. (See *Calculi killers,* page 244.)

Eat less or none at all

- Meat (once per day or less, to cut down on protein)
- Cheese (contains calcium)
- Beets
- Spinach
- Chocolate
- Tea (contains oxalate)
- Carbonated soft drinks (contain phosphorus)

Urinary tract infection

UTIs affect people of all ages and are among the most common urologic disorders. UTIs are 10 times more common in females than males.

What causes UTI?

Explain that a lower UTI, such as urethritis and cystitis, involves the urethra, bladder, or both. Lower UTI results from infection by bacteria.

Upper UTI (called pyelonephritis) affects the kidneys. It usually results from bacterial infection from normal intestinal and fecal flora that grow readily in urine.

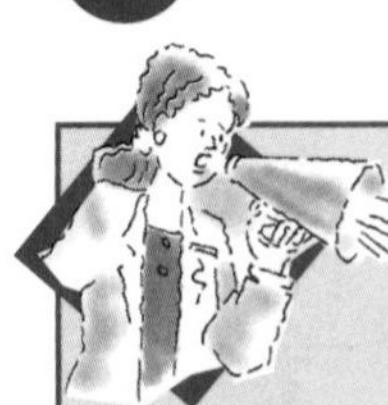

Listen up!

Calculi killers

Teach your patient about invasive and noninvasive procedures to remove calculi.

Extracorporeal shock-wave lithotripsy
Explain that extracorporeal shock-wave lithotripsy successfully removes calculi in 75% of patients with ureteral calculi. Tell the patient scheduled for this procedure that while he sits in a large water tank or tub, the water transmits high-pressure shock waves into the body. Alternatively, he lies on a stretcher over a water-filled cushion; the cushion, containing a shock electrode and reflector, is coupled to the stretcher by a layer of ultrasonic gel and placed against the patient's lower back. Explain that the procedure using the water-filled cushion can be performed with a sedative-analgesic rather than a general anesthetic because improved shock generators keep shock-wave intensity high but below the patient's pain threshold. The goal is to crush the stone small enough to be passed in the urine.

Endoscopic stone manipulation
Tell the patient that this procedure is used to remove small calculi (less than ⅜" [1 cm] in diameter) in the lower ureter. Using a cystoscope, the doctor inserts special loops or basket catheters into the ureter to capture and remove the calculus.

If the doctor is unable to remove the calculus, he may leave a loop or ureteral catheter in place to dilate the ureter for later manipulation. He may also leave a ureteral catheter in place after the procedure to prevent obstruction from edema.

Ultrasonic endoscopy
Inform the patient scheduled for ultrasonic endoscopy that, in this procedure, the trapped calculus is fragmented with an ultrasonic probe and then removed by suction. A J-stent (a catheter that helps to pass the calculus and drain urine) is usually left in place until after discharge.

Percutaneous ultrasonic lithotripsy
Tell the patient that this procedure (also called percutaneous nephrolithotripsy) removes kidney or upper ureteral calculi. Explain that the doctor uses an electrohydraulic or ultrasonic probe to fragment larger calculi with electrical or ultrasonic energy. He removes larger fragments with a basket catheter and smaller pieces with continuous suction through a nephroscope.

Laser lithotripsy
Explain that this procedure directs laser light through a ureteroscope to the calculus, where strobe-light pulsations create tiny shock waves. These pulsations fragment calculi without damaging the ureteral wall.

Chemolysis
Describe how this procedure uses drugs to break up calculi. Tell the patient that the drugs are delivered through a nephrostomy tube to renal calculi or through a catheter to bladder and ureteral calculi. Hemiacidrin is used for struvite dissolution, and sodium bicarbonate for uric acid dissolution.

Surgery
Before the advent of lithotripsy, surgical removal of renal calculi was the major mode of therapy. Today, however, surgery is performed on only about 1% to 2% of patients.

If the patient requires surgery to remove calculi, reinforce the doctor's explanations and answer any questions. Depending on the type and location of the calculi, surgery may involve pyelolithotomy, ureterolithotomy, nephrolithotomy, percutaneous nephrostomy, or nephrectomy.

Symptoms of upper or lower UTI may develop rapidly (if at all) over a few hours or a few days.

What happens in lower UTI?

Explain that lower UTIs usually produce the following symptoms:

- urinary urgency and frequency
- dysuria
- bladder cramps or spasms
- itching
- a feeling of warmth during urination
- nocturia.

Males may complain of urethral discharge. If the bladder wall is inflamed, the patient may also have fever and hematuria. Other common symptoms include abdominal pain or tenderness over the bladder, chills, flank pain, low back pain, malaise, nausea, and vomiting.

What happens in upper UTI?

Upper UTI causes the following symptoms:

- urinary urgency and frequency
- burning during urination
- dysuria
- nocturia
- hematuria.

The urine may appear cloudy and have an ammonia or fishlike odor. Other typical signs and symptoms include a temperature of 102° F (38.9° C) or higher, chills, flank pain, anorexia, and fatigue.

What else?

Although symptoms may resolve without treatment, residual infection is common, and symptoms are likely to recur.

What's at risk?

Warn that failure to observe treatment guidelines can lead to serious complications, such as chronic pyelonephritis, a leading cause of end-stage renal disease. Other kidney damage may occur from chronic UTIs — especially if the patient has a neurogenic bladder, which permits urine retention and consequent infection.

Teaching about tests

Laboratory tests may include urinalysis and culture (to reveal signs of infection and the disease-causing agent), smear and stain of urethral discharge, and CBC. If the patient must collect a urine specimen at home, advise her to put it in a sealed container placed within a plastic bag and store it in the refrigerator to keep bacteria from multiplying. She should take it to the laboratory within 1 hour.

Hey, it's an X-ray!

Discuss radiographic tests, such as KUB radiography, excretory urography, and voiding cystourethrography. KUB radiography—an abdominal X-ray study—shows the position of the kidneys, ureters, and bladder and possible abnormalities. Depending on KUB findings, other studies are usually conducted. (See *Teaching patients about renal and urologic tests,* pages 223 to 225.)

Teaching about activity and lifestyle

Tell the patient that she needn't restrict most activities. She should, however, avoid prolonged bicycling, motorcycling, and horseback riding. These activities may promote urine reflux and may damage the urinary tract.

Let me suggest a few changes

Suggest lifestyle changes to help the patient cope with her condition and fight recurrent UTIs. (See *Living with a UTI.*)

Teaching about diet

Advise the patient to consume additional fluids—up to 14 glasses (3.5 qt [3.5 L]) of water daily—to flush out bacteria. Encourage her to eat foods and drink fluids with a high acid content to acidify her urine and inhibit urinary tract bacteria. High-acid foods include meats, nuts, plums, prunes, and whole-grain breads and cereals. High-acid drinks include cranberry and other fruit juices. (See *Culinary cautions.*)

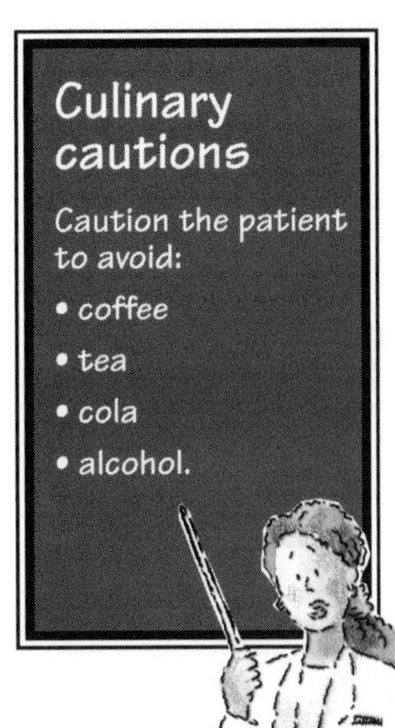
Culinary cautions
Caution the patient to avoid:
• coffee
• tea
• cola
• alcohol.

Teaching about medications

A single-dose or short-term antibiotic usually kills or controls infection and relieves symptoms by rapidly sterilizing the urine. Urge the patient to have her urine analyzed again 1 to 3 days after treatment starts, to check the drug's effectiveness. If she has frequent UTIs, tell her she may require long-term, low-dose antibiotic prophylaxis.

Other antibiotics, such as sulfonamide and urinary tract antiseptics, may be used to treat UTIs. The doctor

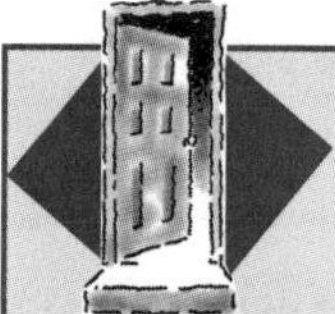

No place like home

Living with a UTI

Here's some advice to help your patient cope with a urinary tract infection (UTI) and prevent it from occurring again.

Until the very end
Tell the patient to take her prescribed medicine exactly as her doctor directs. Warn the patient not to stop taking her medicine just because she feels better. She should finish the prescription to kill all infection-causing organisms. Otherwise, she runs the risk that the infection will come back.

Soothe me
Tell the patient to lay a warm heating pad on her abdomen and sides to soothe any pain and burning sensations. Suggest that she try a warm sitz bath, or that she ask her doctor to prescribe a pain reliever.

It's only sensible
Encourage the patient to practice sensible hygiene. For example, tell her to wipe from front to back each time she goes to the bathroom. This reduces the chance that bacteria from bowel movements will enter her urinary tract.

Dress code
Tell the patient to:
- change her underpants daily
- wear cotton undergarments — cotton permits ventilation, which deters bacterial growth
- avoid tight slacks that prevent air circulation.

Shower power
Encourage the patient to take showers instead of baths because bacteria in the bath water can enter her urinary tract. Tell her to avoid bubble baths, bath oils, perfumed vaginal sprays, and strong bleaches and detergents when doing laundry. These products can irritate her perineal area, which may trigger bacteria growth and infection.

Don't hesitate
Tell the patient to urinate frequently (every 3 hours) to completely empty her bladder. Tell her to use the bathroom as soon as she senses the need. Delayed urination is a major cause of UTIs. Also, advise her to urinate after sexual relations. This will help rid her urinary tract of bacteria.

Pick up the phone
Tell the patient to call her doctor right away if she suspects a new or repeated UTI. Also, tell her to call the doctor if she notices such symptoms as an increased urge to urinate, increased urination (especially at night), pain when she urinates, or bloody or cloudy urine.

may prescribe a nonnarcotic analgesic to treat pain related to the UTI.

Teaching about surgery

Surgery may be recommended to correct an obstruction that causes recurrent UTIs. Common obstructive disorders include calculi, tumors, and benign prostatic hyperplasia.

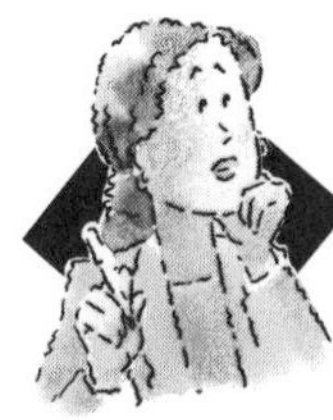

Quick quiz

1. When teaching a patient with acute renal failure, tell him his condition will likely be treated with:

A. antibiotic therapy and regulation of fluid intake.
B. extracorporeal shock-wave lithotripsy.
C. a combination of activity restrictions, medication, dietary changes, and treatment of the underlying cause.

Answer: C. Treatment might also include dialysis and surgery.

2. If the patient is going to receive hemodialysis, teach him that this procedure involves:

A. inserting a catheter into the peritoneal cavity to instill dialysate.
B. circulating the patient's blood through a dialyzer.
C. removing part or all of the kidney.

Answer: B. The patient's blood exits the body through a catheter or fistula. The blood then circulates through a dialyzer that removes waste products. The patient's blood is then returned to his body.

3. Teach the patient with a neurogenic bladder that the purpose of treatment is to:

A. maintain bladder function.
B. prepare the patient for dialysis.
C. keep the bladder free from kidney stones.

Answer: A. Other goals are to prevent infection and incontinence.

Scoring

If you answered all three items correctly, amazing! You approached this chapter with the power of a high-pressure shock wave pulverizing a renal calculus.

If you answered two items correctly, congratulations! There are no significant obstructions to your ability to teach patients about renal and urologic disorders.

If you answered fewer than two correctly, don't sweat it! Modifications in your activities, lifestyle, or diet aren't necessary. Simply review the chapter.

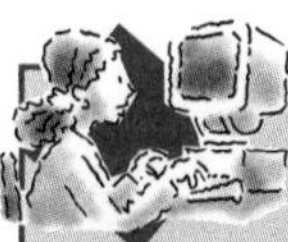

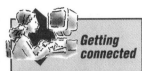

Getting connected

Kidney info on-line

For more information about renal disorders, direct the patient to the following Web sites:

- American Association of Kidney Patients (www. aakp.org)
- National Kidney Foundation (www.kidney.org)
- National Institute of Diabetes and Digestive and Kidney Diseases (www. niddk.nih.gov).

8

Endocrine disorders

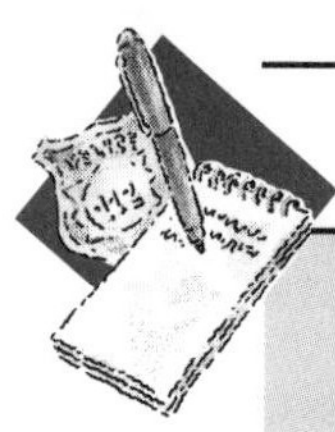

Just the facts

In this chapter, you'll learn how to teach patients with the following endocrine disorders:

- ♦ diabetes mellitus
- ♦ hyperthyroidism
- ♦ hypothyroidism
- ♦ hypoglycemia.

Diabetes mellitus

More than 10 million Americans have diabetes mellitus. Another 5 to 6 million may have the disease without even knowing it. Treatment for diabetes mellitus usually involves major, permanent lifestyle changes.

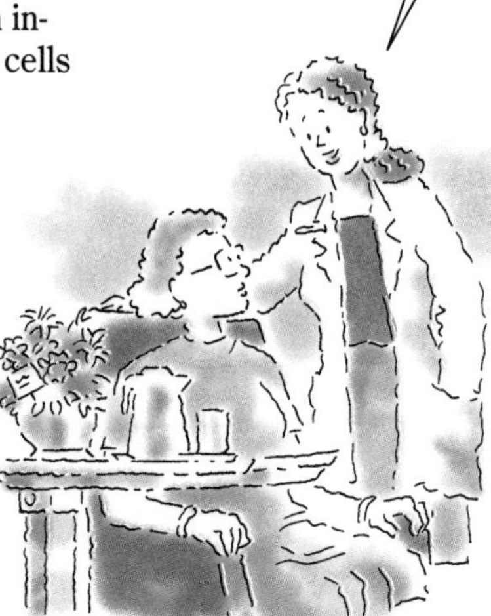
To manage your diabetes, you'll need to make major changes in your lifestyle.

What is it?

Tell the patient that diabetes mellitus is a chronic disorder caused by failure of the pancreas to produce enough insulin to control blood glucose levels or failure of the cells to make efficient use of the insulin produced.

There are two common forms of diabetes:

1. type 1, formerly called insulin-dependent diabetes mellitus
2. type 2, formerly called non-insulin-dependent diabetes mellitus, which accounts for more than 90% of all cases of diabetes mellitus and is the predominant disease form occurring in the elderly.

Type 1 diabetes usually appears before age 30...

Type 1: Sudden onset

Inform the patient with type 1 diabetes that it can develop at any age but typically appears before age 30. Its onset is usually sudden. Mention that this form of diabetes may result from a genetically determined autoimmune disease or from a viral infection that destroys the insulin-producing pancreatic beta cells. Point out to the patient that, because his pancreas doesn't produce sufficient insulin in response to elevated blood glucose levels, he needs daily insulin injections to control diabetes and prevent ketoacidosis.

Type 2: Gradual onset

Tell the patient with type 2 diabetes that this disease form can occur at any age, but is more likely to appear in middle age or later. Because its onset is gradual and symptoms are often vague, many cases go undiagnosed and untreated. Inform him that his body is producing insulin, but that a defect in insulin synthesis and release from beta cells or insulin resistance in the peripheral tissues causes his blood sugar level to rise. Mention that type 2 diabetes has a strong genetic component and is often associated with being overweight.

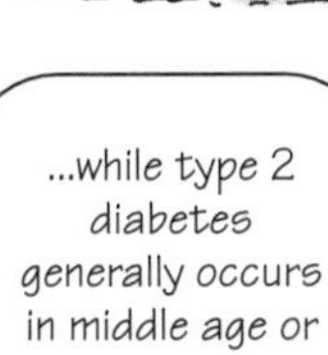
...while type 2 diabetes generally occurs in middle age or later.

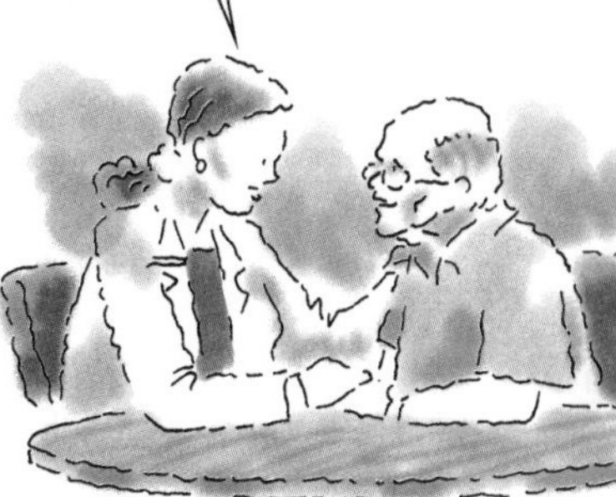

What's at risk?

No matter which diabetes form your patient has, emphasize that complying with treatment can help prevent severe — even fatal — complications. (See *It gets complicated.*)

Teaching about tests

For a patient with suspected diabetes, the diagnostic tests ordered will depend on his signs and symptoms. However, tell the patient that taking several blood samples will be necessary. Describe what he can expect from venipuncture as well as from tests that will measure blood glucose levels. Typical tests include:

- fasting plasma glucose
- random plasma glucose
- oral glucose tolerance
- glycosylated hemoglobin. (See *Teaching patients about endocrine tests,* pages 252 and 253.)

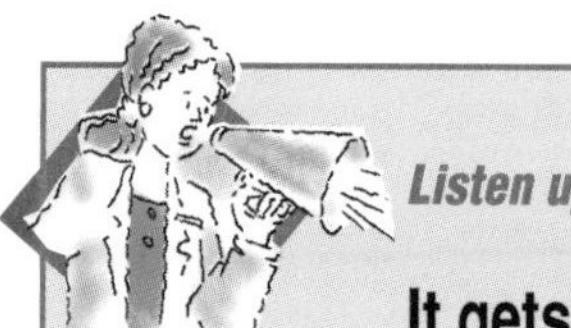

Listen up!

It gets complicated

There are several common complications stemming from diabetes.

DKA: Dangerous but reversible

Diabetic ketoacidosis (DKA) is a complication seen primarily with type 1 diabetes. Inform the patient at risk for DKA that this condition is triggered by extremely high blood glucose levels (hyperglycemia). Point out that DKA commonly results from failure to increase the insulin dosage during times of stress (such as illness, infection, or surgery). It also can occur in patients with undiagnosed or untreated diabetes. Explain that DKA may lead to metabolic acidosis and dehydration. Although life-threatening, DKA is reversible.

Hypoglycemia: An error in management

Emphasize that hypoglycemia, another acute complication, usually results from an error in diabetic management — for example, unplanned exercise or delayed or insufficient food intake. Untreated, it can cause seizures, brain damage, coma, and death.

Chronic complications: Insufficient control

Explain that chronic complications of diabetes include retinopathy, neuropathy, kidney disease, cardiovascular disease, and infections. Why these complications develop isn't clearly understood, but diabetes experts suspect that inadequate blood glucose control may be the cause. Stress that by testing his blood glucose levels daily and using these test results to make adjustments, the patient may be able to stabilize the disease and prevent complications.

Teaching about activity and lifestyle

Teach the patient that a balanced program of exercise and rest will help stabilize his blood glucose levels and reduce his insulin requirements. (See *Treatments for diabetes mellitus,* page 254.)

To the letter

Caution the patient to gear the amount of exercise to his food consumption and medication use and to follow his doctor's exercise guidelines to the letter.

Go aerobic

Recommend participating in aerobic exercises such as walking, running, cycling, and swimming to help decrease blood glucose levels.

The 240-milligram limit

Caution the patient to avoid exercising when his blood glucose level is over 240 mg/dl, especially if ketones are

(Text continues on page 254.)

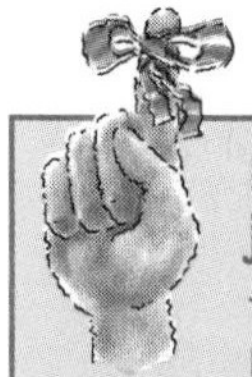

Memory jogger

To remember diabetes diagnostic tests, think *FROG:*

Fasting plasma glucose

Random plasma glucose

Oral glucose tolerance

Glycosylated hemoglobin.

Teaching patients about endocrine tests

Test and purpose	What to teach the patient
Fasting plasma glucose test • To confirm diabetes mellitus • To confirm a low blood glucose level in suspected hypoglycemia • To determine blood glucose level during a hypoglycemic episode	• The patient must not eat or drink anything except water for 12 hours before the test. • Discuss any medications the doctor wants to withhold before the test in order to avoid interference. • A fasting glucose level of 126 mg/dl or greater may indicate diabetes.
Glycosylated hemoglobin test • To assess control of diabetes mellitus	• Performed about every 3 months, this test monitors the patient's blood glucose control during the previous 2 months. • Persistently elevated test results predict a greater risk for developing chronic complications.
I.V. glucose tolerance test • To detect fasting hypoglycemia caused by insulinomas and other tumors	• The doctor prescribes a diet that ensures a daily intake of 150 to 300 g of carbohydrates for 3 days before the test. Then, for 12 hours before the test, the patient must fast. • The patient should avoid caffeine, alcohol, strenuous exercise, and smoking during the fasting and testing periods because these factors can cause misleading test results. • Discuss any medications that must be withheld during the test period. • The test lasts 5 hours; the patient is given an I.V. substance known to stimulate insulin secretion (such as tolbutamide or glucagon). • It's important to report hypoglycemic symptoms immediately. The test will be stopped and he'll be treated promptly if such symptoms occur.
Oral glucose tolerance test • To evaluate the body's response to ingested glucose • To help diagnose reactive hypoglycemia	• The doctor prescribes a diet that ensures a daily intake of 150 to 300 g of carbohydrates for 3 days before the test. For 12 hours before the test, the patient must fast. • The patient should avoid caffeine, alcohol, strenuous exercise, and smoking during the fasting and testing periods because they can cause misleading test results. • Some medications may be withheld during the test period. • The test lasts 5 hours; the patient is given a sweet solution to drink at the start of the test. He should drink all of the solution and notify the doctor or nurse immediately if symptoms of hypoglycemia occur. The interval between ingestion of the glucose solution and onset of symptoms helps determine the patient's type of reactive hypoglycemia.
Radioactive iodine uptake test • To assess thyroid function • To aid diagnosis of hyperthyroidism or hypothyroidism • To help distinguish between primary and secondary thyroid disorders	• This painless test evaluates thyroid function. The patient must fast after midnight before the test. • The patient is given a radioactive iodine capsule or liquid. After 2, 6, and 24 hours, his thyroid is scanned in the X-ray department to determine how much of the substance is present in the thyroid. The amount of radioactivity involved is extremely small and is harmless.

Teaching patients about endocrine tests *(continued)*

Test and purpose	What to teach the patient
Random plasma glucose test • To help confirm diabetes mellitus	• This test measures glucose levels. Fasting isn't necessary. • A glucose level equal to or above 200 mg/dl may indicate diabetes.
Thyroid scan (radionuclide thyroid imaging) • To evaluate the size, structure, and position of the thyroid gland • To evaluate thyroid function, in conjunction with thyroid uptake studies	• This test assesses the thyroid gland for abnormalities. It's painless and won't expose the patient to dangerous radiation levels. • The patient should follow his doctor's guidelines for discontinuing medications before the test. Usually, patients must avoid prescription and over-the-counter medications (particularly multivitamins and cough syrups) for at least 3 days. The patient should also avoid iodized salt, iodinated salt substitutes, and seafood for 3 days before the test. • The patient is given a radioisotope orally or I.V. If he's given the drug orally, his thyroid gland is X-rayed 24 hours later. If he's given the drug I.V., it's X-rayed within 20 to 30 minutes. • Before the X-ray, the patient must remove dentures and jewelry. He's then placed in a supine position with his neck extended. A special X-ray machine called a gamma camera is then placed over his throat to visualize the thyroid gland.
Ultrasonography of the pancreas or the parathyroid, thyroid, or adrenal glands • To evaluate the size and structure of the endocrine gland • To distinguish between a cyst and a solid tumor • To monitor response to therapy	• This test reveals the size and shape of the gland. It takes about 30 minutes and is painless. • For ultrasonography of the pancreas, the patient must fast for 12 hours before the test. This reduces bowel gas, which hinders transmission of ultrasound. • The patient is placed in a supine position. For ultrasonography of the thyroid or parathyroid glands, a pillow is tucked under his shoulder blades to hyperextend his neck. The skin over the gland is coated with a water-soluble gel. Next, the technician moves the transducer over the area to study the gland.

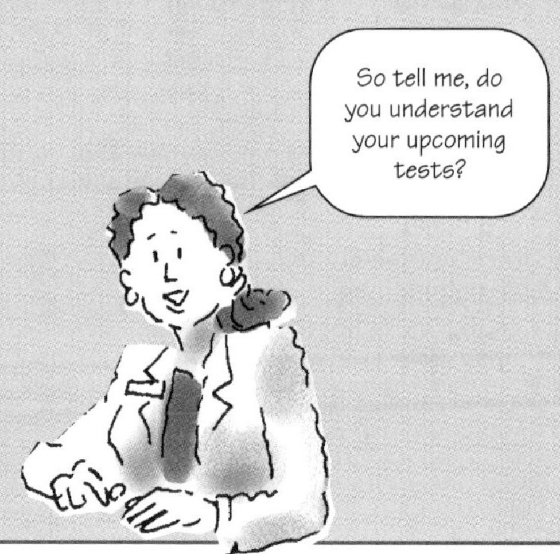
So tell me, do you understand your upcoming tests?

present in his urine, and to avoid extended sessions of anaerobic exercise, such as weight-lifting, because they can increase blood glucose levels. To achieve maximum benefit, instruct the patient to gradually build up to exercising regularly, every other day, for 40 to 60 minutes at a time.

Treatments for diabetes mellitus

- Controlled activity and diet
- Medication (insulin, an oral antidiabetic drug, or glucagon)
- Blood and urine testing along with other self-care measures

Before, during, and after

Tell the patient to ask the doctor how high his heart rate can safely go during the most intense part of the workout. If his doctor advises, instruct him to monitor his heart rate by taking his pulse before, during, and after exercise. Many doctors recommend using perceived exertion to adjust exercise intensity. For example, a common recommendation is that the patient exercise hard enough that he becomes slightly short of breath and perspires, but not so hard that he can't talk.

Just in case

Warn the patient always to carry a source of simple carbohydrates and a medical identification bracelet that gives his name, medical condition, and medications — in case he becomes hypoglycemic while exercising. Also, advise him to eat a snack before exercising, if appropriate.

Exercise don'ts

If the patient is taking insulin, advise him not to inject it into a part of his body that he'll use during exercise. Instruct him to avoid exercising at the peak of insulin activity or before meals, and caution him to refrain from drinking alcohol before exercise. Also tell him never to exercise alone.

Complete stop

Instruct the patient to stop exercising immediately if he experiences any of the following symptoms:

- chest pain
- severe dyspnea
- palpitations
- dizziness or weakness
- nausea.

If any of these symptoms persist, he should contact his doctor at once.

Teaching about diet

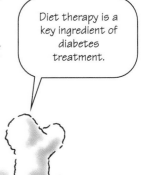

Diet therapy is a key ingredient of diabetes treatment.

Because diabetes affects metabolism, diet therapy is a key component of the treatment plan. Stress the importance of carefully following the prescribed diet to prevent rapid blood glucose changes. Make sure the patient understands his specific meal plan, and urge him to stick to it. Advise him to eat about the same number of calories each day and to spread out his meals and snacks evenly.

Encourage the patient to consult a nutritionist to help adapt the meal plan to his lifestyle, preferences, and income. If appropriate, discuss investigative diet therapy to help control blood glucose levels. (See *Carbohydrate counting,* page 256.)

Diet alone

If the patient has type 2 diabetes, explain that diet alone may control his blood glucose levels. Simply reducing his sugar intake can lower the amount of glucose he produces.

Weight reduction

If the patient is overweight, emphasize the importance of weight reduction. Explain that an obese person must produce more insulin to control his glucose levels than does a person of normal weight. Discuss ways to decrease calorie intake.

Teaching about medication

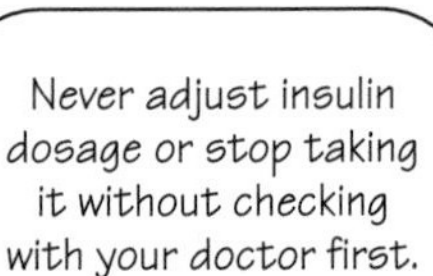

Drugs used to treat diabetes mellitus include:

- insulin
- oral antidiabetic drugs
- glucagon.

Insulin

If the patient will be taking insulin, explain that this drug helps control blood glucose levels but that it's not meant to replace a proper diet. Then outline the types of insulin available — rapid-acting, intermediate-acting, and long-acting. Caution the patient not to change the insulin type or brand without first consulting his doctor.

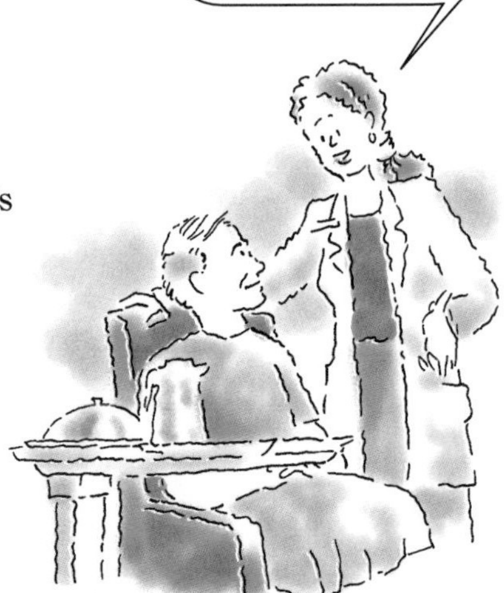

Inject here

Show the patient how to draw up insulin in a syringe and how to give himself a subcutaneous injection. Tell him that the best insulin injection sites are:
- the abdomen (except around the navel and at the waistline)
- the outer area of the upper arm
- the front and the sides of the upper thighs
- the buttocks. (See *Rotating insulin injection sites.*)

Keep with the program

Also, impress upon the patient the importance of adhering to the prescribed medication regimen. Tell him always to take his insulin on schedule and never to adjust the dosage or stop taking the drug without his doctor's approval because his blood glucose level could rise rapidly.

Brand loyalty

Also caution him to always use the same insulin, syringe, and needle brands and to be sure that the syringe corresponds with his insulin concentration. For instance, syringes for U-100 insulin should say U-100 on the package.

Avoid alcohol

Stress the need to avoid alcohol by explaining that alcohol increases insulin's hypoglycemic effect. Point out that changing food or fluid intake or taking over-the-counter drugs can affect insulin requirements.

Cool storage

Advise the patient to keep extra bottles of insulin in the refrigerator and never to let his insulin freeze. If refrigeration isn't possible, tell him to keep the insulin as cool as possible (below 86° F [30° C]) and to shield it from heat and light. Insulin kept at room temperature should be used for 30 days and then discarded. Warn him not to shake the insulin excessively.

Speak up

Finally, tell the patient to report the following adverse effects to the doctor:
- difficulty breathing
- frequent or severe hypoglycemic or hyperglycemic symptoms
- generalized itching
- redness, swelling, stinging, or itching at injection sites.

Carbohydrate counting

Planning meals with consistent amounts of carbohydrates is one of the most effective ways to achieve tight control of blood sugars.

Within 2 hours

Carbohydrates (starches and sugars in food) account for most of the increase in blood glucose levels after meals. Generally, 90% to 100% of carbohydrates are converted to blood glucose within 2 hours. Only about half of the proteins and little of the fat we eat appear as glucose.

Taking control

Patients with type 2 diabetes often limit the amount of carbohydrates eaten to minimize the after-meal rise in blood sugar level. Those with type 1 diabetes can learn to calculate the correct dose of insulin for any meal or snack by counting grams of carbohydrate.

Oral antidiabetic drugs

If the patient is taking an oral antidiabetic drug, explain that it will help regulate his blood glucose levels by increasing insulin secretion and decreasing cellular insulin resistance. Emphasize that oral antidiabetic drugs augment diet therapy and don't replace it. Caution him never to adjust the dosage or stop taking the drug without his doctor's approval.

New on the scene

Until recently, the only oral antidiabetic drugs approved for use in the United States were sulfonylureas, such as glipizide, glyburide, and tolazamide. However, three new oral drugs — metformin (Glucophage), acarbose (Precose), and troglitazone (Rezulin) — are now available. These drugs may be administered alone or given in combination with sulfonylurea therapy.

Take before meals, avoid alcohol

Warn the patient taking oral antidiabetic drugs to avoid alcohol because it may cause a disulfiram reaction (severe nausea, vomiting, and sweating) or a hypoglycemic reaction. Advise him to take the oral antidiabetic drug before meals to avoid possible GI upset.

Sound the alarm

Tell the patient to call the doctor if he has any of the following adverse reactions:

- stomach fullness
- facial flushing
- headache
- heartburn
- nausea
- rash
- vomiting
- jaundice.

He should also notify the doctor if he's ill or under increased stress because these conditions may increase his insulin needs. The doctor may adjust the dosage accordingly or prescribe insulin.

Combination of the two

If the patient takes both insulin and an oral antidiabetic drug, make sure he understands the purpose of combining these drugs. (See *Combination of the two,* page 258.)

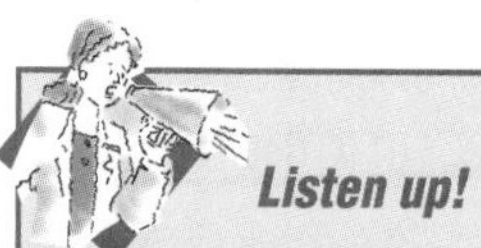

Listen up!

Rotating insulin injection sites

Whether the patient administers his insulin by needle or by insulin pump, he'll need to rotate the injection sites.

Why, why, why?
Explain that rotating the site for injecting insulin reduces injury to the skin and underlying fatty tissue and prevents swelling, lumps, and a buildup of scar tissue.

Rotating the injection site can also minimize a slow insulin absorption rate caused by fibrous tissue growth and decreased blood supply due to repeated injections in one area.

Point out that site rotation can also offset changes that exercise causes in insulin absorption. Exercise increases blood flow to the body part being exercised, thereby increasing the insulin absorption rate. That's why the patient shouldn't inject himself in an area about to be exercised. (For example, he shouldn't inject himself in the thigh before walking or riding a bike.)

Combination of the two

Explain to the patient the purpose of taking both insulin and an oral antidiabetic drug, when to take these medications, and what type of diabetes they're designed to manage.

Correcting deficiency and resistance

Patients take a daily supplemental dose, usually of an intermediate or long-acting insulin, to correct their insulin deficiency. Then they take an oral antidiabetic drug to correct peripheral insulin resistance (oral antidiabetic drugs act principally by enhancing peripheral cell sensitivity to insulin).

Timing

Usually, they take the oral antidiabetic drug 30 minutes before meals and the insulin as a small dose at bedtime. This timing takes advantage of increased peripheral cell receptivity resulting from the effects of the oral antidiabetic drug used during the day.

Who benefits?

Combined therapy works best for patients with type 2 diabetes who don't respond to oral drugs alone or who require large doses of insulin (more than 100 units a day). Because the oral antidiabetic drug increases cellular sensitivity to insulin, the insulin dosage can then be reduced. This therapy doesn't help patients with type 1 diabetes, who characteristically have total insulin deficiency, not insulin resistance.

Glucagon

For the patient taking insulin, explain that glucagon, a drug administered to treat hypoglycemic crisis, raises the blood glucose level when the patient can't take oral glucose. (See *That queasy feeling.*)

Teach the family how to administer glucagon subcutaneously. Also advise them to:

- check the expiration date regularly
- keep the correct type of syringes available.

When to inject

Make sure the patient knows the signs and symptoms of hypoglycemia. (See *Signs of hypoglycemia.*)

Advise the patient that hypoglycemia can be prevented by avoiding:

- overexertion
- inadequate food intake
- excessive insulin.

That queasy feeling

Warn the patient and his family that nausea and vomiting may occur after taking glucagon, so the patient should be turned on his side after the drug is given. Instruct them to call the doctor immediately if the patient has difficulty breathing, develops a rash, or doesn't respond to glucagon.

Teaching about self-care

Diabetes mellitus probably makes more demands on patient compliance than any other medical condition. Here's what to teach your patient about self-care.

Self-monitoring

Stress that checking blood glucose levels regularly, even every day, is crucial to diabetes management. If your patient or a family member can learn the technique, blood glucose self-monitoring can be a valuable management tool. (See *Write it down.*)

By the meter

If appropriate, teach the patient how to use a blood glucose meter. Also teach him how to test his urine for ketones when he's hyperglycemic or ill. Besides explaining how to interpret the results, describe what he should do if results are abnormal.

Preventing infection

Point out that breaks in the skin can increase the risk of infection. Instruct the patient to check his skin daily for cuts and irritated areas, and to see his doctor, if necessary. To avoid infection, advise the patient to follow these steps:
- bathe daily with warm water and a mild soap
- afterward, apply a lanolin-based, alcohol-free lotion to prevent dryness
- pat his skin dry thoroughly, taking extra care between the toes and in any other areas where skin surfaces touch
- always wear cotton underwear to allow moisture to evaporate and help prevent skin breakdown.

Not too hot, not too cold

Advise the patient to avoid extreme temperature changes to reduce the risk of infection (especially in the respiratory tract). Advise the patient of measures to take during illness. (See *Managing diabetes during illness,* page 260.)

On the job

Instruct the patient to be especially careful to avoid accidents. Also discuss possible job hazards; if he's likely to cut or bruise himself on the job, advise him to wear sturdy clothing and shoes and to be extremely cautious. Teach him how to treat cuts or bruises if they do occur. Even a

Signs of hypoglycemia

- Diaphoresis
- Dizziness
- Headache
- Palpitations
- Trembling
- Impaired vision
- Hunger
- Difficulty waking up
- Irritability
- Personality changes

Write it down

Encourage the patient to keep a diary of meals, exercise, medications, self-monitored blood glucose levels, and any symptoms of hypoglycemia. Reviewing this daily record helps him understand how meals and activities affect his blood glucose levels.

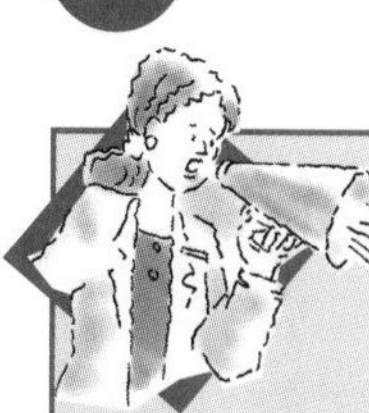

Listen up!

Managing diabetes during illness

Minor illnesses — a cold, a flu, an infection, or an upset stomach — can drastically alter a diabetic patient's ability to control his blood glucose level. As his body attempts to compensate for the stress of an illness, his blood glucose level may rise to dangerous levels. Undetected and untreated, high blood glucose levels during illness may result in life-threatening complications, such as diabetic ketoacidosis and hyperosmolar hyperglycemic nonketotic syndrome.

Personal sick day plan

Advise the patient to prepare a personal sick day plan with his doctor before he becomes ill. Provide him with these general guidelines to follow when he's ill:

- Make sure that you take prescribed diabetes medicine even if you're not able to eat.
- Rest and drink plenty of fluids.
- Even if you're not eating regularly, replace solid foods containing starch and sugar (such as bread and fruit) with liquids containing sugar (such as fruit juices and soft drinks).
- Test your blood glucose level at least every 4 hours.
- Test your urine for ketones.

Tell 'em

Call the doctor promptly if:

- your blood glucose level is consistently higher than 250 mg/dl
- your urine ketone test result is moderate or high
- you think you might have an infection.

relatively minor injury, such as a stubbed toe, can be serious for a diabetic; he could develop an infection from impaired circulation. Also, recommend use of a night-light or flashlight if he habitually goes to the bathroom in the middle of the night.

Watch out

Tell the patient not to use a hot-water bottle or heating pad; he may burn himself because of reduced sensation. Also, teach him the signs and symptoms of impaired circulation, such as dependent edema, pallor, numbness and tingling (paresthesia), and hair loss on the affected limb.

Special problems

Diabetes can affect a patient's health in a number of ways. Discuss measures to prevent diabetes-related health problems.

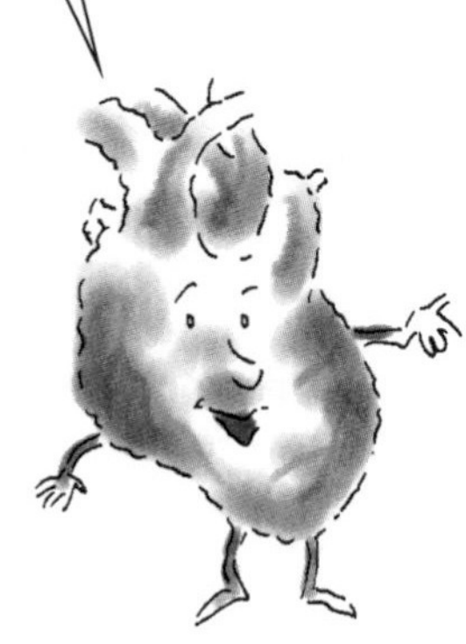
If your patient has diabetes mellitus, I need special care.

From the heart

Inform the patient that diabetes raises his risk of heart disease. Recommend that he take care of his heart by maintaining normal weight, exercising regularly (based on the doctor's recommendations), and eating a low-fat, high-fiber diet to help control his blood pressure and cholesterol levels.

Easy on the eyes

Instruct the patient to have his eyes examined by an ophthalmologist at least once each year. He can detect damage that could cause blindness before symptoms appear. Stress that early treatment may prevent further damage.

If your patient has diabetic retinopathy with vision loss, make sure the booklets and other teaching aids you give him have large type. Urge him to read under a strong light.

Brushing up

Tell the patient to schedule regular dental checkups and follow good home care to minimize dental problems, such as gum disease and abscesses, that may occur with diabetes. Tell him to report these symptoms in his gums or teeth to the dentist immediately:

- bleeding
- pain
- soreness.

Tell him to brush his teeth after every meal and to floss daily. If he wears dentures, he should clean them thoroughly every day and make sure that they fit properly.

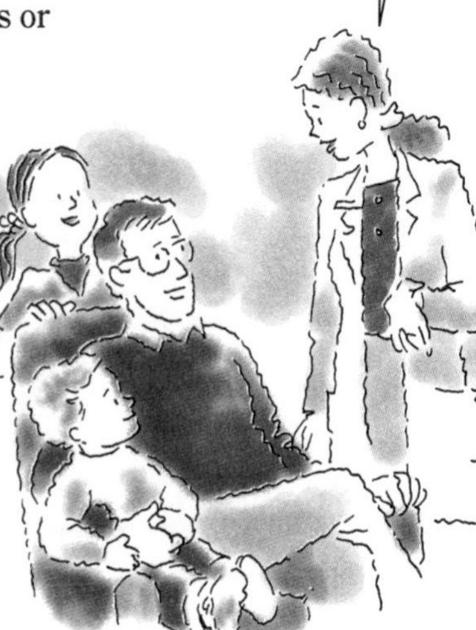
Have your eyes examined by an ophthalmologist at least once a year.

Be sweet to your feet

Inform the patient that diabetes can reduce blood flow to the feet, dulling their ability to feel heat, cold, and pain. Instruct him to follow his doctor's or nurse's instructions on daily foot care and necessary precautions to prevent foot problems. (See *How to treat your feet,* page 262.)

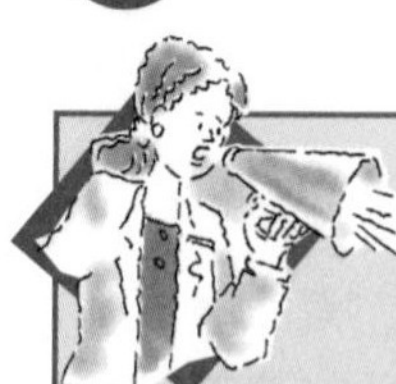

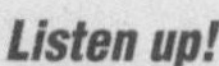

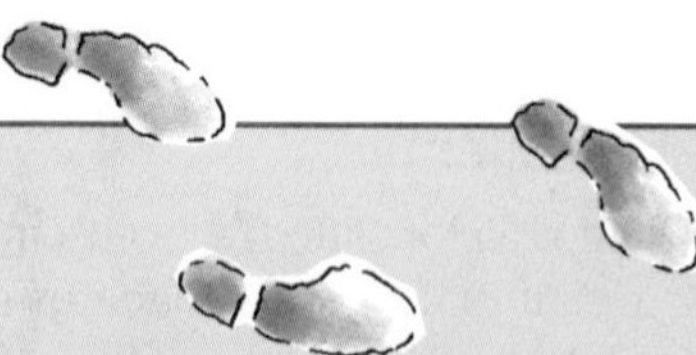

Listen up!

How to treat your feet

Teach your patient that, because he has diabetes, his feet require meticulous daily care. Explain the reason: Diabetes can reduce blood supply to the feet, so even a minor foot injury, such as an ingrown toenail or a blister, can lead to dangerous infection. Because diabetes also reduces sensation in the feet, the patient can burn or chill them without feeling it.

Make it routine

Go over the following routine with the patient:

- Advise the patient to wash his feet in warm, soapy water every day. To prevent burns, instruct him to use a thermometer to check the water temperature before immersing his feet.
- Emphasize that he must dry his feet thoroughly by blotting them with a towel and making sure to dry between the toes.
- Tell him to apply oil or lotion to his feet immediately after drying, to prevent evaporating water from drying his skin. Point out that lotion will keep his skin soft, but caution him not to put lotion between his toes.
- If his feet perspire heavily, advise him to use a mild foot powder. Tell him to sprinkle it lightly between his toes and in his socks and shoes.
- Tell the patient to file his nails, not cut them. Instruct him to file them to be even with the ends of his toes—not shorter than the ends or rounded at the corners. If his nails are too thick, tough, or misshapen to file, he should consult a podiatrist. Also, tell him not to dig under toenails or around cuticles.
- Recommend exercising the feet daily to improve circulation. Tell him to sit on the edge of the bed and point his toes upward and then downward 10 times, and then to make a circle with each foot 10 times.

Protein check

Tell the patient that the doctor will check his urine routinely for protein, which can signal kidney disease. Urge him not to delay telling his doctor if he has symptoms of a urinary tract infection (burning, painful, or difficult urination or blood or pus in the urine).

Tell the patient to see his doctor regularly so that he can detect early signs of complications and start treatment promptly.

Be aware

Help your patient prevent diabetic ketoacidosis or hyperosmolar hyperglycemic nonketotic syndrome by teaching him to recognize its early signs and symptoms and taking immediate and appropriate action. Advise him to test regularly for urine ketones and perform home glucose monitoring. (See *Danger! Cramping, nausea, vomiting.*)

Sexual and reproductive issues

Mention that diabetic patients, particularly men, may experience sexual dysfunction such as impotence. Encourage the patient to discuss any sexual problems he may be having.

Discuss problems of pregnancy with female diabetics. If your patient is already pregnant, refer her to a specialist who cares for diabetic women of childbearing age.

Danger! Cramping, nausea, vomiting

Tell the patient to call the doctor right away if he has any of the following danger signals:

- cramping
- nausea
- vomiting
- headache
- dizziness
- rapid breathing
- shortness of breath
- muscle and joint aches
- increased urination
- thirst
- visual disturbances.

Going somewhere?

Tell the patient who travels for business or vacation to make plans for meals and medication beforehand. He should also pack his insulin and syringes separately.

Advise him to carry his diabetes supplies with him so they don't get lost. When flying, for instance, he should pack his insulin and syringes in a carry-on bag, not in checked luggage. Also instruct him to carry extra insulin and syringes and to protect insulin from excessive heat and cold. When traveling by car, caution him not to leave his insulin in a parked car.

Names and numbers

To help the patient cope with all aspects of diabetes management, provide the names and phone numbers of appropriate resources, such as the American Diabetes Association.

Hyperthyroidism

Although chronic, hyperthyroidism can be a relatively benign condition if the patient complies with therapy. To encourage compliance, you'll need to explain that thyroid hormone overproduction can be curbed by medication or other treatments. You'll want to emphasize that such measures will allow the patient to lead a nearly normal life.

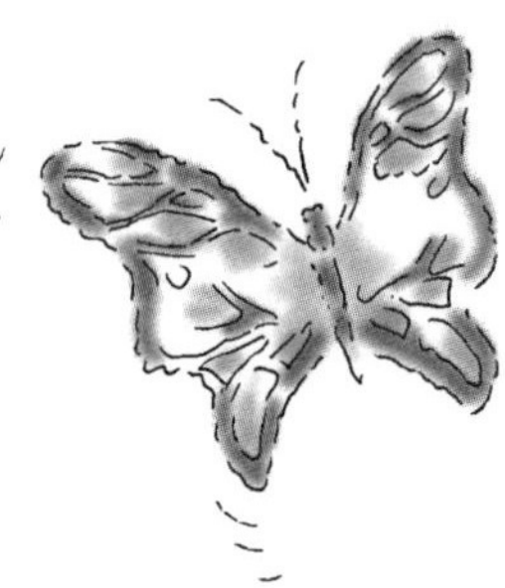

What is it?

Explain that hyperthyroidism results from excessive production of thyroid hormone. Point out that this hormone is produced by the thyroid, a butterfly-shaped gland in the front portion of the lower neck. Tell the patient that overproduction of thyroid hormone accelerates all bodily functions and activities. The condition is more common in women than men.

Where does it come from?

Point out that hyperthyroidism's exact cause is unknown. Explain to the patient that the condition has four main forms:

- Graves' disease is the most common, and may be related to an immune defect that causes formation of abnormal antibodies. It may follow an emotional shock, stress, or infection.
- In toxic nodular goiter, one or more thyroid nodules become hyperproductive. This condition is more common in older women with preexisting goiter.
- Autoimmune thyroiditis (Hashimoto's disease) may cause initial hyperthyroidism before developing into hypothyroidism.
- Factitious hyperthyroidism results from excessive amounts of thyroid hormone medications.

What are its symptoms?

Inform the patient that elevated thyroid hormone levels increase the rate at which the body uses energy. This can lead to signs and symptoms that affect all body systems. (See *Signs of hyperthyroidism.*)

- Cardiovascular effects of hyperthyroidism include hypertension and tachycardia, which can then lead to flushing, palpitations, and heart failure.
- Central nervous system effects include emotional instability, irritability, difficulty concentrating, and insomnia.
- Other signs and symptoms are fine hand tremors, weight loss, and fatigue.

Signs of hyperthyroidism

- Weight loss
- Muscle wasting
- Muscle weakness and tremors
- Fatigue
- Dyspnea
- Breast enlargement
- Palpitations
- Increased appetite
- Irritability and nervousness
- Exophthalmos, lid lag
- Profuse sweating
- Heat intolerance
- Fine, straight hair

It's Graves' disease!

- Uniformly enlarged thyroid gland (goiter)
- Infiltrative ophthalmopathy
- Infiltrative dermopathy

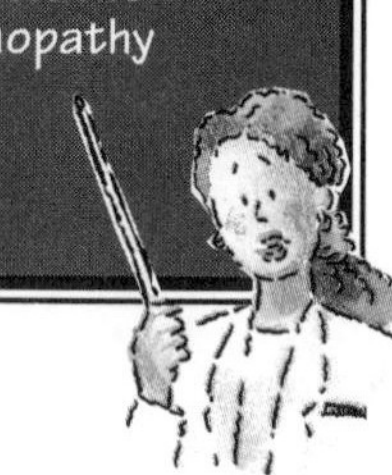

What's at risk?

Encourage compliance with the treatment regimen by pointing out that untreated or poorly managed hyperthyroidism can lead to severe complications.

For example, thyroid storm, an acute complication, can be fatal without prompt treatment. In thyroid storm, the patient's metabolic rate rapidly accelerates, severely taxing the functions of all body systems. Body temperature may rise as high as 106° F (41° C); heart and respiratory rates increase dramatically. Total systemic collapse becomes imminent.

Explain that compliance can also forestall common chronic complications of hyperthyroidism, such as cardiac dysfunction, weight loss, and GI problems.

Treatment goals

Explain to the patient that treatment for hyperthyroidism aims to restore the basal metabolic rate to normal as soon as possible and then to maintain the normal rate. The specific treatment approach depends on the cause, the patient's age, disease severity, and any existing complications.

Teaching about tests

Tell the patient that tests commonly used to evaluate thyroid function include:

- blood tests
- thyroid scan
- ultrasonography
- radioactive iodine uptake test. (See *Teaching patients about endocrine tests,* pages 252 and 253.)

Explain that blood tests require a small blood sample drawn by venipuncture at regular intervals. Studies will be done on thyroid hormone itself or on its by-products found in the blood.

Teaching about activity and lifestyle

Inform the patient that excessive exertion will worsen her symptoms. Encourage her instead to engage in less strenuous activities and to rest frequently. Keep in mind that this may be difficult because of the patient's accelerated metabolic rate. (See *Treatment goals;* and *Living with hyperthyroidism,* page 266.)

Teaching about diet

Stress the importance of following the prescribed diet to prevent nutritional deficiencies, such as vitamin A and B deficiencies. Advise the patient to eat well-balanced meals each day, plus snacks, so that her calorie intake can keep pace with her rapid calorie expenditures. If appropriate, arrange for nutritional counseling. (See *Stay away from....*)

Stay away from...

- Caffeine
- Food with yellow or red dyes
- Food with artificial preservatives

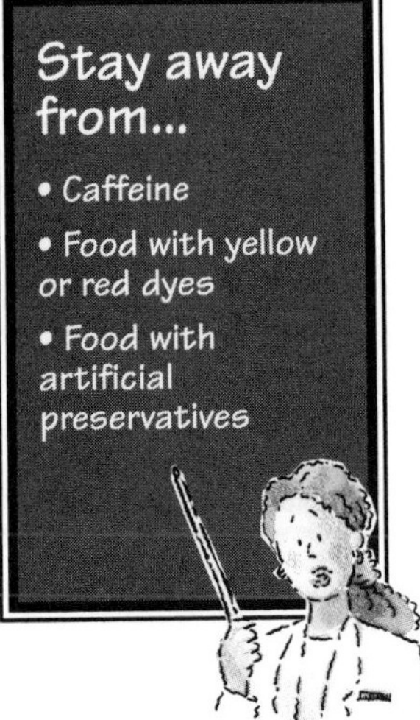

Teaching about medication

Teach the patient about thyroid hormone antagonists and propranolol, if prescribed, to control cardiac effects. Also

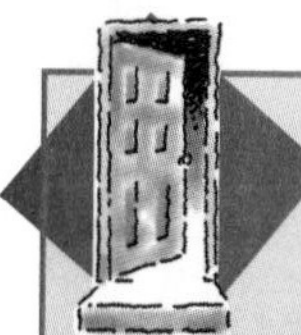

No place like home

Living with hyperthyroidism

Here's some good advice to help your patient live with hyperthyroidism.

Less stress

Advise the patient to avoid stressful situations, which can exacerbate irritability. Recommend keeping environmental stimulation to a minimum. For example, advise the patient to avoid watching television programs or movies that may cause her to become excited or upset. Reassure the patient and family members that behavioral changes, such as irritability, anxiety, lack of concentration, and fatigue, stem from hyperthyroidism and will subside with treatment.

Eye care essentials

If ophthalmopathy is present, teach the patient the essentials of good eye care. Advise her to wear sunglasses and to avoid irritating her eyes. If eyedrops are ordered, show her how to instill them. Instruct her to limit her fluid and salt intake to minimize fluid retention, because such retention will worsen exophthalmos.

Suggest that the patient sleep with her head elevated to prevent fluid accumulation behind the eyes. Instruct her to notify her doctor at once if she experiences visual changes such as blurring. Advise her to visit an ophthalmologist regularly.

teach about other prescribed drugs such as tranquilizers to control irritability and hyperactivity.

Avoiding aspirin

Caution the patient to avoid taking aspirin and any aspirin-containing drugs because they increase the metabolic rate.

Teaching about radioactive iodine therapy

The doctor may recommend radioactive iodine therapy if thyroid hormone antagonists prove ineffective. If the patient is scheduled for this treatment, explain that it reduces thyroid hormone production by destroying thyroid tissue.

Reassure the patient that the procedure is painless and won't harm other body tissues. Make sure she understands the risk of hypothyroidism, which can result from excessive destruction of thyroid tissue and may occur several months to 1 year after treatment. Assure her that exposure to this small amount of radioactivity doesn't cause cancer. (See *After radioactive iodine therapy.*)

It usually works

Inform the patient that symptoms of hyperthyroidism should subside after radioactive iodine therapy. If they don't, she may need a second round of therapy.

Teaching about surgery

Surgery may be recommended if the patient has a very large goiter or can't receive radioiodine. In subtotal thyroidectomy, more than 80% of the thyroid is removed, significantly reducing the gland's ability to produce thyroid hormone.

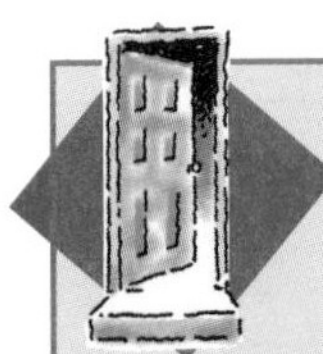

No place like home

After radioactive iodine therapy

Although radioactive iodine therapy is a safe treatment, the patient will need to follow instructions to prevent any harm to herself or others.

Eating and drinking

Inform the patient that she can eat what she likes but must use disposable plates, cups, and utensils for 48 hours after the treatment. Urge her to drink plenty of fluids (about 2 qt [2 L]) for those 48 hours to help remove the radioactive iodine from her body.

Using the bathroom

The patient's urine, feces, saliva, and perspiration will be slightly radioactive for 48 hours after therapy. She may use the family bathroom to urinate or defecate, but should flush the toilet three times to make certain all waste is discarded. Tell her to wash her hands thoroughly afterward.

Bathing and laundering

If the patient takes a shower or bath within 48 hours after treatment, tell her to rinse the shower stall or tub after each use. Instruct her to wash her clothes, towels, and washcloths separately from those of family members.

She can brush her teeth and resume other normal mouth care. Remind her, though, to make sure to rinse and drain the sink when she's finished.

Contact with others

Caution the patient to avoid close contact with infants, children, and pregnant women for 1 week after therapy. For safety's sake, she should sleep alone and avoid kissing or sexual intimacy for 48 hours after the treatment. After that, she may resume a relationship unless the doctor gives other instructions.

If the patient is breast-feeding, she must stop. The doctor will tell her when she can start again.

When to call the doctor

Instruct the patient to call her doctor immediately if she vomits within 12 hours after therapy. Tell her to flush the vomit down the toilet and, if possible, wear gloves while cleaning up. (She should discard the gloves in a plastic bag after use.) Warn her to discourage other people from coming in contact with the vomit. If they do, however, they should wash their hands thoroughly.

If the patient gets a fever and feels restless or upset within 48 hours of therapy, she should call her doctor right away. Also tell her to call the doctor if her neck feels tender. The doctor may prescribe medicine to make her more comfortable.

If the patient is scheduled for subtotal thyroidectomy, review with her the following steps:

- Instruct her to increase her calorie intake before surgery to regain weight. (Surgery may have to be delayed until the patient gains back any weight she lost.)
- If a special preoperative diet (such as a high-protein diet) has been ordered, explain its purpose and urge strict compliance.
- Remind the patient to avoid caffeine and other stimulants that will aggravate her condition.
- Explain the purpose of preoperative thyroid medication: to suppress secretion of thyroid hormone so that an excessive amount isn't released during surgery.
- Explain that iodine preparations may also be ordered to diminish blood flow to the thyroid, thereby minimizing bleeding during surgery.

Before...

Before surgery, review preoperative and postoperative procedures. Explain preoperative preparation of the incision site. Tell the patient that the incision will be made in the lower neck.

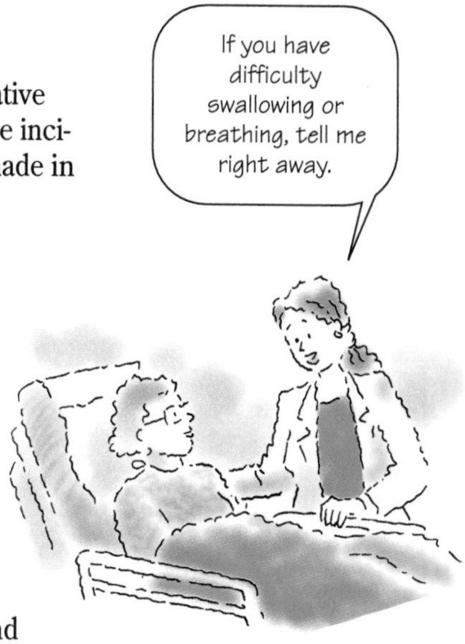

...and after

Show the patient how to avoid putting stress on her incision postoperatively by placing her hands behind her neck for support whenever she wants to turn her head. When rising to a sitting position, she should support her head with a pillow and put her hands together behind her head. If she has difficulty swallowing, she should report it immediately. This problem may indicate hemorrhage or swelling, which could interfere with breathing. Mention that cold drinks and ice will help relieve discomfort and that she'll be on a soft diet temporarily.

If you have difficulty swallowing or breathing, tell me right away.

As little as possible

Tell the patient that her voice will be checked periodically for hoarseness after surgery. Advise her to talk as little as possible during the first few days postoperatively. If she has difficulty breathing, she should report it at once; oxygen may have to be administered. Tell her she can expect to be out of bed on the first day after surgery.

Rest assured

Reassure the patient that she'll receive pain medication postoperatively. Inform her that sutures or surgical clips are usually removed on the second postoperative day, just before discharge.

Going home

To help prepare the patient for discharge, teach her how to take care of her incision at home. Make sure she understands the importance of getting adequate rest and nutrition during recovery. Tell her to promptly report signs or symptoms of infection or hypothyroidism to her doctor.

Set realistic goals

Help patients set realistic goals. Attainable goals can motivate learning, but "impossible dreams" can discourage learning efforts.

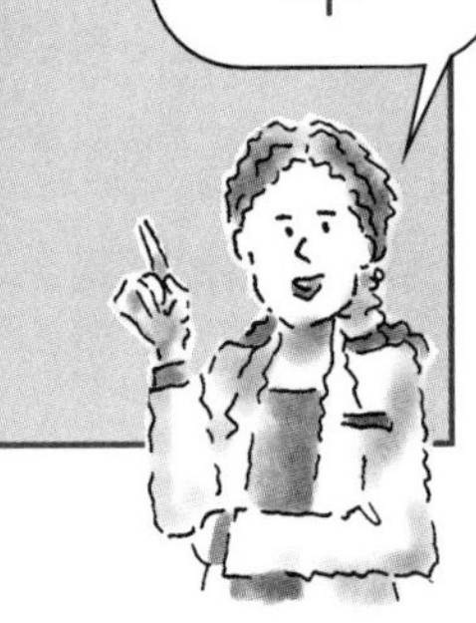

Hypothyroidism

In this chronic disorder, which affects more women than men, the thyroid gland fails to secrete sufficient thyroid hormone. If left untreated or managed improperly, hypothyroidism can have devastating effects. Both acute and chronic complications may occur, affecting the quality of the patient's life and possibly even shortening her life span. That's why it's important for you to teach the patient about the chronic nature of her disorder.

What's the bottom line?

Most important, stress the need to comply with lifelong thyroid hormone replacement therapy. Other areas to cover include diet and activity precautions and possible adjunctive care measures.

What is primary hypothyroidism?

Primary hypothyroidism results from gradual destruction of vital thyroid tissue. In the absence of goiter, its most common cause is radioactive iodine therapy or surgery. When goiter is present, its most common cause is Hashimoto's disease, in which lymphocytes mistake normal thyroid cells for foreign cells and destroy them.

What is secondary hypothyroidism?

Secondary hypothyroidism, which is rare, results from destruction of pituitary tissue responsible for producing thyroid-stimulating hormone (TSH), or thyrotropin. Without TSH, the thyroid gland can't produce thyroid hormone.

What are the effects?

Describe how hypothyroidism affects the body. For example, explain that thyroid hormone deficiency decreases the body's ability to use energy. As a result, cells don't function effectively and use up what little energy is available to them. This causes the patient to tire easily. Besides fatigue, the patient may experience a variety of other symptoms. (See *Signs of hypothyroidism.*)

Signs of hypothyroidism

- Lethargy
- Forgetfulness
- Cold intolerance
- Constipation
- Weight gain (without increased calorie intake)
- Muscle aches and weakness
- Rough, thick, scaly skin
- Dry, coarse, thin, brittle hair
- Facial edema, blank facial expression
- Thick tongue, slow speech

What's at risk?

To underscore the importance of complying with therapy, discuss the complications that might occur if hypothyroidism is poorly managed or left untreated. Myxedema, for example, may develop gradually. In early stages, it produces generalized symptoms, such as fatigue and lethargy. Later, it causes cool, dry skin along with decreased sweat and oil production, thinning of scalp hair, and loss of body hair.

The patient with myxedema may also develop menstrual irregularities, hearing loss, ataxia, dependent edema, and heart failure. Muscles may increase in bulk but decline in strength, and the patient may have muscle cramps.

Impaired muscle function from myxedema predisposes the patient to constipation and urinary tract infection. Decreased lung expansion heightens the risk of respiratory infection. As myxedema worsens, profound hypotension, bradycardia, hypoventilation, and hypothermia may develop. Stress that without prompt treatment, myxedema can be fatal or can lead to other life-threatening conditions such as coma.

What else is at risk?

Other chronic complications of uncontrolled hypothyroidism, such as atherosclerosis, arise from the accumulation of fatty substances in interstitial tissues as well as from decreased metabolism.

Teaching about tests

Explain that thyroid hormone deficiency is easily confirmed by measuring serum levels of thyroxine and protein-bound iodine.

Additional tests may include a thyroid scan or ultrasonography to evaluate the thyroid's size and structure and a radioactive iodine uptake test to assess gland function. (See *Teaching patients about endocrine tests,* pages 252 and 253.)

Treatment for hypothyroidism

- Dietary restrictions
- Thyroid hormone replacement therapy

Teaching about activity and lifestyle

Because patients with hypothyroidism have so little energy, they tend to be sedentary. As a result, you'll need to encourage the patient to increase her activity level. (See *Treatment for hypothyroidism* and *Living with hypothyroidism.*)

One step at a time

Caution the patient to increase her activity level gradually because she risks pain and impaired muscle function from myxedema. Discuss activities she enjoys and can fit into her lifestyle. (Her doctor will have to provide guidelines for all such activities.)

Teaching about diet

Stress the importance of following dietary restrictions to minimize weight gain, reduce cholesterol intake, and alle-

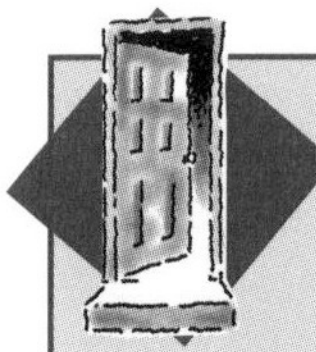

No place like home

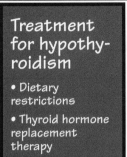

Living with hypothyroidism

Review the signs and symptoms of hypothyroidism with the patient. Tell her to be especially alert for increased lethargy, sensitivity to cold, weight gain, facial and hand puffiness, changes in her skin or hair, and muscle cramps. Instruct her to report any of these changes immediately to her doctor.

A paradoxical precaution

Make sure she's familiar with the signs and symptoms of *hyperthyroidism,* which may develop if her thyroid hormone dosage is too high. These include heat intolerance, increased sweating, nervous activity, difficulty concentrating, frequent defecation, skin changes, apprehensiveness, and irritability.

Check in regularly

Because hypothyroidism is a chronic disorder, encourage the patient to see her doctor regularly for blood tests and physical examinations. Tell her to report any signs or symptoms of infection, such as fever, malaise, diarrhea, and muscle pain. Remind her that hypothyroidism makes her vulnerable to infections.

viate constipation. Remind the patient that thyroid hormone deficiency decreases her body's ability to use sugars and carbohydrates as energy sources. It will also cause her to store fats.

Allow me to recommend our low-in-saturated-fat, low-cholesterol, calorie-restricted, high-fiber, high-protein menu.

Avoid fats...

Advise the patient to avoid foods high in saturated fats and cholesterol. Suggest that she talk with her doctor about whether she can drink alcohol. Explore ways to help her adhere to a calorie-restricted diet. If appropriate, encourage her to join a support group.

...Increase fiber

Also teach the patient how to increase the fiber content in her diet. If she has nonpitting edema, advise her to reduce fluid intake by one to two glasses daily, as prescribed.

Teaching about medication

Thyroid hormone replacement is the primary treatment for hypothyroidism and will help the patient achieve a normal metabolic rate and energy level. Explain that this therapy will be tailored to meet her individual requirements and that she'll need to continue thyroid hormone replacement for the rest of her life. The dosage will depend on the severity of her hypothyroidism.

Finding the right dosage for your needs may take time.

Just the right dosage

Explain that finding just the right dosage for her is a gradual process. This will allow her body to adjust slowly to the changes resulting from the medication, thus helping to prevent complications.

Good advice

Instruct the patient who is taking a thyroid hormone replacement, such as levothyroxine (Levothroid, Levoxine, or Synthroid) or liothyronine (Cytomel), to take the drug exactly as prescribed and not to adjust the dosage or discontinue the drug without her doctor's approval. Advise her to take the medication at the same time every day for uniform absorption. Tell her to store her medication in the original container.

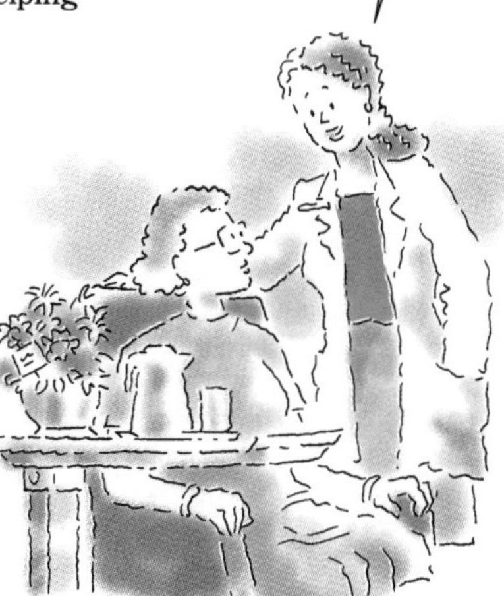

Yikes! Headache, palpitations, hair loss

Instruct her to watch for adverse reactions, including a change in appetite, abnormal bleeding or bruising, chest pain, diarrhea, fever, severe headache, heat intolerance, insomnia, leg cramps, nervousness, palpitations, shortness of breath, rash, sweating, tremors, and weight loss. Mention that constipation, drowsiness, dry skin, headache, menstrual irregularities, nausea, and temporary hair loss may occur. (See *More good advice.*)

> **More good advice**
>
> Caution the patient never to take nonprescription drugs without her doctor's approval. Explain that hypothyroidism slows down her metabolism and thus prolongs drug effects, creating the risk of drug toxicity. Advise her to inform all health care providers of her hypothyroidism so that any prescribed medications (especially narcotics, barbiturates, and digoxin) may be chosen carefully and the dosage reduced appropriately.

Hypoglycemia

Managing hypoglycemia, a chronic disorder, may pose a never-ending challenge to the patient. Besides learning how to recognize the telltale symptoms of a hypoglycemic episode, the patient must master its prompt treatment to prevent possibly irreversible tissue damage. What's more, because hypoglycemia can cause fatigue, difficulty concentrating, and considerable discomfort, he must comply with certain lifestyle changes.

What is it?

Tell the patient that hypoglycemia occurs when glucose, the body's major energy source, isn't being produced fast enough or is being used too rapidly. Mention that a certain amount of glucose must always be present in the blood to meet the energy needs of vital tissues (such as brain cells).

How low does it go?

How low the blood glucose level must fall before triggering a hypoglycemic reaction varies greatly among individuals. Typically, a blood glucose level below 70 mg/dl causes symptoms.

How fast does it fall?

Tell the patient that the nature of his symptoms may reveal how rapidly his glucose level is falling. A rapid decline can result in nervousness, diaphoresis, and an elevated heart rate. A slow decline and levels below 50 mg/dl can cause changes in mental status.

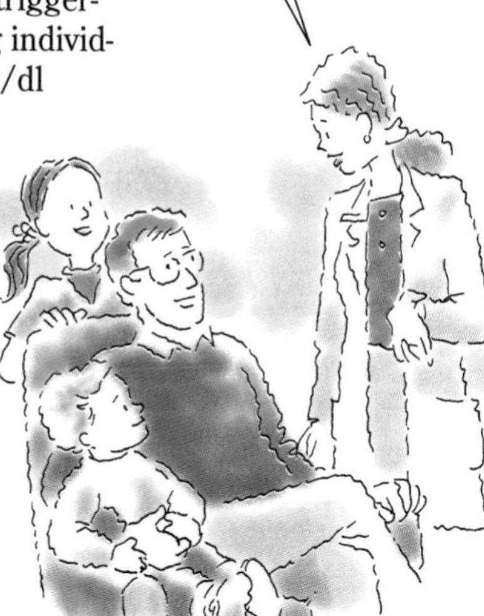
Because of hypoglycemia, you may need to change your lifestyle.

What's at risk?

Emphasize the importance of preventing or promptly treating hypoglycemic episodes to avoid severe complications. (See *Managing a hypoglycemic episode.*) Make sure the patient understands that the key danger with hypoglycemia is that, once it occurs, he may quickly lose his ability to think clearly. If this should happen while he's driving a car or operating machinery, it could cause a serious accident.

What else is at risk?

Explain that brain cells can't survive long without glucose. Prolonged or severe hypoglycemia causes permanent

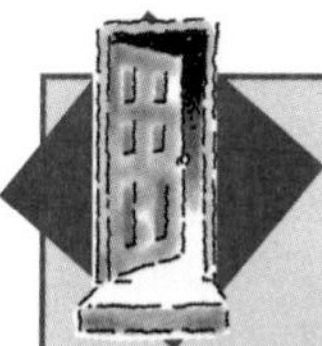

No place like home

Managing a hypoglycemic episode

A sudden hypoglycemic episode may prevent the patient from recognizing his symptoms and taking appropriate action. It may be up to family members or other caregivers to manage the crisis.

In such an emergency, the patient's blood glucose level *must* be raised immediately to prevent permanent brain damage and even death. So tell family members to be sure to keep sources of glucose (sugar) available.

Conscious
If the patient is conscious, give him one of the sources of glucose listed in the chart.

Foods and fluids	Amount
• Apple juice, orange juice, or ginger ale	• 4 to 6 oz (118 to 177 ml)
• Regular cola or other soft drink	• 4 to 6 oz
• Corn syrup, honey, or grape jelly	• 1 tbs
• Hard candy	• 5 to 6 pieces
• Jelly beans	• 6
• Gumdrops	• 10

Unconscious or unable to swallow
If the patient is unconscious or has trouble swallowing, family members should give him a subcutaneous injection of glucagon. Tell family members to check the expiration date on the glucagon kit frequently and replenish the supply as needed. Provide them with instructions as described below.

How to inject glucagon
1. Prepare the glucagon following the manufacturer's instructions included in the kit.
2. Select an appropriate injection site.
3. Pull the skin taut, then clean it with an alcohol swab.
4. Using your thumb and forefinger, pinch the skin at the injection site, then quickly plunge the needle into the skin fold at a 90-degree angle, up to the needle hub. Push the plunger down to quickly inject the glucagon.
5. Withdraw the needle and rub the site with an alcohol swab.
6. Turn the patient onto his side. Because glucagon may cause vomiting, this position reduces the possibility of choking.
7. If the patient doesn't wake up in 5 to 20 minutes, give a second dose of glucagon and seek emergency help. If the patient wakes up and can swallow, family members should give him some sugar immediately (glucagon is effective for only about 90 minutes). Next, family members should call the doctor.

brain damage and could be fatal. (See *Forms of hypoglycemia.*)

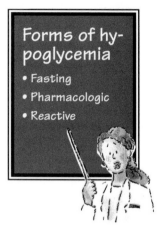

What's reactive hypoglycemia?

Tell the patient with reactive hypoglycemia, also called postprandial hypoglycemia, that his blood glucose level may fall after a meal, resulting in a headache, dizziness, restlessness, mental status changes, and intense hunger. This type of hypoglycemia can occur in patients with rapid gastric emptying and brisk glucose absorption, such as the patient with gastrectomy.

What's pharmacologic hypoglycemia?

Tell the patient with pharmacologic hypoglycemia that his blood glucose level may fall in response to a drug that does one of three things:

increases the amount of insulin circulating in the bloodstream

 enhances insulin action

 impairs the liver's glucose-producing capacity.

The patient's symptoms will depend on whether his blood glucose level is falling slowly or rapidly. (See *Signs of pharmacologic hypoglycemia,* page 276.)

Explain that the most common causes of pharmacologic hypoglycemia are insulin and oral sulfonylureas used to treat diabetes. Other causes include use of beta blockers and excessive ingestion of alcohol.

What's fasting hypoglycemia?

Tell the patient with fasting hypoglycemia that his blood glucose level may fall rapidly but without dropping drastically below normal. He'll experience hunger, weakness, diaphoresis, tachycardia, pallor, anxiety, tremors, and nervousness. These symptoms are usually mild, occurring within a few hours after a meal and resolving quickly with treatment.

Fasting hypoglycemia may result from liver disease or a tumor. For example, a pancreatic tumor called an insulinoma causes excessive insulin secretion. An extrapancreatic tumor can also lead to hypoglycemia, although the mechanism isn't clear. Liver disease interferes with the liver's ability to raise the blood glucose level by gluconeogenesis and glycogenolysis. Other causes of fasting hypoglycemia include adrenocortical insufficiency, growth hormone deficiency, and severe chronic renal failure.

Signs of pharmacologic hypoglycemia

Blood glucose level falls slowly

- Headache
- Dizziness
- Restlessness
- Decreased mental capacity

Blood glucose falls rapidly

- Hunger
- Weakness
- Diaphoresis
- Tachycardia
- Pallor, anxiety
- Tremors
- Nervousness
- Rebound hyperglycemia

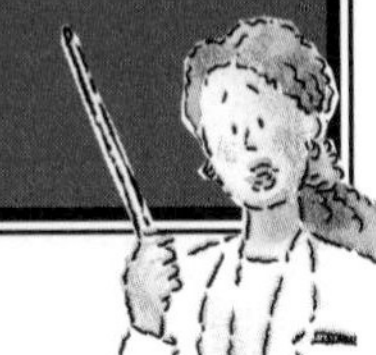

Teaching about tests

Inform the patient that the diagnostic tests ordered depend on whether his symptoms are related to eating or fasting. Once the doctor determines this, he'll order serial blood glucose studies such as a fasting plasma glucose test. He may also order an oral glucose tolerance test, an I.V. glucose tolerance test, and a C-peptide assay. (See *Teaching patients about endocrine tests,* pages 252 and 253.)

Fact finder for fasting hypoglycemia

Explain that a C-peptide assay helps diagnose fasting hypoglycemia. It also differentiates fasting hypoglycemia caused by an insulinoma (a tumor that secretes insulin) from fasting hypoglycemia caused by insulin injections. No preparation is needed.

Teaching about activity and lifestyle

If the patient is obese and has impaired glucose tolerance, suggest ways that he can restrict his calorie intake and lose weight. If necessary, help him find a weight-loss support group. (See *Living with hypoglycemia.*)

Teaching about diet

Emphasize to the patient the importance of carefully following his prescribed diet to prevent a rapid drop in his blood glucose level. Discuss his specific meal plan, and encourage him to comply with it. (See *Treatment for hypoglycemia,* page 278.)

Snacking is good...

Advise him to eat small meals throughout the day, and mention that bedtime snacks may be necessary to keep his blood glucose at an even level. Instruct him to avoid alcohol and caffeine because they may trigger severe hypoglycemic episodes.

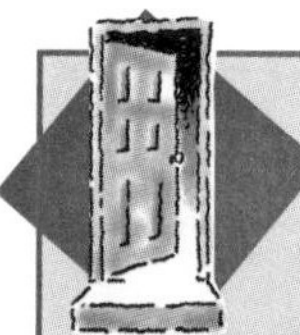

No place like home

Living with hypoglycemia

A large part of the treatment plan for a hypoglycemic patient consists of careful teaching of the patient and his family. Make sure you teach the patient how to prevent a hypoglycemic episode.

Self-awareness

Discuss his lifestyle and personal habits to help him identify possible precipitating factors, such as poor diet, stress, or mismanagement of diabetes mellitus. Explore ways that he can change or avoid these factors.

Stick to the diet

Tell the patient to eat all his meals and snacks at the prescribed time and in the prescribed amounts.

Also instruct him to avoid alcohol and caffeine; they can cause his blood glucose level to drop.

Strictly follow the schedule

If the doctor prescribes medicine to control the patient's hypoglycemia, advise him to follow his schedule strictly. Emphasize that he must take the right amount of medicine at the right time.

Tell him to always check with the doctor treating his hypoglycemia before taking any over-the-counter medicine or any other prescribed medicine. Also tell him to inform the doctor about any new treatments he's receiving for another condition.

Easy does it

Encourage the patient to reduce stress by practicing relaxation techniques, such as deep breathing and guided imagery. Recommend that he change his lifestyle, if possible, by working less and taking more time for hobbies, traveling, and other leisure activities. If necessary, teach the patient stress-reduction techniques and encourage him to join a support group.

Exercise with caution

Instruct the patient to take some precautions when he exercises. For example, he shouldn't exercise alone or when his blood glucose level is likely to drop. He should consume extra calories to make up for those burned.

For example, if he has *fasting hypoglycemia,* his blood glucose level is likely to drop 5 hours or more after a meal. If he has *reactive hypoglycemia,* his blood glucose level will fall 2 to 4 hours after a meal. If he has *pharmacologic hypoglycemia,* he should ask his doctor for guidelines.

If he's a diabetic, tell him not to inject insulin into a part of his body that he'll be exercising during the next few hours.

Carry carbohydrates

Advise the patient to carry a source of fast-acting carbohydrate, such as hard candy or sugar packets, with him at all times.

Know the warning signs

Tell the patient to note what symptoms he typically has before an episode of hypoglycemia. Stress that he should make certain his family, friends, and coworkers know that he has hypoglycemia and that they can also recognize the warning signs. Early recognition can prevent an acute episode.

Alert others

Instruct the patient to wear a medical identification bracelet or carry a medical identification card that describes his condition and what emergency actions to take.

Manage diabetes

For a patient with pharmacologic hypoglycemia caused by insulin or oral antidiabetic drugs, review the essentials of managing diabetes mellitus, if indicated.

Check in

Finally, because hypoglycemia is a chronic disorder, encourage the patient to see his doctor regularly.

...but avoid excess carbos

Tell the patient with reactive hypoglycemia to avoid simple carbohydrates and other foods high in carbohydrates. Such foods load the body with glucose and may stimulate excessive insulin production, triggering a hypoglycemic episode. Help the patient plan low-carbohydrate, high-protein meals by reviewing with him the foods belonging to these food groups. Advise him to add fiber to his diet because it delays glucose absorption from the GI tract.

3 meals a day

Tell the patient with fasting hypoglycemia that he'll need to increase his calorie intake because his body needs more glucose to counteract excessive insulin secretion. Warn him not to postpone or skip meals and snacks because severe and possibly prolonged hypoglycemia may develop. Tell him to call his doctor for instructions if he doesn't feel well enough to eat.

Treatment for hypoglycemia

- Diet to prevent a rapid drop in glucose level
- Drug therapy to control anxiety, delay gastric emptying, alleviate symptoms, and treat tumors
- Possible surgery to remove tumors

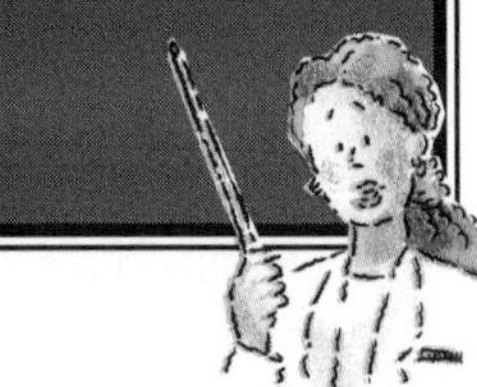

Teaching about medication

Drug therapy may seek to delay gastric emptying and treat tumors.

Delaying gastric emptying

If the doctor prescribes medication to delay gastric emptying in reactive hypoglycemia, teach the patient about possible adverse effects.

Inhibiting insulin release

If the patient has an inoperable insulinoma, explain that diazoxide (Hyperstat) helps treat fasting hypoglycemia by inhibiting insulin release. Together with a high-calorie diet, diazoxide helps maintain adequate blood glucose levels.

Treating a tumor

If the patient will undergo chemotherapy to treat an inoperable tumor, explain the protocol to him and review possible adverse reactions to each drug.

More advice

Advise the patient not to take nonprescription medications such as antihistamines without his doctor's approval. Explain that many nonprescription medications contain ingredients that mask symptoms of decreased blood glucose levels or induce hypoglycemia.

Teaching about surgery

If your patient with fasting hypoglycemia is scheduled for surgery to remove an extrapancreatic tumor or an insulinoma, take the following steps:

- Review with the patient standard preoperative and postoperative procedures.
- After surgery, instruct the patient to notify his doctor if symptoms of hypoglycemia recur.
- Make sure the patient also knows the signs and symptoms of hyperglycemia. (See *Signs of hyperglycemia.*) Hyperglycemia may occur postoperatively if surgery destroys more than 90% of the insulin-producing cells in the pancreas.

Signs of hyperglycemia

- Polydipsia and polyuria
- Increased blood glucose and ketone levels
- Weakness, abdominal pain, generalized aches
- Deep, rapid breathing
- Anorexia, nausea, vomiting

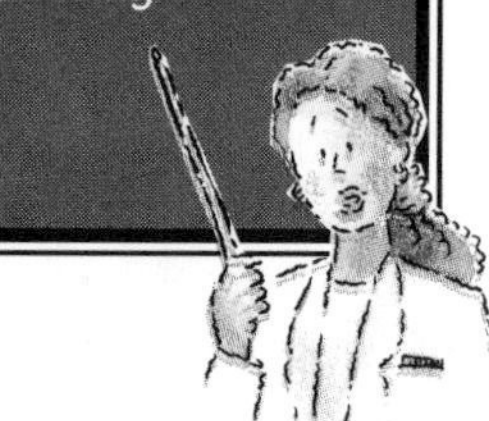

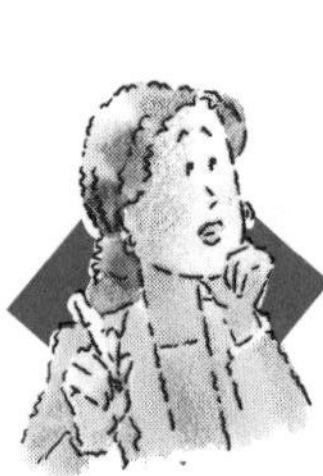

Quick quiz

1. Teach a diabetic patient that type 1 diabetes mellitus differs from type 2 in that:

A. type 1 diabetes requires insulin as treatment.
B. type 2 diabetes requires the use of insulin.
C. type 1 diabetes generally produces insulin resistance.

Answer: A. The person with type 1 diabetes needs daily insulin injections.

2. A patient with diabetes mellitus should be taught that Rezulin and glucophage decrease:

A. insulin resistance.
B. the frequent need for finger sticks.
C. the number of times required to check for urine ketones.

Answer: A. These two drugs decrease cellular insulin resistance.

3. A patient with hyperthyroidism should be taught that he has:

A. a decreased metabolism.
B. an increased metabolism.
C. an increased requirement for thyroid replacement hormones.

Answer: B. Hyperthyroidism is a metabolic disorder resulting from over production of thyroid hormone. With this condition, the patient has an increased metabolic rate.

4. The patient with hyperthyroidism exhibits signs of:

A. facial flushing, exophthalmos, goiter, enlarged breasts, tremors, and fine, straight hair.
B. facial flushing, weight gain, lid lag, goiter, tremors, and thick, dry hair.
C. facial edema, enlarged breasts, tremors, and thick, straight hair.

Answer: A. The signs of hyperthyroidism are facial flushing, exophthalmos, goiter, enlarged breasts, tremors, and fine, straight hair.

5. Expect to teach the patient with hypoglycemia that the signs and symptoms he may experience are:

A. polydipsia, polyuria, and deep, rapid breathing.
B. diaphoresis, trembling, irritability, and headache.
C. shortness of breath, polyuria, weakness, and increased glucose levels.

Answer: B. Other signs and symptoms of hypoglycemia include faintness, palpitations, impaired vision, hunger, difficulty waking up, and personality changes.

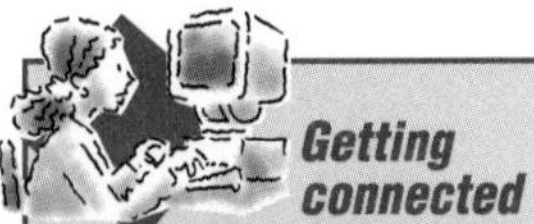

Getting connected

Dialing in to diabetes

For information about diabetes, direct the patient to the following Web sites:

- American Diabetes Association (www.diabetes.org/custom.asp or www.diabetes.org/default.htm)
- National Institute of Diabetes and Digestive and Kidney Diseases (www.niddk.nih.gov).

Scoring

☆☆☆ If you answered all five items correctly, superb! You've got all the signs of being a great patient teacher.

☆☆ If you answered three or four items correctly, great! When it comes to patient teaching, you've got class.

☆ If you answered fewer than three correctly, don't go into shock! Stay cool and review the chapter.

9

Reproductive disorders

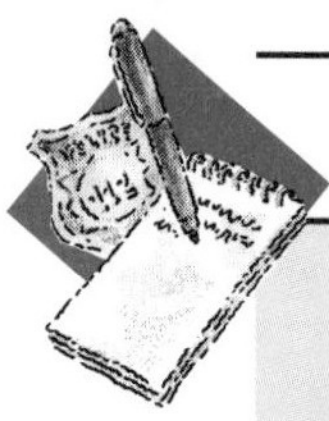

Just the facts

In this chapter, you'll learn how to teach patients with the following reproductive disorders:

- ♦ benign prostatic hyperplasia
- ♦ dysfunctional uterine bleeding
- ♦ endometriosis
- ♦ fibrocystic breast changes
- ♦ pelvic inflammatory disease.

Benign prostatic hyperplasia

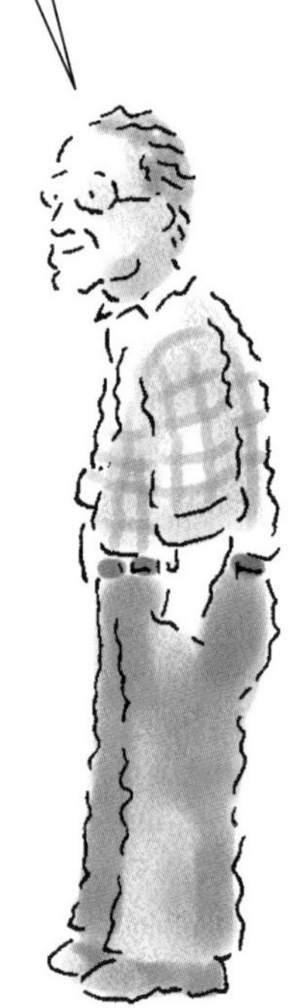

Because BPH affects older men, be prepared for age-related learning barriers.

Benign prostatic hyperplasia (BPH) is a nonmalignant overgrowth of tissue in the prostate. Because it affects older men, when you teach about BPH, be prepared to overcome age-related learning barriers, such as impaired vision and memory, hearing loss, and other physical limitations.

What happens?

Because BPH progresses slowly, a patient may not recognize its symptoms right away. Eventually, though, he'll notice the following symptoms:

- a frequent urge to urinate
- difficulty starting his urine stream
- waking throughout the night to urinate. (See *Tip for a patient with mild BPH,* page 282.)

Is it connected to aging?

Inform the patient that BPH is related to aging and that, by age 70, most men have some degree of prostate enlargement. Explain that the cause of BPH is unknown, but researchers suspect a metabolic or hormonal condition.

What's at risk?

Caution the patient that BPH may lead to complications if it remains untreated. For instance, the patient may notice a decreasing ability to empty his bladder as the enlargement causes resistance to urine flow. This residual urine may lead to urinary tract infection. Ultimately, he may be unable to void. Then he'll experience acute urine retention and increased bladder pressure, which can result in renal damage if untreated.

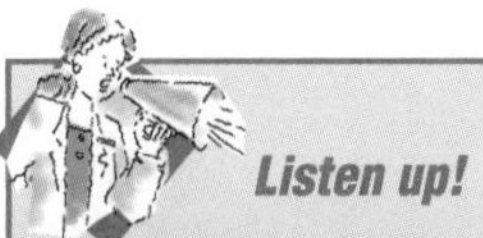

Tip for a patient with mild BPH

Tell the patient with mild benign prostatic hyperplasia (BPH) that he can reduce his need to urinate during the night by:
- decreasing fluid intake in the evening
- decreasing intake of substances that irritate the bladder, such as caffeine and alcohol.

Teaching about tests

Explain the physical examination to the patient. Tell him to expect the following steps:
- The doctor examines the prostate gland by inserting a gloved finger into the patient's rectum.
- He also evaluates the rectal sphincter, which indirectly reflects bladder innervation.
- The doctor observes the patient as he voids to determine the size and force of his urine stream.
- The patient is catheterized immediately after urination to measure postvoiding residual volume.
- The patient may undergo a transabdominal ultrasound of the bladder and a prostatic ultrasound.

Blood and urine tests

Next, explain the blood and urine tests that evaluate BPH. Tell the patient that blood samples will be drawn to measure blood urea nitrogen, serum creatinine, acid phosphatase, and prostate-specific antigen (PSA) levels. PSA levels are elevated in approximately 25% of patients with BPH. PSA is also significantly elevated in patients with prostate cancer.

Urine specimens will also be collected for urinalysis and to check for infection. As ordered, teach the patient about radiologic tests, such as excretory urography, and endoscopic tests, such as cystourethroscopy. (See *Teaching patients about reproductive system tests.*)

(Text continues on page 286.)

Teaching patients about reproductive system tests

The following chart will help you teach your patient about reproductive system tests.

Test and purpose	What to teach the patient
Breast biopsy • To determine if a breast lump is malignant • To determine if a breast lump is a cyst	*Needle biopsy* • The doctor uses a needle to remove a tissue or fluid sample from a breast lump. This simple procedure is commonly performed in the doctor's office. The patient isn't required to restrict food or fluids and will probably receive a local anesthetic. The procedure may take only 5 to 10 minutes. • The doctor cleans the skin of the breast with an antibacterial solution. Then he inserts a needle into the breast lump. Using a syringe, he aspirates a tissue or fluid sample, which he sends to the laboratory for evaluation. The patient will feel some pressure during the procedure. • After the anesthetic wears off, the breast may feel sore or tender for awhile. The doctor will recommend a mild analgesic for pain relief. The patient should watch for and report bleeding, redness, or tenderness at the biopsy site. *Surgical biopsy* • The patient may receive either general or local anesthesia. If she's having general anesthesia, she must fast after midnight before the test. • After she receives a general or local anesthetic, the doctor makes an incision in the breast to expose the mass. He then either incises a portion of tissue or excises the entire mass, sending the specimen to the laboratory for evaluation. After that, the doctor sutures the wound and applies an adhesive bandage. • After the procedure, medical staff check her vital signs frequently and she receives an analgesic to relieve postsurgical pain. She should watch for and report bleeding, tenderness, or redness at the biopsy site.
Breast ultrasonography • To help differentiate a cyst from a solid tissue mass	• This test provides an image of the inside of the breasts and can help detect and evaluate breast lumps. It can't determine if a lump is cancerous. • The patient isn't required to restrict her diet, medications, or activities before the test. She must remove her clothes from the waist up and put on a hospital gown. She should rest quietly during the test so the operator can concentrate on the images. The test is usually painless. • In most facilities, the patient lies on her back while medical staff apply a water-soluble gel to her breast. The test operator glides a handheld transducer back and forth over the breast. The patient will probably be able to see images of her breast on the monitor, but they'll look obscure. • She can resume her normal activities immediately after the test.
Colposcopy • To visualize the cervix and vagina • To evaluate vaginal or cervical lesions • To confirm malignancy after a positive Papanicolaou test	• This test allows close study of the vagina and cervix and, thus, provides more information than a routine pelvic examination. It's safe and painless and takes 5 to 10 minutes. • The patient assumes the lithotomy position. Next, the doctor inserts a vaginal speculum and swabs the cervix to remove any mucus. After viewing the cervix and vagina with the colposcope, he may biopsy areas that appear abnormal. • If a biopsy is performed, the patient should abstain from intercourse and shouldn't insert anything into the vagina until the biopsy site heals.

(continued)

Teaching patients about reproductive system tests *(continued)*

Test and purpose	What to teach the patient
Cystourethroscopy • To diagnose and evaluate urinary tract disorders	• This 20-minute test permits visualization of the bladder and urethra and helps evaluate the degree of prostatic enlargement and urinary obstruction. If a local anesthetic is ordered, the patient may receive a sedative before the test to help him relax. If a general anesthetic is used, he must fast for 8 hours before the test. • The patient lies in a supine position on an X-ray table with hips and knees flexed. Medical staff clean his genitalia with an antiseptic solution and drape him. The doctor administers a local anesthetic, if appropriate, and introduces the cystourethroscope through the urethra into the bladder. Next, he fills the bladder with irrigating solution and rotates the scope to inspect the bladder wall surface. • If the patient receives a local anesthetic, he may feel a burning sensation when the cystourethroscope passes through the urethra. He may also feel an urgent need to urinate as the bladder fills with irrigating solution. • If the patient receives a general anesthetic, his blood pressure, heart rate, and respirations are monitored every 15 minutes for the 1st hour after the test, and then hourly until stable. He should drink plenty of fluids and take prescribed analgesics. He should avoid alcohol for 48 hours after the test. Urinary burning and frequency will soon subside. He must take antibiotics, as ordered, to prevent bacterial infection. He should report flank or abdominal pain, chills, fever, or decreased urine output to the doctor immediately and should notify the doctor if he doesn't void within 8 hours after the test or if bright red blood continues to appear after three voidings.
Dilatation and curettage • To obtain tissue samples from reproductive organs to investigate the cause of bleeding • To detect the spread of cancer into the endometrium	• This test takes about 1 hour. The doctor obtains tissue samples from the uterus, cervix, endometrium, and other sites for laboratory analysis. If the patient has endometriosis, this procedure serves as a test and a treatment, not only determining the cause of abnormal bleeding but possibly also correcting it. • If the patient will have a general anesthetic, she shouldn't eat or drink anything for 8 to 10 hours before the procedure. If she'll be an outpatient, she should arrange for transportation home because she'll be groggy afterward. • The patient lies on her back with feet in stirrups. Then she receives local or general anesthesia. The doctor dilates her cervix and scrapes the uterine lining with a curette. Then he sends tissue samples to the laboratory for microscopic evaluation.
Excretory urography • To determine the size, shape, and position of the kidneys, their internal structures, and perirenal tissues • To evaluate and localize urinary obstruction and abnormal accumulation of fluid • To assess and diagnose complications following kidney transplantation	• This test evaluates the kidneys and urinary tract, and takes about 1 hour. • The patient should drink plenty of fluids and then fast for 8 hours before the test. He may receive a laxative or other bowel preparation before the test. • The patient lies in a supine position on an X-ray table. After injection of a contrast medium, a technician takes X-rays at specific intervals. The technician may place a belt around the patient's hips to keep the contrast medium at a certain level. The X-ray machine will make loud, clacking sounds as it exposes films. He may experience a transient burning sensation and metallic taste when the contrast medium is injected; he should report these and any other sensations to the doctor. • After the test, the patient should report symptoms of delayed reaction to the contrast medium.

Teaching patients about reproductive system tests *(continued)*

Test and purpose	What to teach the patient
Hysterosalpingography • To confirm tubal abnormalities, such as adhesions and occlusion • To confirm uterine abnormalities, such as fistulas, adhesions, and the presence of foreign bodies	• This test confirms uterine and fallopian tube abnormalities, and takes about 15 minutes. • The patient assumes the lithotomy position. Then the doctor inserts a vaginal speculum and swabs the cervix to remove any mucus. Next he inserts a cannula into the uterus and slowly injects a radiopaque dye. If this triggers cramping, the doctor temporarily stops the injection until the cramps subside. After the dye is injected, the uterus and fallopian tubes are viewed fluoroscopically, and radiographs are taken. The test may increase the likelihood of pregnancy; as the dye flows through the tubes, it may break up adhesions, stimulate cilia that promote passage of the ovum, or alter cervical mucus to be more receptive to sperm. • After the test, the patient should report signs of infection, such as fever, pain, increased pulse rate, malaise, and muscle ache.
Laparoscopy • To visualize the pelvic organs • To detect abnormalities of the uterus, fallopian tubes, and ovaries • To determine the extent of endometrial tissue growth and classify the severity of endometriosis • To remove endometrial implants • To confirm diagnosis of pelvic inflammatory disease	• This test allows the doctor to view the pelvic organs through a tubelike apparatus. It takes about 1 hour. • The patient shouldn't eat or drink anything after midnight before the test, unless advised otherwise by her doctor. She'll receive a general anesthetic. The procedure may require an outpatient visit or overnight stay. • The patient lies flat on the examining table with her feet in stirrups. The doctor makes two to four small abdominal incisions and inserts the laparoscope. If minor surgery is necessary (such as to remove an endometrioma or small fibroid tumors), the doctor performs it by passing instruments through one of the incisions. He may inject air into the abdominal cavity to see the internal structures better. • After the test, the patient who has had air injected into her abdominal cavity might experience shoulder pain from air irritating her diaphragm. Abdominal and shoulder pain should disappear within 36 hours. She should lie in a prone position with a pillow under her abdomen and should watch for signs of infection, such as redness, warmth, or increased tenderness at the incision site. She should temporarily refrain from douching and intercourse as her doctor orders.
Mammography • To screen for breast cancer • To investigate palpable and unpalpable breast masses, breast pain, or nipple discharge • To help to distinguish benign breast changes from breast malignancy	• This test is simply an X-ray of the breast. It can be used to screen for breast cancer or to diagnose the cause of a breast complaint. Although the test uses radiation, the amount is negligible. • The patient should tell her doctor if she might be pregnant or is breast-feeding. She may also be asked to avoid using deodorant on the test day (some deodorants contain substances that may interfere with test results). She should avoid lotions, which may make the breast slippery. She must take off her clothing above the waist, put on a gown, and remove jewelry from her neck. • The technician may ask the patient to either sit, stand, or lie still for the test. A technician helps her position her breast on an X-ray plate. Then the technician presses down another plate toward the first one to flatten the tissue. The patient will probably feel a cold sensation where her breast touches the plate and the compression may cause some discomfort. She may be asked to lift her arm or use her hand to hold her other breast out of the way. While the X-ray is being taken, she's told to hold her breath for a few seconds. Then the procedure is repeated for the other breast. • After the test, the patient may resume her normal diet and activities.

(continued)

Teaching patients about reproductive system tests *(continued)*

Test and purpose	What to teach the patient
Pelvic ultrasonography • To visualize pelvic structures • To detect foreign bodies and distinguish between cystic and solid masses (tumors)	• This test takes about 30 minutes. If the patient is pregnant, the test won't harm the fetus. • The patient must drink 6 to 8 glasses of fluid 1½ to 2 hours before the test. She must not void before the test because a full bladder serves as a landmark to define other pelvic organs. • The patient lies on her back while medical staff coat her abdomen with mineral oil. Then the technician guides a transducer over the abdomen to visualize the uterus, vagina, and adjoining organs. • The patient is allowed to empty her bladder immediately after the test.

Teaching about activity and lifestyle

If the patient is prescribed an indwelling urinary catheter, he may need help with catheter care at home. The patient may also need help coping with changes in sexual functioning. (See *Helping the BPH patient cope.*)

Teaching about medication

Discuss the drugs leuprolide acetate (Lupron) and nafarelin acetate, which hold promise for patients who aren't candidates for surgery. Both drugs prevent secretion of gonadotropins (sex hormones). Tell the patient that continuous use of these drugs reduces prostate volume, which may ease urinary frequency and urgency, diminished urine stream, and other signs and symptoms.

New options

A new medication, finasteride, blocks the production of the active form of testosterone, resulting in a reduction of prostate volume, which helps to ease such symptoms as incomplete bladder emptying and urinary frequency. Adverse effects of finasteride include decreased ejaculate volume and reduced libido. These symptoms decrease with time and are reversible with discontinuation of the drug.

Still more options

Other options include the drugs doxazosin and terazosin. These drugs reduce increased muscle tone of the prostate bladder and neck, thereby reducing obstruction and improving urinary outflow. Because these drugs are a first-line treatment, they're an effective combination therapy for men who suffer from BPH and hypertension.

Teaching about surgery

Tell the patient that surgery is the primary treatment for BPH. Describe two types of surgery to remove some or all prostatic tissue: transurethral resection (TUR) and open prostatectomy.

For either operation, explain that the patient may be placed on a low-residue diet before surgery and that the night before surgery he may receive a cleansing enema. The doctor typically prescribes antibiotics, usually 500 mg of erythromycin and 1 g of neomycin every 4 hours for 24 hours before surgery.

Transurethral resection

If the patient is having a TUR, tell him that the surgeon passes a small endoscopic instrument into the urethra to visualize the obstructing prostatic tissue. Then instruments to trim away the enlarged portion of the gland are inserted through the endoscope.

Less time and less pain

Explain that TUR typically takes less time, requires a shorter hospital stay, and produces less postoperative pain than an open prostatectomy. If the prostate gland is extremely large, however, TUR isn't feasible and an open procedure is usually necessary.

Open prostatectomy

During an open prostatectomy, the surgeon makes one of three incisions to expose and remove the obstructing prostatic tissue: suprapubic, retropubic, or perineal.

After surgery

The patient has an indwelling catheter for several days after surgery. The catheter is connected to a continuous flu-

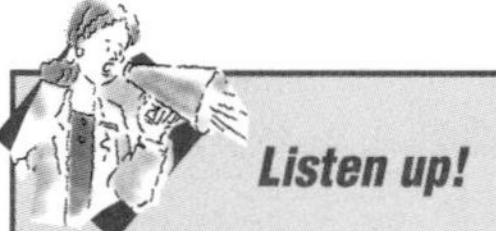

Listen up!

Helping the BPH patient cope

Here are a few last items to discuss with your patient with benign prostatic hyperplasia (BPH) before discharge.

Catheter care

If the patient will be discharged with an indwelling catheter in place, make sure that he knows how to care for the catheter. Tell him when to return to the health care facility for catheter removal.

Concerns about sexuality

Rarely, a patient experiences temporary or permanent impotence after surgery. More commonly, a patient may still be able to have an erection but will become sterile because his semen is expelled backward into the bladder instead of being ejaculated. Reassure the patient that seminal fluid in the bladder does no harm; it's simply eliminated in the urine. If he has problems adjusting sexually, refer him and his partner to a reputable counselor.

id irrigation system to ease the passage of blood clots. Tell him to expect blood in his urine for several days afterward.

When bleeding subsides

Inform the patient that as soon as the bleeding subsides, the catheter is removed. Warn him that bladder spasms may occur while the catheter is in place, but that medication can be given to provide relief. Following catheter removal, he may experience a sensation of heaviness in the pelvic region, urinary urgency, burning during urination, difficulty controlling urination, and the reappearance of some blood in the urine. Tell him that these effects subside with time.

Dysfunctional uterine bleeding

Dysfunctional uterine bleeding can be frightening and puzzling to a patient. She may ask you questions such as "What's happening to my body?" and "Do I have cancer?" Such questions will require you to provide not only information, but also emotional support. Most importantly, you'll need to reassure her that dysfunctional uterine bleeding is common and treatable.

What is it?

Explain to the patient that dysfunctional uterine bleeding is characterized by excessive and irregular uterine bleeding for which no organic cause can be found. Inform her that bleeding is judged abnormal based on:

- amount
- time of occurrence
- duration.

What is true dysfunctional bleeding?

True dysfunctional uterine bleeding results from a disruption in the hormones that regulate the menstrual cycle and estrogen-progesterone secretions, which, in turn, causes endometrial abnormalities and abnormal bleeding. Explain that this hormonal disruption has four variations. Either the body produces:

- no progesterone (resulting in nonovulatory dysfunctional uterine bleeding)

Causes of pseudodysfunctional uterine bleeding

Local disorders

- Uterine fibroids
- Cervicitis
- Pelvic inflammatory disease
- Ovarian tumors

Endocrine and systemic disorders

- Adrenal dysfunction
- Diabetes mellitus
- Hypothalamic or pituitary disorders
- Thyroid dysfunction
- Idiopathic thrombocytopenic purpura
- Leukemia
- Systemic lupus erythematosus
- Renal or hepatic disease
- Obesity

Drugs

- Anticoagulants
- Oral contraceptives
- Possibly digitalis glycosides

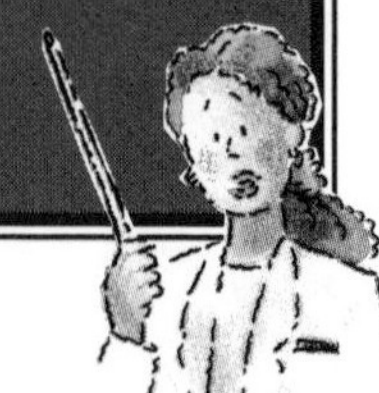

- too little progesterone (resulting in irregular endometrial ripening)
- too much progesterone or slow withdrawal of progesterone (resulting in irregular endometrial shedding)
- too little estrogen and no progesterone (resulting in endometrial atrophy).

What is pseudodysfunctional bleeding?

Pseudodysfunctional uterine bleeding, on the other hand, results from local disorders, endocrine or systemic disorders (or both), and certain drugs. (See *Causes of pseudodysfunctional uterine bleeding.*)

What's at risk?

Emphasize that untreated dysfunctional uterine bleeding can cause anemia. Urge the patient to report changes in breathing rate, dizziness, light-headedness, fatigue, and sweating to her doctor. Point out that hemorrhage from dysfunctional uterine bleeding can be life-threatening.

Teaching about tests

Tell the patient to expect a thorough physical and gynecologic examination. Warn her that, because dysfunctional uterine bleeding can stem from many causes, the doctor may order several diagnostic tests, including dilatation and curettage, a test in which tissue samples are scraped from the uterine lining.

Blood and urine tests

Inform the patient that blood and urine tests may provide clues about her health. For instance, they can tell whether she has anemia or abnormal levels of follicle-stimulating hormone, luteinizing hormone, prolactin, or testosterone. Thyroid function and glucose tolerance tests can determine whether a systemic disease is causing the bleeding.

Other tests may include a complete blood count (CBC), platelet count, prothrombin time, activated partial thromboplastin time, lupus erythematosus preparation (to rule out systemic lupus erythematosus), and an antinuclear antibody test (to rule out a connective tissue disease).

Diagnostic procedures

In addition to dilatation and curettage, the doctor may perform endometrial biopsy, hysterosalpingography, hysteroscopy, laparoscopy, or pelvic ultrasonography. (See *Teaching patients about reproductive system tests,* pages 283 to 286, and *Treating dysfunctional uterine bleeding.*)

Teaching about activity and lifestyle

In your teaching, help the patient understand the consequences of dysfunctional uterine bleeding. The patient may feel depressed or discouraged, especially if the cause of her bleeding has been difficult to diagnose. If she needs a hysterectomy, she might feel even more depressed after surgery because of abrupt hormonal fluctuations. (See *Coping with depression.*)

Teaching about medication

If the patient has pseudodysfunctional uterine bleeding from pelvic inflammatory disease, the doctor may prescribe antimicrobial therapy. If the patient has true dysfunctional uterine bleeding, explain that the doctor commonly prescribes hormonal therapy.

Various hormonal combinations and amounts are used to treat dysfunctional uterine bleeding, depending on the underlying disorder.

Failure to ovulate

For patients who don't ovulate or have irregular ovulation, estrogen and progesterone may help the endometrium develop normally and stimulate ovulation. Estrogen supplements stimulate the endometrium during the menstrual cycle's proliferative phase. Progesterone supplements, such as medroxyprogesterone (Provera) or norethindrone (Micronor), promote secretory development of the endometrium.

Irregular endometrial ripening

For irregular endometrial ripening, the doctor may prescribe progesterone. However, this drug should be prescribed cautiously because, if the patient is in the first 4 months of pregnancy, fetal abnormalities may result.

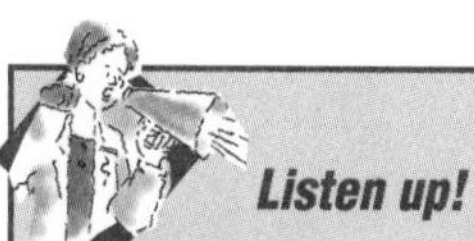

Treating dysfunctional uterine bleeding

Explain that as soon as the doctor determines the cause of uterine bleeding, appropriate treatment can start. Treatment usually follows one of two paths:

1. For true dysfunctional or pseudodysfunctional uterine bleeding, drug therapy is customarily used, unless the patient has cancer or is pregnant.
2. For bleeding caused by fibroids, uterine cancer, or uterine prolapse, a hysterectomy may be performed.

Irregular endometrial shedding

For irregular endometrial shedding, the doctor may prescribe a monophasic, biphasic, or triphasic oral contraceptive. Explain that:

- a monophasic drug supplies the same hormonal formula for 21 days
- a biphasic drug supplies two different formulas for 21 days
- a triphasic drug supplies three different formulas for 21 days.

Endometrial atrophy

For endometrial atrophy, indicating both estrogen and progesterone deficiencies, the doctor usually prescribes an oral contraceptive such as estrogen with progestin (Enovid, Ovulen). Reinforce the doctor's instructions on how to take the drug. Explain that withdrawal bleeding similar to a normal menstrual period should occur after she takes the last tablet.

Listen up!

Coping with depression

Reassure the patient with dysfunctional uterine bleeding that depression and irritability are common but temporary. Encourage her to express her feelings and ask questions. Counsel her family about mood swings, encouraging them to respond calmly and with understanding. Refer the patient and her family to a source of support and information.

Teaching about surgery

Explain that hysterectomy involves removing the uterus either abdominally or vaginally, depending on the disorder that is causing the problem. (See *Three types of hysterectomy.*)

Before surgery...

Inform the patient that she won't be allowed any food or fluids after midnight before surgery, she must shower with an antibacterial soap, and she may have to douche. She may also be given a cleansing enema. The morning of surgery, an indwelling urinary catheter is inserted, and an I.V. line is started. Shortly before surgery, the patient receives a sedative.

...and after

Tell the patient that she'll return from surgery with a perineal pad in place. Inform her that she can expect some abdominal pain; advise her not to wait until the pain is intense to ask for medication. Show her how to do leg exercises to prevent thromboembolism, and explain that she'll need to get out of bed and walk several times each day.

Three types of hysterectomy

- Total (removal of the entire uterus)
- Subtotal (removal of part of the uterus, leaving the cervical stump intact)
- Radical (removal of the uterus, upper vagina, cervix, and parametrial tissue)

From clear liquid to solid foods

Let her know that she'll still have an I.V. line in place and will be allowed nothing by mouth until she has bowel sounds and is passing gas or air; then her diet will progress from clear liquids to solid foods, as tolerated. (See *After surgery*.)

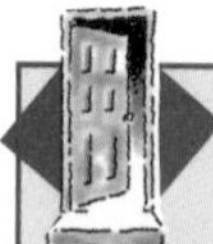

No place like home

After surgery

Review home care measures with your patient.

Coping with complications
Discuss signs of complications she should report and how to clean her wound to prevent infection.

Check daily
Instruct her to check vaginal discharge daily, explaining that small spots of blood or brownish staining are normal and may last about 1 week. Instruct the patient to report bleeding that resembles a menstrual period, severe cramping, or hot flashes.

Do's and don'ts
Urge the patient to walk or exercise regularly as tolerable. Caution her not to exercise too vigorously or to lift heavy objects. Emphasize that she shouldn't use a tampon, douche, engage in sexual intercourse, or insert anything into her vagina for 6 weeks. To prevent constipation, suggest a diet high in fiber or tell her to drink plenty of fluids.

Endometriosis

Start your teaching by reassuring the patient that endometriosis isn't life-threatening or cancerous (rarely, an endometrial mass may become malignant).

What is it?

Explain that endometriosis is a benign growth of endometrial tissue (the tissue that makes up the uterus's inner membrane) outside the uterus.

What happens?

Tell the patient that tissue growths, also known as endometrial implants, are usually confined to the pelvic area but can appear anywhere in the body. Explain that hormones secreted during the menstrual cycle influence this misplaced tissue, causing profuse menstrual bleeding and, sometimes, pain in the lower abdomen, vagina, posterior pelvis, and back.

How painful is it?

Typically, the patient feels suprapubic pain (pain above the pubic arch) that begins several days before menses and lasts possibly throughout menstruation. Associated symptoms include dyspareunia and painful bowel movements. As the tissue grows and spreads, it irritates and scars surrounding structures, leading to fibrosis, with adhesions and blood-filled cysts.

What causes it?

Inform the patient that the definitive cause of endometriosis is unknown, although several theories exist. Endometriosis is currently thought to stem from abnormal metabolic and immunologic activity.

What are the risk factors?

Tell her that although the causes of endometriosis are controversial, the risk factors are indisputable. Women with short menstrual cycles (fewer than 27 days) and long menstrual periods (more than 7 days) are prone to the disease. Also at risk are women who have a family history of the disease, give birth late in life, or have a retroflexed (tilted) uterus.

Who does it affect?

From 5% to 10% of all women develop endometriosis in their lifetime. Most commonly, diagnosis occurs between ages 25 and 29. Race doesn't affect the prevalence of the disorder.

What's at risk?

Urge the patient to comply with prescribed treatment because this may help prevent or postpone such complications as:

- infertility
- ruptured endometrioma (an ovarian cyst composed of endometrial cells)
- anemia.

Explain to the patient that endometrial implants cause inflammation. Consequently, fibrosis (scar tissue and adhesions) usually involves the fallopian tubes, ovaries, uterus, bladder, and intestine, binding these organs and contributing to infertility. Also inform her that excessive bleeding during menstruation may lead to anemia.

Teaching about tests

Teach about diagnostic procedures to detect and confirm endometriosis, including a pelvic examination, abdominal palpation, and laparoscopy. (See *Teaching patients about reproductive system tests,* pages 283 to 286.)

Small and bluish

Inform the patient that the doctor will take her history and then perform an internal pelvic examination to look for endometrial implants, which appear as small bluish areas on the cervix and in the vagina.

Then he'll check the uterosacral ligaments and cul-de-sac for nodules and tenderness, the ovaries for enlarge-

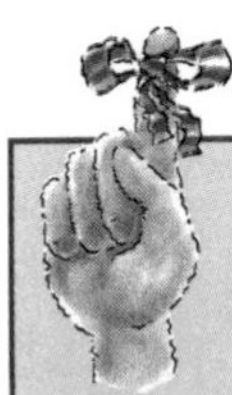

Memory jogger

To help your patient remember the procedures to diagnose endometriosis, think *PAL* — your friends in fighting this disease:

Pelvic exam

Abdominal palpation

Laparoscopy.

ment and tenderness, and the adnexa for fullness and nodules. He will also palpate over the uterus to check its position and, if necessary for accuracy, will palpate through the rectum.

Inform the patient that the doctor occasionally orders other tests, such as a barium enema, cystoscopy, or cul-de-sac aspiration, to pinpoint sites of endometrial tissue growth. (See *Treating endometriosis*.)

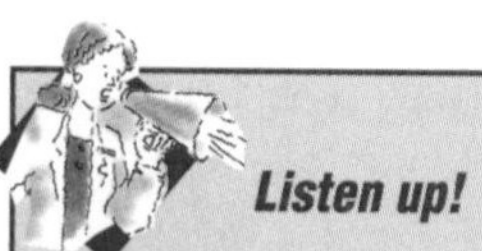

Listen up!

Treating endometriosis

Explain that treatment for endometriosis usually begins conservatively, then progresses to more aggressive measures as needed.

Factors affecting treatment for endometriosis include:

- patient's age
- desire to bear children
- disease stage
- severity of symptoms.

Medication, surgery, or both

Common treatments include medications to relieve pain, reduce inflammation, and suppress ovulation, or surgery to remove endometrial implants and adhesions. Alternatively, the doctor may recommend combined therapy: medication to shrink the implants, allowing easier surgical removal. This treatment may also prevent adhesions.

Teaching about activity and lifestyle

In your teaching, include information to help the patient cope day-to-day with the physiologic and emotional aspects of this disorder. (See *Tips for women with endometriosis.*)

Teaching about medication

Tell the patient that the doctor may prescribe analgesics and anti-inflammatory drugs to relieve symptoms and reduce inflammation. Examples include ibuprofen (Advil, Motrin), mefenamic acid (Ponstel), and naproxen (Anaprox). Inform her that hormonal agents, such as oral contraceptives or androgens, may be the primary treatment.

Oral contraceptives

Point out that oral contraceptives treat endometriosis, not just its symptoms. Explain that suppressing ovulation with oral contraceptives has the same effect as pregnancy, which helps resolve endometriosis or cause remission.

A state of pseudopregnancy

Tell the patient that the doctor usually prescribes low-dose oral contraceptives for 6 to12 months, depending on her response, to reduce menstrual flow and endometrial implants. The oral contraceptives create a state of pseudopregnancy, which causes atrophy of endometrial implants. Mention that this therapy may improve her condition only temporarily.

Good advice

Because oral contraceptives may cause breast tenderness, dizziness, headache, and nausea, advise the patient to take safety precautions. For example, if she feels dizzy, she shouldn't drive a car.

Androgens

Explain that danazol (Danocrine), a steroid, lowers estrogen production and stops ovulation and menstruation, which induces pseudomenopause. As a result, endometrial cells atrophy, improving endometriosis. The patient can start this therapy immediately after a menstrual period. Tell her that she'll probably take danazol twice daily for 6 to 9 months.

Possibly irreversible

Make sure that she understands danazol's possible adverse effects. (See *Adverse effects of danazol,* page 296.) Explain that these effects result from the drug's androgenic effects and that some effects may be irreversible.

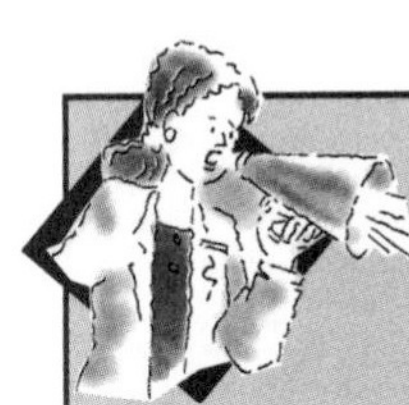

Listen up!

Tips for women with endometriosis

Provide your patient with the following tips about endometriosis.

Doing away with dyspareunia
If your patient has dyspareunia, suggest that she take an analgesic or apply a vaginal lubricant before sexual intercourse. Also suggest that she use a superior or side-lying position for greater control over pressure exerted during intercourse to help prevent dyspareunia.

Asking about anemia
If the patient feels exceptionally weak and tired or has other symptoms suggesting anemia, urge her to discuss this with her doctor. Advise her to include iron-rich foods in her diet and to get adequate rest.

Getting group support
Finally, help the patient cope with endometriosis by acquainting her with a support group. If she asks for help in dealing with endometriosis-related infertility, refer her to a support group such as Resolve for infertile couples.

Straight talk about pregnancy
If you're teaching a young woman with mild endometriosis who wants to have children, tell her the following:

- More than 50% of patients with mild-to-moderate endometriosis are able to become pregnant.
- Pregnancy delays the progression of endometriosis, but it doesn't always cure the disorder.
- Hormonal changes associated with pregnancy cause the implants to soften and atrophy.
- Don't postpone pregnancy because infertility is a common complication of endometriosis.

Drugs to reduce estrogen levels

If the doctor prescribes nafarelin or a similar drug to reduce circulating estrogen levels, tell the patient that reduction of circulating estrogen levels induces pseudomenopause. Nafarelin is thought to be as effective as danazol in halting the progression of endometrial implants.

Forewarned

Make sure that the patient understands how this drug works, and warn her about adverse effects related to low estrogen levels, including bone loss, decreased libido, hot flashes, and vaginal dryness.

Adverse effects of danazol

- Acne
- Decreased breast size
- Edema
- Flushing
- Mild hirsutism
- Sweating
- Voice deepening
- Clitoral enlargement
- Weight gain
- Depression
- Dizziness
- Fatigue
- Light-headedness

Teaching about surgery

Explain that the goal of surgery is to remove as many endometrial implants, adhesions, or endometriomas as possible and still preserve healthy, functioning tissue. Answer questions about anesthesia, and tell the patient how to follow preoperative and postoperative procedures to prevent complications and ensure recovery. (See *Surgery for endometriosis.*)

Therapeutic laparoscopy

Inform the patient that the doctor may remove endometrial implants found during diagnostic laparoscopy. Then explain how the surgeon may combine laparoscopy with such procedures as electrocautery, cryosurgery, or laser surgery to remove the implants. (See *Without a knife.*)

Laparotomy

If the doctor can't treat the patient during laparoscopy, he may perform a laparotomy. In this procedure, the surgeon makes an abdominal incision to open the pelvic cavity, and may remove implants or cysts.

Benefits

Explain that cyst removal typically relieves dysmenorrhea, abnormal bleeding, and dyspareunia and preserves the remaining tissue. Preserving tissue helps to maintain reproductive function, with minimal scarring and adhesions.

Without a knife

Tell your patient that during laparoscopy the surgeon may remove endometrial implants and adhesions by inserting special instruments through two to four tiny incisions.

Laser surgery

Laser energy can destroy deep-seated, widespread implants and adhesions. Focused through the laparoscope, this beam travels to the target tissue and raises the tissue's intracellular water temperature to the flash point. In turn, the tissue vaporizes, and the intense heat coagulates blood vessels. The vapor is removed by suction through the laparoscope.

Cryosurgery

To destroy tissue by freezing, the surgeon uses the laparoscope to introduce a probe into the target area. Then he instills a refrigerant (such as liquid nitrogen or Freon) to produce intracapillary thrombosis and tissue necrosis.

Electrocautery

The surgeon uses laparoscopy to apply to implants a small wire loop heated by a steady, direct electrical current. Doing so de-

Hysterectomy and bilateral salpingo-oophorectomy

For widespread endometriosis in a patient who accepts the loss of fertility, who's beyond childbearing age, and whose disease doesn't respond to drug therapy, the doctor may recommend total hysterectomy and bilateral salpingo-oophorectomy. Explain that this surgery prevents recurrent endometriosis by removing the uterus, cervix, fallopian tubes, and ovaries.

Addressing aftereffects

Discuss the aftereffects of surgery, including decreased estrogen levels leading to bone loss, decreased libido, hot flashes, and vaginal dryness. Then, if appropriate, discuss possible treatments, such as estrogen replacement therapy, which reduces the severity of these effects.

Presacral neurectomy

For severe pain with endometriosis, the doctor may perform a presacral neurectomy.

Good news and bad

Make sure the patient understands that this procedure relieves pain by removing a nerve, but that it doesn't cure endometriosis. Also explain that after this operation she may have decreased bowel and bladder control and heav-

Surgery for endometriosis

- *Therapeutic laparoscopy* — removing endometrial implants using a laparoscope
- *Laparotomy* — removing endometrial implants through an incision in the abdomen
- *Hysterectomy and bilateral salpingo-oophorectomy* — removing the female reproductive organs
- *Presacral neurectomy* — removing a nerve to relieve endometrial pain

ier menstrual periods because of vasodilation. If appropriate, teach bowel and bladder retraining techniques.

Fibrocystic breast changes

Tell the patient that fibrocystic breast changes are alterations in the breasts (such as swelling, lumpiness, and cysts) that occur during the menstrual cycle.

Is it dangerous?

Emphasize that the condition is benign. Also stress how common it is: about 50% of all women have signs and symptoms of fibrocystic breast changes, and 90% of all women have tissue changes characteristic of the condition.

Is it cancer?

In teaching about fibrocystic breast changes, your first priority is to reassure the patient that this condition isn't cancerous. Tell the patient that only women with certain histologic changes have an increased risk of developing cancer; emphasize that the vast majority of women with fibrocystic breast changes have no increased risk of breast cancer.

Is it a disorder?

Many medical experts don't consider fibrocystic breast changes a disorder at all. Because of the condition's benign nature, they've dropped the use of pathologic terms, such as "fibrocystic breast disease," to describe it.

Even so, the patient's symptoms must be taken seriously. If she has lumpy breasts, plan to prepare her for diagnostic tests. If she has breast discomfort, expect to review treatment measures.

How is it recognized?

Explain that signs and symptoms differ among patients. The most common complaints are lumpy, tender, and painful breasts, but cysts or nipple discharge may also be present.

Inform the patient that an increase in fibrous tissue also may cause breast lumpiness — but again, this change does

It's a cycle

Point out the cyclic nature of most signs and symptoms and their close relationship to the menstrual cycle or menopause. Mention that they usually worsen just before the menstrual period and improve afterward. Explain that the patient's symptoms often increase as she approaches menopause, while, ironically, the condition improves following menopause.

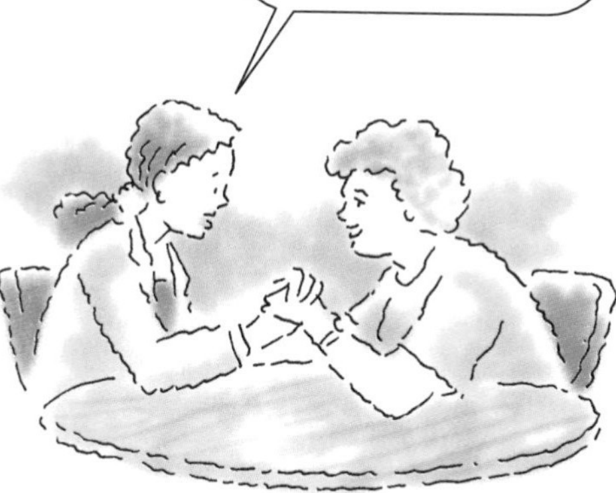
Fibrocystic breast changes are benign and very common. Most likely, you have no increased risk of breast cancer.

not indicate breast cancer. In some patients, fibrocystic breast changes are associated with nipple discharge. If so, advise the patient to see her doctor, particularly if the discharge is spontaneous, persistent, or unilateral.

A full, aching feeling

Tell the patient that estrogen levels increase during the follicular phase of the menstrual cycle, causing fluid retention and glandular tissue proliferation. As breast tissue stretches to accommodate the excess fluid, the patient may experience breast discomfort, often described as a full, aching feeling. (See *It's a cycle.*)

Nerve irritation and inflammation

Breast discomfort may also result from nerve irritation and inflammation associated with edema and fibrocystic breast changes. Typically, the upper outer quadrants of both breasts become painful in the week before menstruation. Reassure the patient that this discomfort usually subsides with the start of her menstrual period.

Through the life span

Symptoms of fibrocystic breast changes typically change with age. Discuss with the patient what to expect at each stage of aging. (See *Fibrocystic breast changes through the life span.*)

Where does it come from?

Inform the patient that the cause of fibrocystic breast changes is unknown. However, most researchers agree that ovarian hormones are involved. Fibrocystic breast changes may result from abnormal hormone production or from hypersensitive breast tissues that overrespond to normal hormone levels. Mention that fibrocystic breast changes are more common in women with early menarche, late menopause, and irregular or anovulatory cycles. Women with fibrocystic breast changes also are more likely to have symptoms of premenstrual syndrome.

Fibrocystic breast changes through the life span

If your patient has fibrocystic breast changes, explain how the symptoms are likely to change as she ages.

Late teens to early 30s
Common signs and symptoms of fibrocystic breast changes include breast tenderness and fullness with minimal lumpiness in the week before menstruation.

Late 30s to mid-40s
Breast pain typically increases and lasts longer during the menstrual cycle. Increasing breast nodularity prompts many women to seek medical evaluation.

Late 40s and 50s
A woman may experience increasing discomfort and the sudden onset of painful single or multiple lumps.

Teaching about tests

Tell the patient that fibrocystic breast changes seldom cause complications, although the signs and symptoms may progress. Rarely, a patient who undergoes biopsy for a benign breast lump is found to have atypical hyperplasia (an abnormal increase in tissue).

This clinical finding, combined with a family history of breast cancer, does increase the risk of breast cancer. If the patient has atypical hyperplasia, advise her to seek close follow-up care.

Expect an exam

Teach the patient that the diagnostic workup begins with a medical history and physical examination. Explain that the doctor will examine her breasts for lumps, tenderness, and other signs and symptoms. Other tests may include mammography, ultrasonography, needle aspiration, and breast biopsy. (See *Teaching patients about reproductive system tests,* pages 283 to 286.)

Teaching about activity and lifestyle

Provide the patient with insight on how to cope with her condition in daily life. (See *Living with fibrocystic breast changes.*)

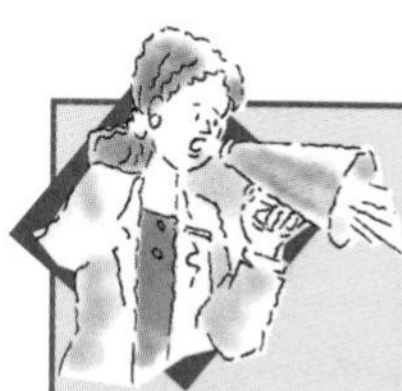

Listen up!

Living with fibrocystic breast changes

Here are some additional teaching points for helping women cope with fibrocystic breast changes.

Once a month

Encourage the patient to perform monthly breast self-examinations. Although the patient with fibrocystic breasts may be no more prone to breast cancer than other women, her lumpy breasts may make it harder to detect a malignant tumor.

Timing

Advise her to examine her breasts at the same time during each menstrual cycle — ideally, 2 or 3 days following her menstrual period — so that she doesn't become confused by her normal cyclic fibrocystic changes. Instruct her to contact her doctor if she notices any new or unusual lumps or increased tenderness.

Additional support

Advise the patient to wear a support bra — even while sleeping — when she experiences breast discomfort. Point out that a support bra is especially important during exercise.

...and more support

To help her cope with the condition, refer her to an organization such as OncoLink (reach them on the Internet at www.oncolink.upenn.edu) that can provide further information and support.

Teaching about diet

Advise the patient to cut down on salt in the week before her menstrual period. Explain that reducing salt intake can help prevent the fluid retention that causes breast discomfort. Instruct her not to add salt to foods during cooking or at the table. Also caution her to avoid the many processed foods with hidden salt. Other treatment approaches include the use of vitamin E and thiamine. (See *Hold the pickles,* page 302.)

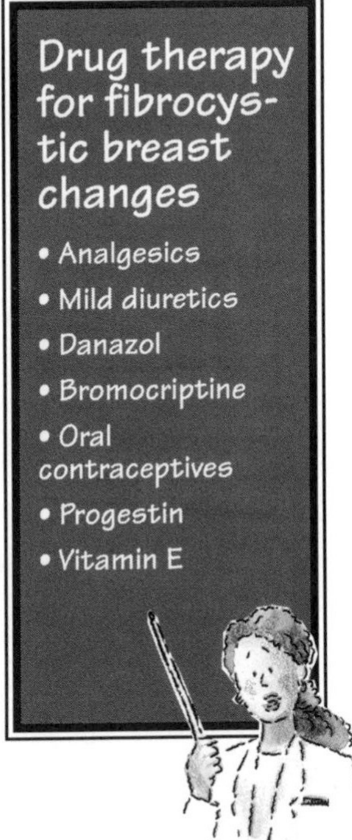
Drug therapy for fibrocystic breast changes
• Analgesics
• Mild diuretics
• Danazol
• Bromocriptine
• Oral contraceptives
• Progestin
• Vitamin E

Teaching about medication

Explain that medication use varies for each patient, depending on her signs and symptoms. (See *Drug therapy for fibrocystic breast changes.*)

For minor pain

If the patient suffers breast discomfort, suggest that she talk to her doctor about taking aspirin or acetaminophen during the week before her menstrual period.

A mild diuretic

The doctor also may prescribe a mild diuretic, such as chlorothiazide (Diuril), during this time. Explain that the diuretic may relieve breast fullness by reducing the amount of fluid in the body. Caution the patient about the potential effects of fluid and electrolyte imbalance.

For severe pain

If the patient has severe breast pain that can't be relieved by conservative measures, the doctor may prescribe danazol (Danocrine), a steroid. Danazol reduces hormonal stimulation of the breast, thereby helping to reduce breast pain and nodularity.

Caution the patient that danazol can cause harsh adverse effects. (See *Adverse effects of danazol,* page 296.)

Helpful but not without a down side

A prolactin blocker, bromocriptine mesylate (Parlodel) helps some women, but it also causes adverse reactions. Caution the patient that possible adverse reactions include dizziness, headache, and nausea. Like danazol, bromocriptine is usually reserved for patients with severe pain.

Partaking of the pill

Oral contraceptive use (estrogen-progestin combinations) or progesterone therapy helps to relieve breast tenderness in some patients. For example, medroxyprogesterone acetate (Provera) blocks estrogen's effects on the breast. If the doctor prescribes Provera, reinforce instructions on when to take it — typically on days 15 through 25 of the menstrual cycle. Inform her of potential adverse effects.

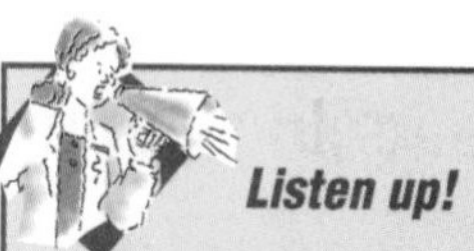

Listen up!

Hold the pickles

List the salt-laden foods that the patient with fibrocystic breast changes should avoid, such as pickles, canned soups, bacon, baked goods, and commercially prepared foods.

I can't prove it but...

Mention that some patients notice that their signs and symptoms subside when they avoid foods and medications containing caffeine and other methylxanthines. If the patient wants to try this treatment, recommend diet changes to eliminate methylxanthines. However, point out that this treatment isn't medically proven.

Teaching about surgery

As a last resort, the patient may need to have a cyst surgically removed. Usually, this operation is necessary only if a cyst can't be aspirated or if a solid mass remains after aspiration. Tell the patient that the procedure is usually done under local anesthesia in an outpatient unit.

Pelvic inflammatory disease

Tell the patient that pelvic inflammatory disease (PID) is an infection of the female genital tract. Because PID is commonly transmitted sexually, your teaching challenges may include helping the patient talk openly about her sexual history and encouraging her to avoid sex during treatment and to adopt safe-sex practices following treatment.

You'll also need to urge the patient to contact her sexual partners so they can be checked for infection and treated, if necessary. Make the patient aware that, if not properly treated, PID can permanently damage her reproductive system, causing infertility and other complications.

What causes it?

Specify the risk factors for PID. (See *Risk factors for PID.*) Because of their recipient role during intercourse, women are more likely to receive an infection from their partner than to transmit it. In addition, the warmth and moistness of the vagina provide a medium for bacterial growth.

How does it happen?

Inform the patient that bacteria may invade the fallopian tubes and ovaries from distant sources of infection, as in tuberculosis, or from adjacent infected areas, as may occur in appendicitis or inflammatory bowel disease.

More commonly, bacteria ascend from the vagina and cervix. Infection by this route may result from normal genital bacteria or from sexually transmitted bacteria, such as *Neisseria gonorrhoeae* and *Chlamydia trachomatis.*

Risk factors for PID

- Beginning sexual activity at an early age
- Multiple sex partners
- History of sexual disorders
- Certain types of contraception
- Avoidance of contraception entirely

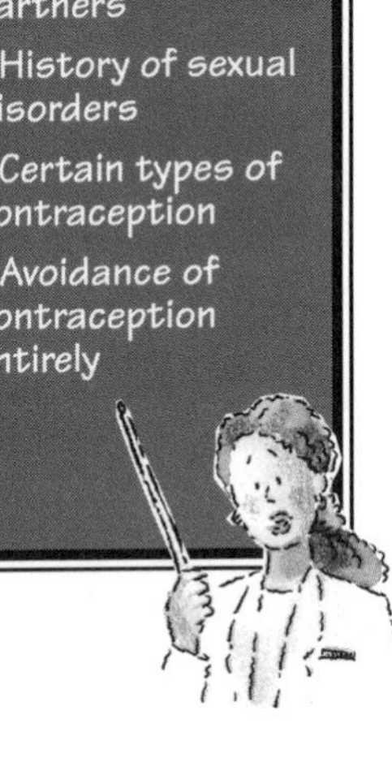

What are the effects?

Explain that the most common symptom of PID is lower abdominal pain; however, it's also possible to be asymptomatic. (See *Diagnosing PID,* page 304.)

What's at risk?

Complications may include recurrent or chronic PID, pelvic peritonitis, chronic pelvic pain, tubo-ovarian abscess, periappendicitis, perihepatitis, infertility, and ectopic pregnancy. Point out that compliance with antibiotic therapy is essential to prevent serious, permanent complications.

Teaching about tests

Explain to the patient that various tests may be ordered to confirm PID's cause, identify the causative microorganisms, and select antibiotic therapy.

Basic tests

For example, you'll teach the patient about baseline laboratory studies, including a CBC and erythrocyte sedimentation rate. She may also have a pelvic examination to obtain a sample of endocervical secretions for a Gram stain. Tell the patient that this test will help select the appropriate antibiotic. If appropriate, describe other tests, such as culdocentesis, laparoscopy, and ultrasonography.

Culdocentesis

If the doctor orders culdocentesis to obtain secretions for a Gram stain and culture, tell the patient that this test involves the insertion of a needle through the vagina and aspiration of fluid in an area called the cul-de-sac (a small pouch that lies between the lower portion of the uterus and the rectum). Tell her that this painless test takes about 30 minutes. Mention that positioning is the same as for any pelvic examination.

Laparoscopy

Explain that laparoscopy takes 15 to 30 minutes and may be used to inspect pelvic structures to help detect abnormalities of the uterus, fallopian tubes, and ovaries. Inform the patient that this test may reveal erythema, edema, or seropurulent exudate to confirm the diagnosis of PID.

Ultrasonography

Inform the patient that the doctor may order pelvic ultrasonography. Explain that this test takes about 30 minutes and may be performed using an ultrasound wand inserted into the vagina or held over the abdomen to visualize the pelvic structures.

Teaching about activity and lifestyle

Instruct the patient to get extra rest to help resist infection. If she requires surgery, explain that she may have activity restrictions afterward. Most important, instruct the patient on how to avoid future infection, including the importance of adopting safer sexual practices, such as making sure sexual partners use condoms. (See *PID points.*)

Teaching about medication

Explain that antibiotic therapy begins immediately after collection of culture specimens to prevent progression of PID. Tell the patient that drug therapy will be reevaluated when laboratory results are available (in 24 to 48 hours).

Details about drug therapy

Inform the patient that the preferred therapy for PID includes cefoxitin, ceftriaxone, doxycycline, and clindamycin. One of these may be used as a single drug therapy or in combination with another. Emphasize to the patient that she should take her medication at the same time every day for the prescribed duration. Tell her to take it with adequate amounts of fluid (8 oz [237 ml]). If GI upset occurs, she should take the drug with food. Tell her to report diarrhea, vomiting, and nausea.

Diagnosing PID

Symptoms that must be present:

- abdominal tenderness
- history of pelvic pain
- cervical motion tenderness
- adnexal tenderness (ovaries, fallopian tubes, and uterine ligament).

Plus at least one of these:

- fever of 100.4° F (38° C) or higher
- purulent vaginal discharge
- abnormal vaginal bleeding
- leukocytosis
- white blood cells and bacteria in peritoneal fluid
- inflammatory mass
- elevated erythrocyte sedimentation rate
- gram negative diplococci or *Chlamydia trachomatis.*

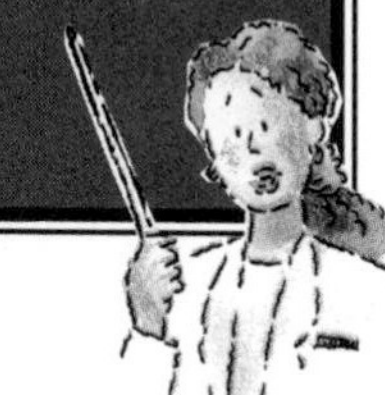

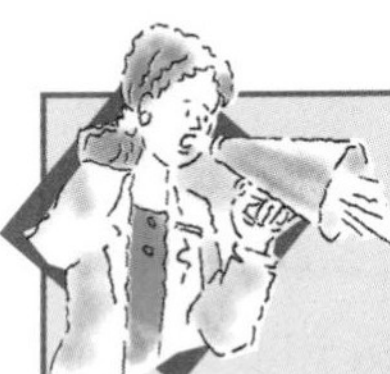

Listen up!

PID points

Here are some important points to share with the patient with pelvic inflammatory disease (PID).

Wait

Advise the patient with PID to avoid sexual activity until she has completed the medication course and remains free from all signs of infection. If PID results from a sexually transmitted disease, advise her to avoid sexual activity with any infected partners until after they're treated.

Do's and don'ts

Teach the patient how to reduce the risk of reinfection (PID has a 25% recurrence rate). Because bacteria may reenter the cervix from the vagina, warn her to avoid inserting anything into her vagina, such as fingers, tampons, or douches. Stress that she seek immediate medical care for recurring symptoms.

More do's and don'ts

Advise the patient to reduce the risk of contracting a sexually transmitted disease. Strongly encourage her to use condoms with a vaginal spermicide or a diaphragm for contraception, but to avoid using an intrauterine device. If she becomes pregnant, encourage early prenatal care because PID increases the risk of ectopic pregnancy.

Reacting to a rash

Explain to the patient that if she develops a rash when exposed to sunlight or ultraviolet light, she should stop taking the drug and call the doctor immediately. He may prescribe alternative therapy.

In the hospital

If the patient is hospitalized, teach her that treatment consists of I.V. drug therapy for at least 4 days, followed by oral drug therapy after discharge to complete the 10- to 14-day regimen.

Teaching about surgery

Inform the patient that if she fails to respond to antibiotic therapy or exhibits signs of tubo-ovarian abscess, leakage, or rupture, she'll undergo laparotomy.

Removing infected tissue

Explain that the surgeon makes an abdominal incision to enter the pelvic cavity. Then he removes the infected tissues. Be sure to prepare the patient for the possibility that removal of the infected tissues may involve her uterus, ovaries, and fallopian tubes.

6 weeks off

After laparotomy, instruct the patient to check the incision site for signs of infection, such as redness, swelling, or discharge. Tell her to resume activities as tolerated but to avoid heavy lifting or other strenuous activities for about 6 weeks.

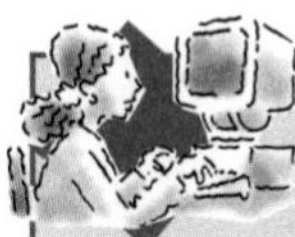

Getting connected

PID on-line

For more information about pelvic inflammatory disease (PID), direct the patient to the PID section of the National Institutes of Health Web site (www.niaid.nih.gov/factsheets/stdpid.htm).

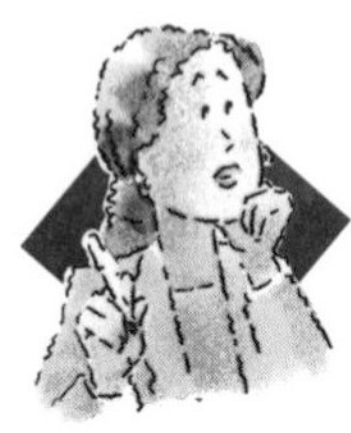

Quick quiz

1. Tell the patient with an enlarged prostate that he may experience:

A. irregular bowel movements.
B. urine retention.
C. lower abdominal pain.

Answer: B. Because the prostate is enlarged, the urethra can be obstructed, causing incomplete emptying of the bladder.

2. Explain to the patient with endometriosis that this disorder results from growth of endometrial tissue:

A. inside the uterus.
B. outside the uterus.
C. inside the ovaries.

Answer: B. Endometriosis is the growth of endometrial tissue outside the uterus.

3. In your patient teaching, emphasize that endometriosis is a:

A. benign disorder.
B. chronic disorder.
C. sexually transmitted disease.

Answer: A. Endometriosis is a benign disorder that isn't life-threatening or cancerous.

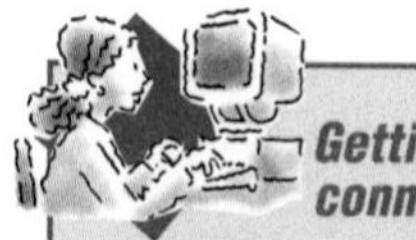

Getting connected

Endometriosis on the net

For information about endometriosis, direct the patient to the Endometriosis Association Web site (www.endometriosisassn.org).

Scoring

If you answered all three items correctly, great!
You're learning the answers at a remarkable rate!

If you answered two correctly, don't moan or whine.
It's easy to see, your mistakes are benign.

If you answered fewer than two correctly, don't be blue.
Just sit down with this chapter for a quick review.

Cancer

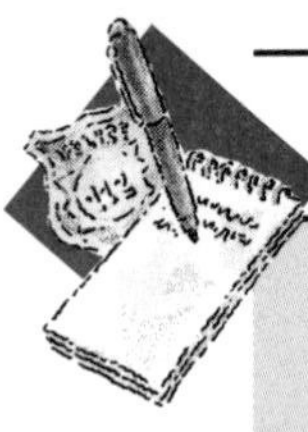

Just the facts

In this chapter you'll learn:

- how to teach patients with recently diagnosed cancer
- how to teach patients with recurring cancer
- how to teach about diagnostic tests for cancer
- how to teach about cancer treatments.

Teaching about cancer

The diagnosis of cancer threatens every patient's sense of well-being. Patients commonly experience disbelief, fear, isolation, and confusion. What's more, they may have misconceptions mixed with realistic concerns about the disorder, its treatment, and its prognosis.

Cancer is characterized by cells that grow and multiply uncontrollably.

Ups and downs

When cancer recurs, the effect may be even more shattering. Affected patients may suffer disbelief and guilt compounded by despair or rage. Commonly, their first reaction is "How can this be happening to me again?" Some patients may have put their past experiences with cancer behind them. As a result, the impact of its recurrence may be more profound than that of the initial diagnosis. Other patients, in contrast, may not be surprised when cancer recurs. Still, they'll endure emotional ups and downs as they adjust to the diagnosis.

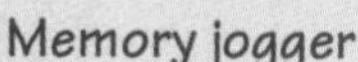

Memory jogger

Early detection of cancer offers the best chance for cure. But how can patients know what to look for? Teach them to remember the word *CAUTION*. It will help remind them of cancer's warning signs:

- **C**hange in bowel or bladder habits
- **A** wound that doesn't heal
- **U**nusual bleeding or discharge
- **T**hickening or lump in a breast or testicle or elsewhere
- **I**ndigestion or difficulty swallowing
- **O**bvious change in wart or mole
- **N**agging cough or hoarseness.

If the patient notices any of these signs, he should report them to his doctor.

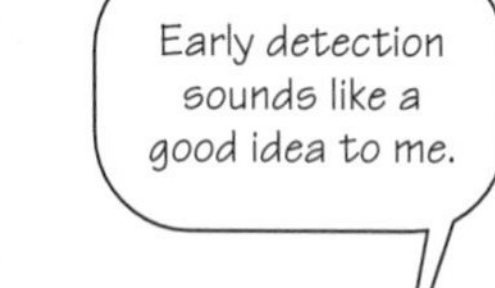
Early detection sounds like a good idea to me.

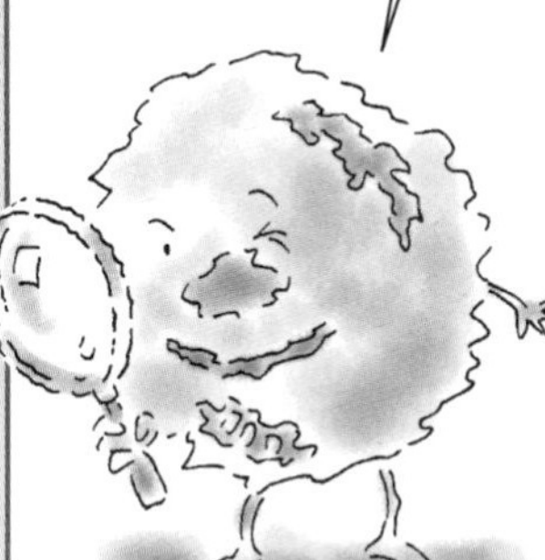

Recently diagnosed cancer

Help your patient adjust to a recent diagnosis of cancer by giving him only the information he needs, requests, or seems ready to learn. Answer his questions specifically, but don't bombard him with details.

Clear, accurate, factual, sensitive

Pay attention to the way you present information. A patient who has endured weeks of tension before learning the diagnosis may interpret vague descriptions or broad reassurances as an attempt to avoid discussing death. Provide clear, accurate information in a factual but sensitive way, and give the patient time to absorb what you tell him.

Let it sink in

Remember, some patients respond to stress by hearing only what they want to hear. A patient who repeats the same questions or remembers only part of what you tell him may need more time to absorb the information. He may also need to hear certain information repeated. Reassure him that he'll be working with health care workers dedicated to treating his disease.

Tell me what you know about cancer.

Discussing the patient's perception

Find out what your patient knows about cancer, its diagnosis, and its treatment. By understanding his perception of cancer, you can set learning goals to fill knowledge gaps and correct misconceptions. Ask your patient about his experience with other people who have had cancer. This may affect his attitude about his diagnosis. For example, a patient whose neighbor died of colorectal cancer may perceive this type of cancer as invariably fatal.

Common fears

Determine the patient's response to what the doctor has told him. Cancer patients commonly experience fear about their condition or treatment. (See *Common cancer fears.*) Never dismiss the patient's feelings. Determine whether the patient needs professional counseling or other help. If necessary, consult a more experienced colleague or a professional counselor. (See *Let's clear this up,* page 310.)

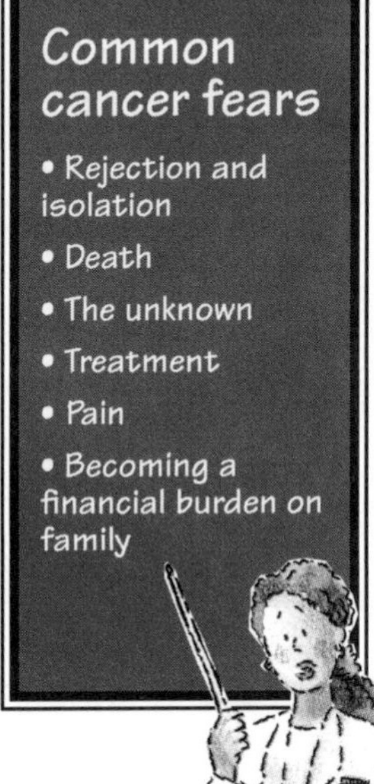

Common cancer fears
• Rejection and isolation
• Death
• The unknown
• Treatment
• Pain
• Becoming a financial burden on family

Discussing the disorder

Tell the patient that cancer refers to a group of disorders characterized by cells that grow and multiply uncontrollably and have the capacity to invade and metastasize to other sites. Discuss with him details regarding his particular type of cancer. (See *Cancer teaching points,* pages 311 to 315.)

Tumors

If the patient has a tumor, explain that as cancer cells continue to multiply, the tumor grows. A localized tumor remains confined to a specific area. A metastatic tumor invades neighboring tissues or spreads to other sites — most commonly the lungs, liver, bones, and brain.

Let's clear this up

Help the patient by correcting misconceptions. Sometimes a patient's misconceptions about cancer and its treatment are far more disturbing than the facts. Common misconceptions include:

- Cancer is always fatal.
- Cancer is always excruciatingly painful.
- Cancer is contagious.
- Cancer always causes disfigurement.

Cancer isn't always fatal

Cancer survival rates have improved consistently since the turn of the century. Today one of every two cancer patients will be cured.

Cancer isn't always excruciatingly painful

Many patients can recall one or more friends or relatives who suffered painful cancer deaths. If your patient has a type of cancer that doesn't usually produce pain, such as basal cell carcinoma, reassure him that he needn't fear pain.

On the other hand, if he has a painful cancer, such as metastatic bone cancer, discuss methods for controlling pain, such as heat, massage, distraction, surgery, radiation, and drugs. Inform him that these relief-giving methods — used alone or in combination — can be very effective.

Cancer isn't contagious

Tell your patient that even though cancer is widespread, no evidence indicates that cancer is an infectious disorder.

Cancer doesn't always cause disfigurement

Cancer dramatically alters a patient's body image. However, cancer and its treatment don't always cause disfigurement. Many of the surgeries performed today are less invasive and cause much less disfigurement than surgeries used in the past. For example, when possible, a lumpectomy is used to treat breast cancer instead of a mastectomy.

If cancer destroys external body tissues or requires disfiguring surgery, help your patient prepare by discussing the procedure and the possibilities for reconstructive surgery. Be aware that even if your patient's cancer doesn't change his physical appearance, he may still feel that his condition sets him apart from others.

Leukemia

If your patient has leukemia, explain that this cancer originates in the bone marrow, where blood cells are made. As the cancer cells grow, they crowd out and inhibit the growth of platelets, white blood cells, and red blood cells. Eventually, the cancer cells spill into the bloodstream and travel throughout the body.

Lymphoma

If your patient has lymphoma, explain that this cancer arises in the lymph system, a network of glands, vessels, and organs that provides a major defense against infection. The lymphatic vessels carry the cancer cells throughout the body. (See *Factors linked to cancer development,* page 316.)

(Text continues on page 315.)

Cancer teaching points

Look below for specific topics to discuss with your cancer patients.

Bladder cancer

Teach the patient:

- about tests, such as cystoscopy, biopsy, urinalysis, excretory urography, retrograde cystography, pelvic arteriography, computed tomography (CT) scan, and ultrasonography
- about treatments, such as transurethral resection, transurethral fulguration, intravesical therapy, radical cystectomy, partial cystectomy, external radiation therapy, and chemotherapy
- about investigational treatments, such as photodynamic therapy and intravesicular administration of interferon alfa and tumor necrosis factor
- about care for the urinary stoma, including proper skin-cleaning technique and how to prepare and apply the pouch
- with a urinary stoma to avoid heavy lifting and contact sports
- to empty the urinary drainage pouch when it is one-third full or every 2 to 3 hours
- to contact other resources, such as the American Cancer Society and The United Ostomy Association, for further support and information
- undergoing a radical cystectomy and urethrectomy to expect to be impotent, although a subsequent penile implant may make sexual intercourse possible (Viagra, a new prescription drug, also treats impotence.)
- undergoing a radical cystectomy to expect removal of the uterus, fallopian tubes, ovaries, and anterior vaginal wall and surrounding fascia
- undergoing external radiation treatment to expect 4 to 6 weeks of therapy, along with various adverse effects.

Breast cancer

Teach the patient:

- about tests, such as mammography, needle biopsy, surgical biopsy, estrogen receptor assays, and ultrasonography
- about treatments, such as lumpectomy, simple mastectomy, and radical mastectomy
- how to perform coughing and deep-breathing exercises to prevent pulmonary complications
- how to perform pain management techniques and to request pain medications as needed
- to get out of bed and ambulate postoperatively
- with a mastectomy about the incisional drain or suction device used to remove accumulated serous or sanguineous fluid
- to exercise her hand and arm regularly and avoid activities that may cause infection in the hand or arm in order to prevent lymphedema
- about breast prostheses
- to ask her doctor about the possibility of reconstructive surgery
- that breast surgery doesn't interfere with sexual function and that she may resume sexual activity as soon as she desires after surgery
- that she may experience phantom breast syndrome after surgery.

Lung cancer

Teach the patient:

- about tests, such as chest X-ray, sputum cytology, CT scan, bronchoscopy, and needle biopsy
- about surgical treatments, such as lobectomy, radical lobectomy, and pneumonectomy
- about procedures, such as radiation therapy and chest tube insertion
- how to perform coughing and deep-breathing exercises
- undergoing radiation therapy to wear loose clothing and avoid exposure to the sun and harsh ointments on the chest
- to try to quit smoking, if appropriate. (Refer the patient to the American Cancer Society or other sources of support and information.)

Colorectal cancer

Teach the patient:

- about tests, such as tumor biopsy, digital rectal examination, Hemoccult test, proctoscopy, sigmoidoscopy, colonoscopy, CT scan, barium X-ray, and carcinoembryonic antigen test
- about treatments, such as tumor resection, radiation therapy, and chemotherapy
- to expect to have a nasogastric tube and nothing to eat for a few days
- how to care for the colostomy, including proper skin cleaning technique and how to prepare and apply the pouch
- with a colostomy that, if flatus, diarrhea, or constipation occurs, to eliminate foods from the diet that may have caused it and to try to reintroduce them later
- to resume physical activities as long as there is no threat of

(continued)

Cancer teaching points *(continued)*

Colorectal cancer *(continued)*
injury to the stoma or surrounding abdominal muscles, but to avoid heavy lifting
- to have yearly colon cancer screenings.

Acute leukemia
Teach the patient:
- about tests, such as bone marrow biopsy, blood counts, and lumbar puncture
- about treatments, such as chemotherapy, bone marrow transplantation, granulocyte injections, platelet transfusions, red blood cell transfusions, and antibiotic, antifungal, and antiviral drugs
- how to recognize signs and symptoms of infection (fever, chills, cough, sore throat) and abnormal bleeding (bruising, petechiae) and how to stop such bleeding (pressure, ice to area)
- with neutropenia to avoid patients with infections and contact with flowers, raw meat, and uncooked fruits and vegetables
- how to perform proper oral hygiene to help prevent ulceration, such as by using a soft toothbrush, cutting down on the use of commercial mouthwashes, and avoiding hot, spicy foods
- to include the family in the patient's care as much as possible.

Hodgkin's disease
Teach the patient:
- about tests, such as lymph node biopsy, bone marrow biopsy, liver biopsy, mediastinal biopsy, spleen biopsy, chest X-ray, abdominal CT scan, lung scan, and bone scan
- about treatments, such as radiation therapy, chemotherapy, and combined chemotherapy and radiation therapy

Endometrial cancer
Teach the patient:
- about tests, such as endometrial biopsy, cervical biopsy, endocervical biopsy, fractional dilatation and Schiller's test, physical examination, chest X-ray, CT scan, excretory urography, cystoscopy, blood studies, electrocardiography, proctoscopy, and barium enema studies
- about treatments, such as total abdominal hysterectomy and bilateral salpingo-oophorectomy, radiation therapy, intracavitary irradiation, chemotherapy, and irradiation, surgery, and progestational agents
- undergoing lymphadenectomy and total hysterectomy about the drainage system in place after surgery
- who is premenopausal and undergoing an oophorectomy that the procedure will result in menopause
- how to perform coughing and deep-breathing exercises and how to use an incentive spirometer
- undergoing internal radiation:
  - that the procedure requires a 2- to 3-day hospital stay, a bowel preparation, and nothing by mouth the night before treatment
  - that she will be in a private room
  - about safety precautions taken by health care workers, such as distance and shielding after the radioactive source has been implanted
  - to limit her movement while the source is in place
- undergoing external radiation:
  - that treatment is generally given 5 days per week for 4 to 6 weeks
  - that the skin will be marked with permanent ink to enable the treatment beam to be lined up in the exact location at each treatment
  - that pelvic radiation may cause diarrhea, and to take antidiarrheals as prescribed by her doctor
  - to keep the radiation site dry, avoid wearing clothes that rub against the area, and avoid using heating pads, alcohol rubs, or any skin creams
  - that, unless undergoing a total pelvic exenteration, the vagina remains intact and, once she recovers, sexual intercourse is possible.

Esophageal cancer
Teach the patient:
- about tests, such as X-ray of the esophagus with barium swallow and motility studies, endoscopy, punch and brush biopsies, and exfoliative cytologic tests
- about treatments, such as surgical resection, radiation, chemotherapy, and combined radiation therapy and chemotherapy
- about palliative treatments, such as endoscopic dilatation or gastrostomy and jejunostomy tube placement for enteral feedings, how to administer tube feedings, and care for the feeding tube and insertion site
- about postoperative care, including gastrostomy tubes, the closed chest drainage system, and NG suctioning
- to eat in the Fowler's position to help prevent aspiration.

Cancer teaching points *(continued)*

Gastric cancer

Teach the patient:

- about tests, such as barium X-rays of the GI tract with fluoroscopy, gastroscopy with fiberoptic endoscopy (for gastroscopic biopsy)
- about treatments, such as subtotal gastrectomy, total or near-total gastrectomy, radiation therapy, and chemotherapy
- undergoing surgery to expect an NG tube postoperatively
- undergoing a partial gastrectomy that he may eventually be able to eat normally
- undergoing a total gastrectomy
  - to expect a slow recovery and only partial return to a normal diet
  - to eat small, frequent meals upon recovery
- to perform coughing and deep-breathing exercises and how to use an incentive spirometer
- undergoing gastrectomy:
  - about dumping syndrome
  - about the need to take a vitamin and iron replacement for the rest of his life
- undergoing radiation therapy to eat high-calorie, well-balanced meals
- to contact a home health agency or hospice, if appropriate.

Malignant brain tumor

Teach the patient:

- about tests, such as stereotactic surgery and tissue biopsy, skull X-ray, brain scan, CT scan, magnetic resonance imaging (MRI), cerebral angiography, and lumbar puncture
- about treatments, such as tumor resection, radiation therapy, and chemotherapy
- to avoid Valsalva's maneuver or isometric muscle contractions postoperatively because they increase intracranial pressure
- to contact occupational and physical therapists, as needed.

Teach the family:

- what to do if the patient has a seizure.

Cervical cancer

Teach the patient:

- about diagnostic tests, such as Papanicolaou test, colposcopy, and staining with Lugol's solution or Schiller's solution
- about tests to detect metastasis, such as lymphangiography, cystography, and various scans
- about treatment for preinvasive lesions, such as total excisional biopsy, cryosurgery, laser destruction, conization, and hysterectomy
- about treatment for invasive carcinoma, such as radical hysterectomy, radiation therapy, combined surgery and radiation therapy, chemotherapy, and combined radiation and chemotherapy
- undergoing cryosurgery:
  - that the procedure will take approximately 15 minutes
  - that the doctor will use refrigerant to freeze the cervix
  - that she may experience abdominal cramps, headache, and sweating, but will feel little pain
- undergoing laser therapy that the procedure will take approximately 30 minutes and may cause abdominal cramping
- undergoing biopsy, cryosurgery, or laser therapy:
  - to expect discharge or spotting for about 1 week afterward
  - not to douche, use tampons, or engage in sexual intercourse for 1 week after the procedure
  - to watch for and report any signs of infection
  - to have a follow-up Pap smear and a pelvic examination within 3 months after the procedures and periodically thereafter as instructed by the doctor
- undergoing a hysterectomy about all postoperative procedures
- undergoing internal radiation:
  - that the procedure requires a 2- to 3-day hospital stay, a bowel preparation, a povidone-iodine vaginal douche, a clear liquid diet, insertion of an indwelling urinary catheter, and nothing by mouth the night before the implantation
  - that she'll have less contact with staff and visitors while the implant is in place because of the risk of exposure to radiation
  - that she'll have a private room and must lie flat and limit her movement while the implant is in place
  - that she may elevate the head of her bed slightly if this is more comfortable
- undergoing external radiation therapy:
  - that it usually continues for 4 to 6 weeks
  - about the need to report adverse effects to the doctor
  - to avoid during therapy people with obvious infections.

(continued)

Cancer teaching points *(continued)*

Testicular cancer
Teach the patient:
- about diagnostic tests, such as testicular palpation, transillumination, excretory urography, urinary or serum luteinizing hormone levels, lymphangiography, ultrasonography, abdominal CT scan, and surgical excision and biopsy
- about tests to indicate testicular tumor activity, such as serum alpha-fetoprotein level and serum beta-human chorionic gonadotropin level measurements
- about treatments, such as orchiectomy and retroperitoneal node dissection, radiation, chemotherapy, and autologous bone marrow transplantation
- undergoing an orchiectomy:
  - that sterility and impotence may not result from unilateral orchiectomy
  - that most surgeons don't remove the scrotum
  - that a testicular prosthesis can correct any anatomic disfigurement
  - about postoperative procedures, such as ice application to the scrotum for the first day after surgery and use of a scrotal athletic supporter while ambulating.

Oral cavity cancer
Teach the patient:
- about tests, such as biopsy, CT scan, chest X-ray, and bone scan
- about treatments, such as surgical excision, radiation therapy, chemotherapy, and combined chemotherapy and radiation therapy
- about treatment to prevent premalignant disease from becoming a malignant carcinoma, such as carotene and 9 cis-retinoic acid
- who smokes or drinks alcohol to quit, and refer him to the appropriate resources
- about possible adverse effects of radiation therapy, such as mucositis, dysphagia, long-term loss of taste, or decreased tongue mobility
- good mouth care techniques.

Prostate cancer
Teach the patient:
- about tests, such as digital rectal examination, serum prostate-specific antigen test, ultrasonography, biopsy, MRI, CT scan, excretory urography, and serum acid phosphatase levels
- about treatments, such as total prostatovesiculectomy, prostatectomy, external radiation therapy, interstitial radiation, androgen deprivation and estrogen administration, and chemotherapy
- about experimental therapies, such as hyperthermia, cryosurgery, and high-intensity focused ultrasonography, as appropriate
- about possible adverse effects of surgery (such as impotence and incontinence) and radiation
- about use of the drug Viagra to treat impotence
- how to do perineal exercises one to ten times each hour preoperatively (Have him squeeze his buttocks together, hold this position for a few seconds, then relax.)
- about postoperative care:
  - that antispasmodics will be given to relieve bladder spasms
  - that an indwelling urinary catheter with an irrigation system will be in place postoperatively
  - to report any pain or bladder fullness
- undergoing a perineal or retropubic prostatectomy that urine leakage after catheter removal is normal and will subside
- undergoing hormonal therapy to report adverse effects, such as gynecomastia, fluid retention, nausea and vomiting, and thrombophlebitis, to the doctor
- undergoing radiation therapy to report any adverse effects such as proctitis, diarrhea, bladder spasms, and urinary frequency
- undergoing internal radiation:
  - that he may develop cystitis in the first 2 to 3 weeks
  - to drink at least 2 L of fluid per day.

Chronic granulocytic leukemia
Teach the patient:
- about tests, such as the test for Philadelphia chromosome, leukocyte alkaline phosphatase levels, complete blood count (CBC), serum uric acid levels, bone marrow aspirate or biopsy, and CT scan
- about treatments, such as aggressive chemotherapy, as well as ancillary treatments, such as local splenic radiation or splenectomy, leukapheresis, and prompt treatment of infections
- with persistent anemia to plan for rest periods throughout the day
- to take precautions to help prevent bleeding such as using a soft bristle toothbrush and electric razor

(continued)

Cancer teaching points *(continued)*

Chronic granulocytic leukemia *(continued)*

- with splenomegaly to eat small, frequent meals, and take a stool softener or laxative as needed to ease abdominal discomfort
- how to perform coughing and deep-breathing exercises
- to watch for and immediately report signs and symptoms of infection, including fever over 100° F (37.8° C), chills, redness or swelling, sore throat, and cough
- to watch for signs of thrombocytopenia, to immediately apply ice and pressure to any external bleeding site, and to avoid aspirin and aspirin-containing compounds because of the risk of increased bleeding.

Chronic lymphocytic leukemia

Teach the patient:

- about tests, such as CBC and bone marrow aspiration and biopsy
- about treatments, such as chemotherapy, prednisone, local radiation treatment, and allopurinol
- to report any signs and symptoms of infection: temperature over 100° F, chills, and redness or swelling of any body part
- to watch for and report any signs of thrombocytopenia and anemia, such as black tarry stools, easy bruising, nosebleeds, bleeding gums, pale skin, weakness, fatigue, dizziness, and palpitations
- not to use aspirin or aspirin-containing products
- to avoid contact with obviously ill people
- about the importance of follow-up care, frequent blood tests, and taking all medications as prescribed.

Basal cell carcinoma

Teach the patient:

- about tests, such as incisional or excisional biopsy and histologic studies
- about treatments, such as curettage and electrodesiccation, topical 5-fluorouracil, microscopically controlled surgical excision, irradiation, cryotherapy, and chemotherapy
- to avoid excessive sun exposure and use a strong sunscreen or sunshade to protect his skin
- to relieve local inflammation from topical fluorouracil with cool compresses or corticosteroid ointment
- with noduloulcerative basal cell epithelioma to wash his face gently when ulcerations and crusting occur to prevent bleeding
- to periodically examine his skin for precancerous lesions.

Squamous cell carcinoma

Teach the patient:

- about tests such as excisional biopsy
- about treatments, such as wide surgical excision, electrodesiccation and curettage, radiation therapy, and chemotherapy
- how to perform proper wound care, including keeping the wound dry and clean
- to avoid excessive sun exposure and wear protective clothing
- to use a strong sunscreen (including on the lips) when outdoors and to apply it 30 to 60 minutes before sun exposure
- to periodically examine the skin for precancerous lesions.

Malignant melanoma

Teach the patient:

- about diagnostic tests such as skin biopsy with histologic examination
- about tests to determine metastasis, such as chest X-ray, bone scan, and CT scan of the chest, abdomen, or brain
- about treatments, such as surgical resection, regional lymphadenectomy, adjuvant chemotherapy and biotherapy, and radiation therapy
- about investigational treatment, such as isolated limb perfusion for management of malignant melanomas of the extremities
- what to expect before and after surgery, including what the wound will look like and what type of dressing he'll have
- about the need for follow-up care to detect recurrence
- with metastatic disease to take regularly scheduled analgesics
- about measures to prevent the disease, such as avoiding overexposure to the sun, using a sunblock or sunscreen, and examining the skin periodically.

Discussing the prognosis

Most cancer patients maintain hope for a cure as long as they live. Try to help your patient form realistic expectations of treatment without supporting or providing false hope. Stress that, although cure rate statistics help to determine which treatments are usually most effective, his individual response to treatment matters most. Inform him of other options if his initial treatment fails.

Helping the patient in remission

A patient whose cancer has been removed surgically or who is in remission may also experience emotional turmoil. He may feel a combination of relief and anxiety about resuming his occupation or lifestyle. He may also feel anxious during periodic checkups. Encourage him to express his feelings and concerns. Also teach him to recognize possible signs of recurrence, such as weight change, bleeding, and continuing pain.

Helping the patient in advanced stages of cancer

A patient whose cancer progresses to an advanced or terminal stage may become increasingly discouraged and depressed. He's likely to sleep for long periods, refuse food and visitors, and express sadness and hopelessness. You can help this patient by:

- supporting him as he comes to grips with the prospect of his death
- encouraging him to reflect on his past accomplishments to help him find purpose in his life and view death from a peaceful perspective
- providing privacy so he and his family can share their feelings and resolve any lingering conflicts (Remember, sometimes a patient is more prepared than his family to face death.)
- discussing hospice care, as appropriate, with the patient and his family.

Factors linked to cancer development

- Genetic predisposition
- Chemical carcinogens
- Radiation
- Tobacco and alcohol
- Certain dietary elements

Recurrent cancer

A patient whose cancer recurs may experience some of the same emotions he felt when his cancer was first diagnosed. However, there's a difference: He has already faced cancer, endured treatment-related discomfort, seen his lifestyle disrupted, and probably come to grips with his mortality.

Such a patient may believe, "I've coped with this before; I can do it again." Alternatively, if his memories of treatment discourage or frighten him, he may wonder,

"Will the treatment really work this time?" or "How can I go through this again?"

Tests can be troubling

The patient's apprehension about treatment can be aggravated by an exhaustive series of tests to outline the cancer's stage and metastasis. He's likely to feel alone and anxious as he awaits the results. You'll need to tailor your teaching to meet his special needs for information and support.

Discussing recurrent cancer

Indicate to the patient that even though his treatment aimed to destroy his original cancer, a few cells too small for detection may have survived. When these cancer cells multiply, they're detected, and the patient is diagnosed with recurrent cancer. Recurrence usually refers to the return of cancer at the same site, such as colon cancer that recurs in the colon. Point out that the recurrent cancer is the same type as the original cancer no matter where it appears.

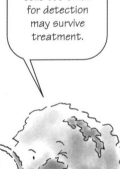

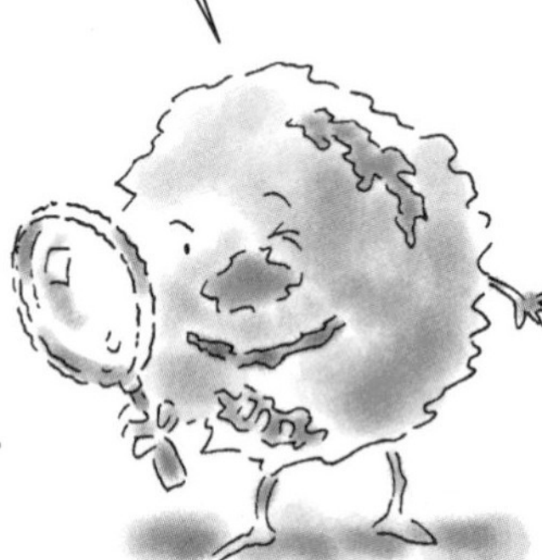
A few cancer cells too small for detection may survive treatment.

From one site to another

If the patient had a tumor, explain how cells can break away and travel through the lymphatic system or bloodstream to start new cancer growths. This spread of the cancer from one site to another is called metastasis. For example, if breast cancer recurs in the lung, it's not lung cancer, but breast cancer that has spread, or metastasized, to the lung.

Discussing the patient's perception

Patients with recurrent cancer usually express expectations about how they'll handle their disorder, based on their past experiences. Ask your patient about his first bout with cancer. How did he cope with the disorder before? What, if anything, would he like to do differently this time?

Weighing risks

Occasionally, recurrent cancer is treated similarly to the initial cancer, although perhaps more intensively. The patient will probably be familiar with the treatment-related effects he's likely to experience. However, if the doctor recommends a different treatment, make sure your patient knows what to expect. If the patient feels that the treatment's likely risks outweigh its benefits, support his decision to refuse it. In this way, you can provide comfort during a potentially lonesome and frightening time.

Discussing the prognosis

Starting cancer treatment again will tax your patient's spirits as well as his body. That's why your teaching must also emphasize the importance of maintaining hope. At times, the patient may be overcome by fear, anxiety, depression, and rage as he learns to cope with this setback. Encourage him to express such feelings. Stress that a positive attitude may help him control some of his emotional and physical reactions to treatment.

Teaching about tests

Typically, a cancer patient undergoes an array of tests to confirm cancer, to select and monitor treatment, to predict prognosis, and to check for recurrence. He may feel fearful and powerless as he endures these tests and awaits their results. (See *Teaching patients about cancer tests.*)

A sense of control

Your teaching can help the patient throughout the diagnostic workup. By telling him which tests he'll undergo and when, you can help him maintain a sense of control. By clearly explaining test procedures, you can prepare him for what to expect. By teaching him how to recognize and manage possible adverse effects, you can help him assume an active role in posttest care. Also, by answering his questions about test results, you can help him make informed decisions about his future.

What works?

Ask the patient how he learns best — such as by watching and imitating, or by reading and following instructions. Use complementary teaching materials, such as videotapes, photographs, and cartoons.

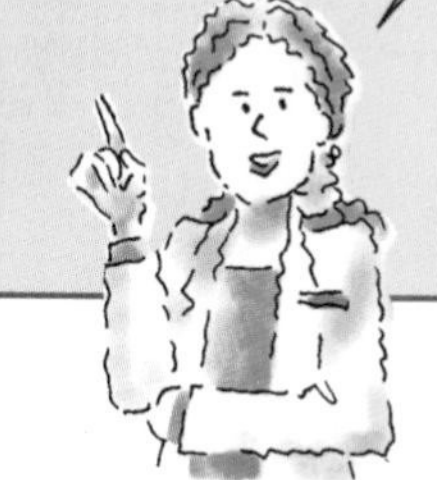

Teaching patients about cancer tests

Test and purpose	What to teach the patient
Blood studies • In suspected cancer, to determine how well the blood delivers oxygen to the body, whether the patient has any infection, and whether the blood clots normally • Specialized blood studies, such as radioimmunoassays, to detect tumor markers and provide information about the extent of malignant disease and treatment effectiveness	• Who will perform the venipuncture and when. • There may be pretest restrictions. For example, the patient may have to fast for 6 hours before having blood drawn for some studies. • The sample can be obtained in minutes. • He may experience brief discomfort from the tourniquet and needle puncture.
Radiographic and imaging tests • To allow visualization of internal structures and guide biopsy procedures • To help detect and localize cancer or identify an underlying disorder	• Although most tests are painless, the equipment may appear frightening at first. • The X-ray machine will make a clacking sound. The patient will feel a mild burning sensation following infusion of the contrast medium. • Most tests don't require dietary restrictions. • The exposure to radiation is minimal.
Cytologic tests • To help detect suspected primary or metastatic disease and assess the effectiveness of treatment	• Most tests are painless. • No dietary restrictions are required.
Histologic tests (tissue examination) • To confirm findings of cytologic tests • To establish a definitive diagnosis • In bone marrow biopsy, to diagnose leukemia, to determine whether cancer has spread to the bone marrow, or to evaluate response to treatment	• Usually, the doctor performs a biopsy to obtain a tissue sample for microscopic examination. • In an *aspiration biopsy,* a tissue specimen is aspirated from the bone marrow, liver, or breast with a flexible or fine aspiration needle, needle guide, and aspiration syringe. An excision refers to surgical removal of an entire lesion from any tissue. • If undergoing local anesthesia, he needn't restrict food, fluids, or medication. He may feel weak or tired after the procedure but may resume his usual activities in 1 or 2 days. • If undergoing general anesthesia, the patient should fast beginning at midnight before the test. • The test takes about 15 to 30 minutes. Pretest blood studies, urinalysis, and X-rays may be required. • If undergoing *open biopsy* (performed in the operating room), the surgeon obtains a tissue specimen and sends it immediately to the laboratory for rapid analysis. If the result of the biopsy is positive for cancer, doctors will try to remove the tumor. Some doctors will perform the procedure in two different surgeries.

(continued)

Teaching patients about cancer tests *(continued)*

Test and purpose	What to teach the patient
Histologic tests (tissue examination) *(continued)*	• If undergoing *bone marrow biopsy,* the procedure may be an aspiration or needle biopsy. *Aspiration biopsy* retrieves a fluid specimen in which bone spicules are suspended. *Needle biopsy* involves removing a core of marrow cells. The sternum, anterior or posterior iliac crest, vertebral spinous process, or tibia may be selected as the biopsy site. The procedure takes only 5 to 10 minutes. Test results are usually known in a few days. • The patient receives a local anesthetic but will feel pressure when the biopsy needle is inserted and a brief, pulling sensation as the marrow is removed. More than one bone marrow specimen may be required. A blood sample is also collected.
Lumbar puncture • To detect cancer cells or infection in the cerebrospinal fluid	• This test usually takes about 45 minutes. • The patient must not eat or drink anything after midnight before the procedure. • The patient receives a local anesthetic. • After the test, he should lie flat for 6 to 8 hours and increase fluid intake to help prevent a headache. • Frequent measurement of vital signs may be required.
Endoscopic tests (laryngoscopy, bronchoscopy, or colonoscopy) • To obtain a biopsy specimen • To visualize internal structures • To perform minor surgery	• Where the test will be done, how long it will last, and what to expect. Many patients find endoscopic tests are uncomfortable and embarrassing. It's common to feel anxious before and during the procedure. • Dietary restrictions may be required before the test. • Bowel cleansing may be required for certain tests such as colonoscopy. • The patient may be sedated to help alleviate discomfort. • Vital signs will be monitored frequently.

Test sequence

Although test selection depends on the patient's history and physical examination findings, the diagnostic workup usually follows this sequence:

First, the doctor will order routine blood and radiologic tests.

Second, cytologic and histologic tests may follow to confirm or rule out malignant disease.

Finally, further special tests, such as computed tomography (CT) scan, magnetic resonance imaging (MRI), and endoscopy, help determine the extent of malignant disease, predict prognosis, select and monitor treatment, and check for recurrence.

As you teach the patient about laboratory and diagnostic tests, explain that many tests are repeated periodically to evaluate response to treatment. Emphasize that repeating a test doesn't necessarily indicate a setback.

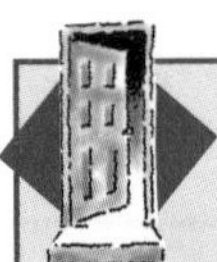

No place like home

Living with cancer

You may need to teach the patient and family members how to perform special procedures, such as tracheostomy care, as well as basic care measures, such as oral hygiene. You'll also need to help the caregiver learn how to avoid or manage stress and burnout. Always stress the importance of maintaining optimal health through good nutrition and hygiene.

You're not alone

Emphasize the many sources of support available to the patient and family. For example, the American Cancer Society may be able to arrange for transportation to and from the hospital or treatment center. Make sure your patient and his family realize that they don't have to face cancer alone.

Teaching about treatments

Whether the patient is scheduled for surgery, chemotherapy, or radiation therapy, he's likely to be apprehensive. After all, he may associate treatment with uncomfortable and, at times, disfiguring adverse effects.

Although you can't expect to eliminate the patient's fear, you can help him adjust to the treatment's effects with appropriate teaching. For example, you could explain to the patient who'll be receiving chemotherapy that not all patients experience uncontrollable nausea and vomiting. In fact, some don't experience any. Also, explain that drugs and diet can minimize or prevent nausea and vomiting. Before radiation therapy, reassure the patient that he'll be protected from potentially harmful effects. When appropriate, put your patient in touch with patients who've had (or are undergoing) similar treatment. (See *Living with cancer.*)

Why?

Tell the patient that the goal of cancer treatment is to destroy malignant cells while minimizing damage to normal ones.

How?

A single treatment or a combination of treatments may be used. Explain that surgery and radiation therapy combat malignant cells locally and regionally, whereas chemotherapy combats them systemically—throughout the body. Treatment selection depends on many factors, including:

- the type of cancer
- its size and location
- the patient's general health.

(See *Is it working?* page 322; and *Teaching about cancer treatment*, page 323.)

Surgery

If your patient will undergo surgery, explain and compare the three major types:

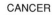

Curative surgery is performed to remove the entire tumor, along with a margin of surrounding tissue and some nearby lymph nodes.

Preventive surgery is performed to remove noncancerous growths that would probably become cancerous if left in place.

Palliative surgery is performed to relieve symptoms such as pain; it doesn't cure cancer.

Surgical techniques

As appropriate, describe the specific surgical technique the patient will experience:

- Local excision involves removing only the malignancy. Usually, this is adequate for most skin cancers, which seldom spread to the lymph nodes.
- Electrosurgery uses a high-frequency electric current—transmitted through a blade, needle, or disk electrode—to cut or coagulate tissue. It's performed for certain skin, mouth, and rectal cancers.
- Cryosurgery involves freezing and destroying a tumor with liquid nitrogen applied with a special probe. It's used most often to treat premalignant disease like cervical intraepithelial neoplasia.

Chemotherapy

This treatment involves the administration of drugs that interfere with cell replication. These drugs are given by mouth, injection into veins, muscles, or spinal fluid, or instillation into a body cavity, such as the bladder and peritoneum. Typically, they're given in specific cycles and sequences, so that the body can recover during the drug-free period.

Tell the patient the type and sequence of drugs that he'll receive and whether they'll be administered in the hospital or at home. Inform the patient of any harmful drug interactions. Usually, food, beverages, and over-the-counter drugs don't influence the safety or effectiveness

Is it working?

Tell the patient that the doctor will check his condition regularly. During these checkups, the doctor may take X-rays to see whether the cancer is shrinking in response to chemotherapy or radiation therapy. Other tests can show any damage that treatment is causing to normal cells.

Feelings

The patient's own reports of how he feels may be the best sign of the treatment's success. Advise the patient to tell the doctor if he notices any decrease in pain, bleeding, or other discomforts associated with cancer.

After the patient completes treatment, the doctor will want to see him regularly—but less often—to see how he's doing and check for cancer recurrence or possible complications of therapy. Encourage the patient to keep follow-up appointments.

of chemotherapy drugs. But you should teach the patient about a few important exceptions. For example, he should avoid aspirin and aspirin-containing products while on chemotherapy.

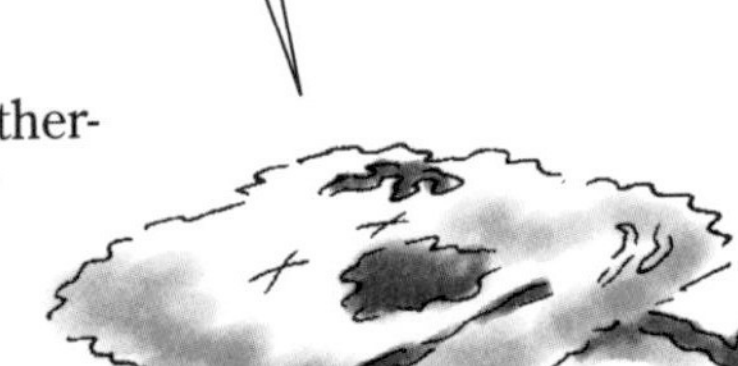
Chemotherapy can also affect normal cells.

Rapidly growing cells beware

Explain that adverse effects may occur during chemotherapy because the drugs can affect any rapidly growing cells in the body — normal cells as well as cancer cells. The normal cells most likely to be affected are in the bone marrow, digestive tract, reproductive organs, and hair follicles. Teach the patient how to manage common adverse effects of chemotherapy.

An individual matter

Make sure that the patient realizes that every person responds differently to chemotherapy. Some people have few or no adverse effects; others have more difficulty. Reassure him that if a drug causes severe adverse effects, the doctor can adjust the dosage or prescribe medications that will treat those adverse effects. Explain that most adverse effects subside before or shortly after treatment ends. However, the fatigue that some patients experience during chemotherapy may linger.

If appropriate, discuss the guidelines for oral chemotherapy. (See *Tips for taking oral anticancer drugs*, page 324.)

Radiation therapy

Bombarding cancer cells with high-level radiation destroys their ability to grow and multiply. Although radiation also affects normal cells, these cells usually recover quickly. Explain to the patient that radiation therapy may be used:
- before surgery, to shrink a tumor
- after surgery (perhaps combined with chemotherapy), to stop the growth of any remaining cancer cells and to prevent recurrence.

Where, who, what type

Make sure that the patient understands when and where he'll receive radiation therapy and who will administer it. Reinforce the doctor's explanation of the procedure, and

Teaching about cancer treatment

- Explain the recommended treatment, including its purpose, procedure, and potential adverse effects.
- Prepare the patient and his family to recognize and manage adverse effects.
- Allow adequate time to answer their questions and provide support.

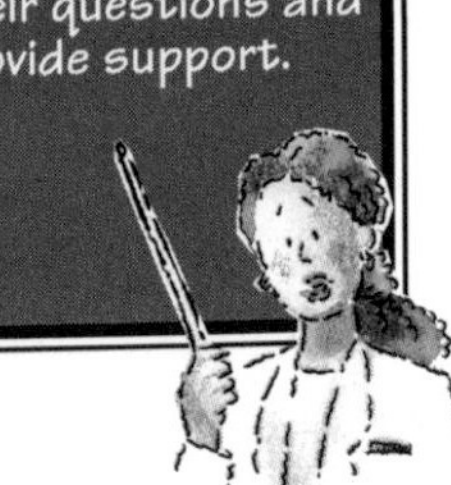

answer any questions. Explain the type of radiation — external or internal — that the patient will receive.

External radiation

In external radiation therapy, a machine directs high-level radiation at the cancer cells as well as at some of the normal surrounding tissue. Explain that one or two visits for treatment planning will be necessary. Also, a simulation test will be performed before therapy to determine the exact location and size of the cancer.

X marks the spot

Tell the patient that he'll be asked to lie still on a table while an X-ray machine locates the area to be treated. Then the skin will be marked with tiny dots of permanent ink that are rarely noticeable to anyone except the treatment team. The marks are needed to line up the treatment beam in the exact location at each treatment. Emphasize to the patient that he mustn't scrub off the ink because it's important to treat the same area each time.

Monday through Friday

Tell the patient that treatments are given as an outpatient. Inform him that most treatment courses are 5 days each week, Monday through Friday, for 4 to 6 weeks.

Be still

Reassure him that special lead shields will be placed between the machine and certain body areas to protect normal tissue and organs. Instruct him to remain still so that the radiation is delivered only to the target area. Reassure him that radiation therapy is painless and won't make him radioactive. Stress that he'll be under close observation during the treatment and need only call out if he wants anything.

The skinny on skin

Teach the patient how to care for the skin in the treatment area. Instruct him not to apply powder, lotion, perfume, topical medication, or extreme heat or cold to the area, and to avoid rubbing the skin. If he must shave the area, tell him to use an electric shaver instead of a razor. Advise him to protect the area from the sun with soft, lightweight clothing and a sunscreen, if his doctor permits. Suggest

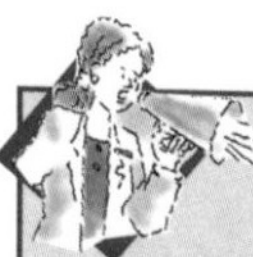

Listen up!

Tips for taking oral anticancer drugs

Advise the patient taking oral anticancer drugs to:

- store pills in a child-proof container
- take the drug at the same time each day to achieve a maximum blood level and foster compliance
- use a syringe to measure liquid medication accurately
- crush pills or open capsules and mix with food or liquids (if recommended)
- place tablets in the freezer for easy splitting
- repeat the dose if vomiting occurs within 20 minutes of taking a dose
- take an antiemetic drug if nauseated and then wait about 20 minutes before taking the anticancer drug
- notify the doctor if he misses doses because of a GI infection.

that he limit activities that might irritate the area, and warn him that the area may be sore or sensitive for some time after therapy.

Be aware of the threat to hair

If the patient has hair in the treatment area, explain that some or all of it may fall out during therapy. Clarify that only hair in the treatment area is affected. Provide reassurance that the hair will probably grow back after therapy. In the meantime, recommend that the patient wear a toupee, wig, hat, or scarf if scalp hair is affected.

Internal radiation

In internal radiation therapy, a small amount of radioactive material may be implanted in a body cavity (intracavitary approach) or directly into the tumor itself (interstitial approach). This provides high levels of radiation to the tumor while sparing most of the normal tissue surrounding it. Explain the type of implant that the doctor will use and where it will be placed. Low-dose internal radiation is usually implanted in the operating room or radiation department and requires hospitalization. Tell the patient how long he'll be hospitalized, and whether he'll be required to stay in a private room.

Time's up

Explain that hospital staff and visitors will need to limit the amount of time they spend in the patient's room to avoid excessive exposure to radiation. If the implant is temporary, tell the patient when it will be removed.

A permanent addition

If the implant is permanent, explain that it will lose a small amount of radioactivity each day, and that only a low level of radiation will remain when the patient leaves the hospital.

The systemic approach

If the patient will receive radiation systemically, explain that radioactive materials in solutions are given orally, I.V., or by instillation. Describe the procedure and any necessary preparation and aftercare.

Check the mood

An overwhelming health problem can leave the patient apathetic about learning. A patient who feels happy about his progress and hopeful about recovery is more likely to be ready to learn.

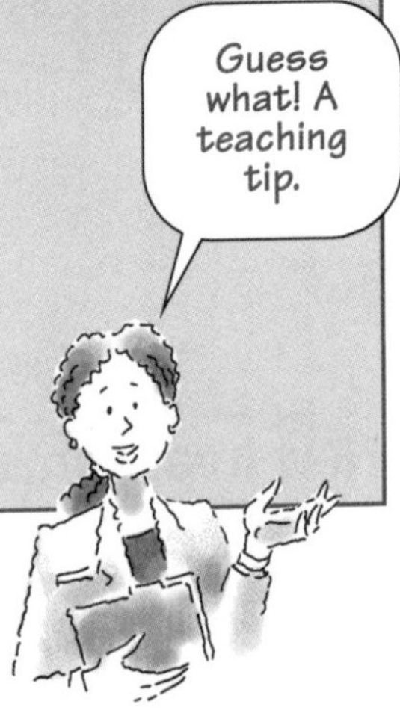
Guess what! A teaching tip.

Managing adverse effects

Whether the patient's receiving external or internal radiation therapy, you'll need to teach him how to manage adverse effects. Tell him to notify the doctor if adverse effects are persistent or especially troublesome, or if he develops fever, cough, or unusual pain. Because chemotherapy, and sometimes radiation therapy, may increase susceptibility to infection, warn the patient to avoid people with colds or other infections during therapy.

Eat well, rest up

In collaboration with the dietitian, teach the patient how to maintain a balanced diet while he's receiving chemotherapy and radiation therapy. Stress that good nutrition is a must, and provide tips to stimulate the patient's appetite if his desire for food lags during therapy. Advise him to get plenty of rest; his body will need extra energy over the course of therapy.

New treatments

Three new treatments are currently under investigation for limited use in cancer treatment:

- bone marrow transplantation
- immunotherapy
- monoclonal antibody therapy.

Bone marrow transplantation

Bone marrow transplantation replaces diseased bone marrow with healthy bone marrow, and thus may enable the patient to manufacture normal blood cells. Whether or not a patient receives a bone marrow transplant depends on his underlying disease, his age and health, and the availability of a compatible donor.

Immunotherapy

Immunotherapy introduces antigens and other substances into the patient's body in an attempt to prod the immune system to recognize and attack cancer cells. Explain to the patient that immunotherapy is used with other treatments such as radiation therapy.

Monoclonal antibody therapy

Explain how monoclonal antibodies help detect and treat cancer. When radioactive tracers are attached to monoclonal antibodies that are specific to selected cancer cells, they can accurately locate areas of that cancer in the body. When used with chemotherapy, these antibodies can destroy cancer cells while leaving normal ones alone. Inform the patient that the use of monoclonal antibodies is still considered experimental.

Looking at alternatives

Fear of the prescribed therapy or feelings of despair as cancer progresses may make a cancer patient consider undergoing alternative therapy. When a patient chooses an alternative treatment, he may refuse prescribed therapy and risk experiencing damaging adverse effects.

If a patient tells you he is considering seeking alternative care, ask him to discuss his concerns about his disorder and its prescribed therapy. If he mentions that he's considering a specific alternative therapy, be willing to discuss it openly. Point out any known medical risks. (See *Three alternatives,* page 328.)

Pain control

Adequate pain control helps to improve the patient's quality of life at every stage of the disease. By teaching the patient what causes pain and how to relieve or reduce it, you can help him control it more effectively.

Where pain comes from

Explain that pain results from the growing cancer's intrusion on normal tissues; it doesn't radiate from the cancer itself, as many people erroneously believe. Pain may also result from diagnostic tests associated with cancer, such as bone marrow biopsy, and from cancer treatments.

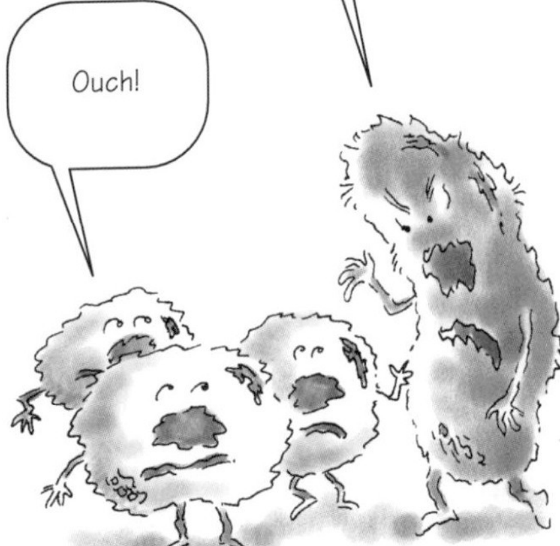
Pain results from the growing cancer's intrusion on normal tissues.
Ouch!

The mind-body connection

Point out that the patient's emotional state can profoundly influence his perception of pain. Fear and anxiety about his body image, financial problems, and the future can worsen pain.

Three alternatives

The following are three examples of common alternative therapies for cancer.

Laetrile

Laetrile is derived from such foods as apricots, peaches, plums, almonds, cloves, and lima beans. Advocates offer the following explanations for laetrile's cancer-curing properties:

- Cancer cells contain an enzyme that releases cyanide from laetrile, and this kills the cancer cells.
- Cancer is a vitamin deficiency, and laetrile provides the missing vitamin B_{17}.

Opponents of this therapy report that testing shows that laetrile isn't an effective cancer treatment. Also, it can cause cyanide toxicity, hypotension, vomiting, and motor disturbances.

Macrobiotic diet

This diet is based on the Eastern philosophy of keeping a proper balance between one's self and the environment. Supporters believe that cancer is related to an increased intake of "yin" or "yang" foods. A macrobiotic diet usually includes cereals, vegetables, and beans, with limited fluids.

Opponents claim that a macrobiotic diet has no proven effect on cancer therapy and may cause diminished levels of essential vitamins, iron deficiency, and anemia.

Shark cartilage

Recently, shark cartilage has received attention in the popular media as an alternative cancer treatment. Proponents claim that shark cartilage inhibits the ability of a tumor to form a blood supply. Without a blood supply, the tumor can't grow.

Opponents argue that there is no research to support use of shark cartilage as cancer treatment. Further, the oral form of cartilage sold in health food stores is digested by gastric acid before it can be absorbed into the bloodstream.

Relieving pain

Discuss ways pain can sometimes be relieved. (See *Techniques for relieving cancer pain.*)

A 3-step ladder

Discuss with the patient medications that may be prescribed in the three-step pain control ladder:

- For mild pain he should take a nonopioid analgesic, such as aspirin, acetaminophen, or a nonsteroidal anti-inflammatory drug such as ibuprofen.
- The second step of the pain control ladder aims at controlling moderate pain that persists or increases with the addition of such prescription drugs as opioids (codeine, hydrocodone, morphine, or oxycodone) or fixed combination drugs (acetaminophen and oxycodone or oxycodone and aspirin).

• In the third step, the aim is to relieve persistent moderate or severe pain by increasing the potency or dose of the opioid.

Around-the-clock

In all of these steps, glucocorticoids or antidepressants may be given as adjuvant therapy for adequate pain control. Inform the patient that the medications should be taken around-the-clock and that supplemental doses may be given as needed for break-through pain.

At home with a narcotic analgesic

If the patient is discharged with a prescription for a narcotic analgesic to control moderate or severe pain, make sure he understands the dosage instructions. If appropriate, demonstrate how to deliver the medication with an infusion pump. Teach the patient how to manage adverse effects of narcotics, such as constipation and drowsiness. (See *Coping with adverse effects of narcotic analgesics.*) Tell him to notify the doctor if adverse effects are persistent or troublesome.

Techniques for relieving cancer pain

- Removing the tumor or decreasing its size through surgery, chemotherapy, or radiation therapy
- Medication
- Distraction
- Relaxation
- Imagery
- Cutaneous stimulation

If these measures fail

- Neurosurgical techniques

Hospice alternative

When all curative medical therapies are discontinued and the patient is receiving only palliative treatment, you may refer him for hospice care. Hospice care may be delivered in the home, in an extended-care facility, or both. The goal is to give the dying patient and his family as much control over his care as possible.

Coping with adverse effects of narcotic analgesics

Here are some tips to help your patient deal with the adverse effects of narcotic analgesics:

- If troubled by constipation, eat high-fiber foods, including cereals, bran products, whole-grain breads, and lots of fruits and vegetables (especially raw ones). Drink eight to ten 8-oz (237-ml) glasses of liquid daily (including water) and ask the doctor for stool softeners and laxatives, if not already ordered.
- For dry mouth, suck on ice or sugarless hard candies and increase fluid intake.
- If nausea and vomiting are a problem, follow the antiemetic treatment prescribed by the doctor.
- If narcotics cause drowsiness, avoid driving or engaging in any activity that requires alertness.
- Contact the doctor to ask about adjusting the narcotic dosage or prescribing another drug.

When discussing hospice care, explain that the hospice nurse will teach the patient and his family how to care for the patient's physical needs and will prepare them emotionally to cope with his approaching death. After the patient dies, the hospice nurse and health care team should maintain close contact with the family to support them throughout the grieving process.

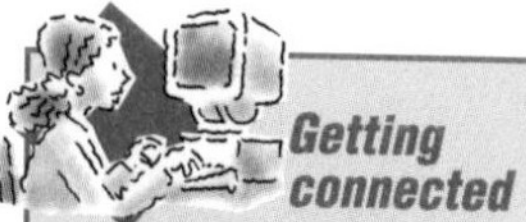

Cancer info on-line

For more information about cancer, direct the patient to the following Web sites:

- American Cancer Society (www.cancer.org)
- Oncolink (www.oncolink.upenn.edu)
- National Cancer Institute (www.cancernet.nci.nih.gov).

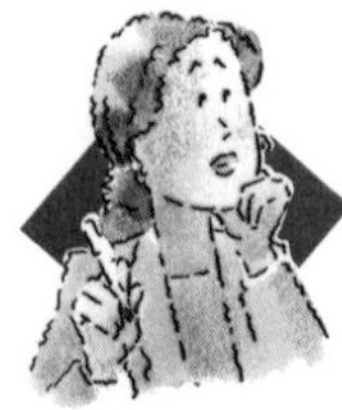

Quick quiz

1. One common misconception about cancer is that:
A. cancer can be caused by environmental factors.
B. cancer is contagious.
C. cancer can be affected by dietary factors.
Answer: B. Although cancer is widespread, no evidence exists that cancer is an infectious disorder.

2. A metastatic tumor is one that:
A. spreads to neighboring tissues.
B. remains localized to one area.
C. shrinks on its own without treatment.
Answer: A. A metastatic tumor invades neighboring tissues and spreads to such sites as the lungs, liver, bones, and brain.

3. Palliative surgery is designed to:
A. remove a noncancerous growth before it becomes cancerous.
B. remove an entire tumor.
C. relieve symptoms, such as pain, without curing cancer.
Answer: C. Palliative surgery is performed to relieve certain symptoms, but doesn't cure cancer.

Scoring

☆☆☆ If you answered two or three items correctly, terrific! Your patient-teaching skills are proliferating with remarkable speed and accuracy.

☆☆ If you answered less than two items correctly, look on the bright side. Early detection is the key to improvement. Now review the chapter once more.

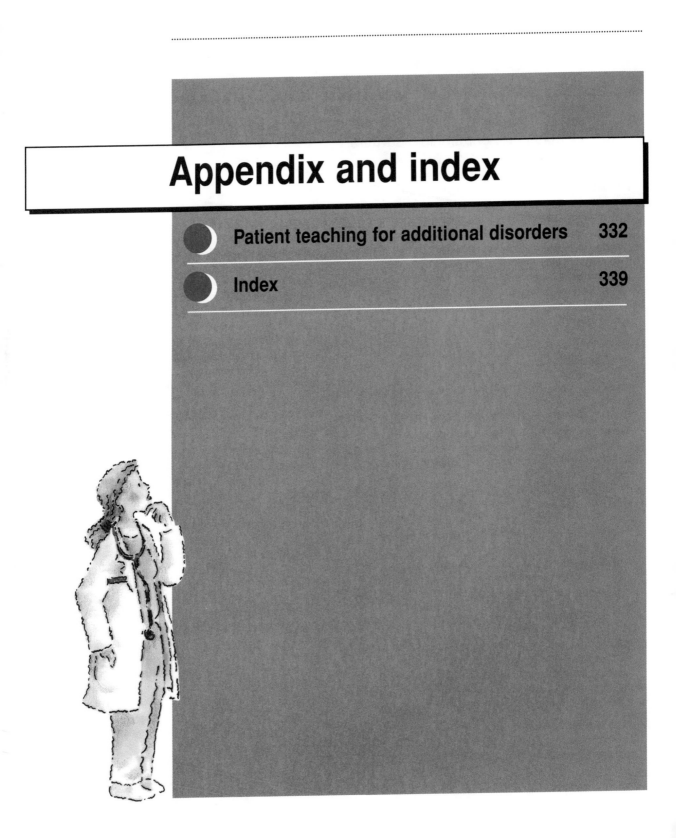

Appendix and index

Patient teaching for additional disorders 332

Index 339

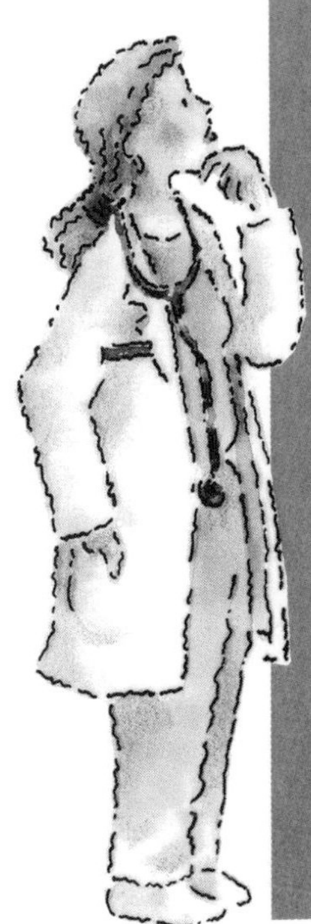

Appendix

Patient teaching for additional disorders

Use the chart below to find teaching guidelines for additional disorders

Abdominal aneurysm

Teach the patient:

- about tests, such as abdominal ultrasonography, anteroposterior and lateral X-rays, computed tomography (CT) scan
- about treatments such as Dacron graft
- about treatments for acute dissection, such as fluid and blood resuscitation and I.V. propranolol or I.V. nitroprusside for blood pressure control
- not to push, pull, or lift heavy objects after surgery until the doctor allows it.

Acute respiratory failure

Teach the patient:

- about tests, such as arterial blood gas (ABG) analysis, chest X-ray, pulse oximetry, and pulmonary artery catheterization
- about treatments, such as oxygen therapy via nasal prong, nonrebreather mask, or Venturi mask
- about treatments for respiratory acidosis, such as mechanical ventilation, high-frequency ventilation, bronchodilators, and corticosteroids
- about antibiotics for infection
- the reasons for suctioning, chest physiotherapy, and blood tests
- not to speak (if intubated) and to explore alternative means of communication
- to avoid smoking and seek antismoking resources
- how to perform coughing and deep-breathing exercises
- how to use the incentive spirometer.

Acute tubular necrosis

Teach the patient:

- about tests, such as urinalysis and blood studies
- about treatments, such diuretics and I.V. fluids
- about treatments for acute renal failure, such as peritoneal dialysis, hemodialysis, electrolyte balance maintenance, and a low-protein, low-potassium diet.

Adult respiratory distress syndrome

Teach the patient:

- about tests, such as ABG analysis, pulmonary artery catheterization, serial chest X-rays, sputum analysis, blood culture, and toxicology
- about testing serum amylase to rule out pancreatitis
- about treatments, such as administration of humidified oxygen by a tight-fitting mask (which facilitates the use of continuous positive airway pressure); intubation and mechanical ventilation with positive end-expiratory pressure; fluid restriction and diuretic therapy; sedatives, narcotics, or neuromuscular blocking agents to decrease oxygen consumption and facilitate ventilation if mechanically ventilated; antimicrobial drugs; nitric oxide; and high-dose corticosteroids if adult respiratory distress syndrome is secondary to fat emboli or chemical injury
- to allow time for recovery and expect a period of weakness
- to avoid overexertion in order to conserve energy and decrease oxygen consumption.

Anaphylactic reaction

Teach the patient:

- about tests, such as skin testing and a scratch test (done first in high risk situations)
- about treatments, such as epinephrine injection, maintenance of patent airway and possibility of intubation, oxygen therapy, cardiopulmonary resuscitation if cardiac arrest occurs (should be taught to family members), volume expanders, and I.V. vasopressors
- to avoid consuming the offending item in any combination or form
- to read food labels before purchasing and check with restaurant personnel about the content of menu items when ordering
- to avoid insect stings by avoiding scented colognes or deodorants and by staying away from open fields and wooded areas during insect season
- to always wear a medical identification bracelet naming allergies
- to carry an anaphylaxis kit whenever outdoors, and when and how to use it.

Aortic insufficiency
Teach the patient:
• about tests, such as cardiac catheterization, chest X-ray, echocardiography, and electrocardiography (ECG)
• about treatments, such as valve replacement surgery, digitalis glycosides, low-sodium diet, diuretics, vasodilators, angiotensin-converting enzyme inhibitors, supplemental oxygen in acute episodes
• to plan for periodic rest in daily routine in order to prevent undue fatigue and to raise legs whenever sitting
• to look for signs and symptoms of decreased cardiac output, such as dizziness, clammy skin, fatigue, and dyspnea, and report these findings to the doctor.

Aortic stenosis
Teach the patient:
• about tests, such as cardiac catheterization, chest X-ray, echocardiography, and ECG
• about treatments such as digitalis glycosides, low-sodium diet, diuretics, oxygen, commissurotomy in children, valve replacement surgery, and percutaneous balloon aortoplasty
• to plan for periodic rest in daily routine and to raise legs when sitting
• to look for signs and symptoms of decreased cardiac output, such as dizziness, clammy skin, fatigue, and dyspnea, and to seek medical attention if these occur.

Appendicitis
Teach the patient:
• about tests, such as white blood cell (WBC) count and radiographic contrast enema
• about treatments such as appendectomy
• about treatments if peritonitis develops, such as GI intubation and antibiotics
• to expect that analgesic administration may be delayed, and that it will be given as soon as possible
• how to decrease pain using Fowler's position
• to notify the doctor if pain is suddenly relieved without medication or surgical treatment.

Cataract
Teach the patient:
• about tests, such as indirect ophthalmoscopy, slit lamp examination, and visual acuity testing
• about treatments, such as surgical lens extraction and implantation of an intraocular lens
• to take safety precautions until the cataract can be removed
• to avoid night driving
• to wear an eye patch for a temporary period after cataract removal
• to expect temporary loss of depth perception and decreased peripheral vision on affected side
• to notify the doctor immediately if sudden eye pain, red or watery eyes, photophobia, or sudden vision changes occur
• to wear dark glasses postoperatively.

Diverticular disease
Teach the patient:
• about tests, such as barium studies, radiography, biopsy to rule out cancer, complete blood count, and stool hemetest (guaiac)
• about the initial treatment for mild GI distress and pain, such as a liquid or bland diet, stool softeners, occasional doses of mineral oil, antibiotics, analgesics, and antispasmodics
• about treatment after pain subsides, such as a high-residue diet and bulk medications
• about treatment for severe illness, such as I.V. fluids and nasogastric (NG) tube for decompression
• to notify doctor of temperature greater than 101° F (38.3° C), abdominal pain that's severe or lasts longer than 3 days, or blood in stool
• to observe recommended dietary changes, such as drinking 2 to 3 qt (2 to 3 L) of fluid per day; increasing high-fiber foods (fresh fruits, vegetables, and whole grain breads); and avoiding foods that are difficult to digest, may lodge in the diverticulum, and cause infection, such as corn and peanuts
• to avoid a fiber-rich diet, which may cause flatulence
• to use stool softeners or take bulk-forming cathartics with plenty of water.

Endocarditis
Teach the patient:
• about tests, such as blood cultures and blood studies
• about treatments, such as I.V. antibiotics for a 4-week course, bed rest, aspirin, and valvular replacement surgery for severe valvular damage
• to report signs of relapse, such as fever and anorexia
• to take prophylactic antibiotics before, during, and after dental work, childbirth, and any genitourinary, GI, or gynecologic procedures

(continued)

Endocarditis *(continued)*

- to recognize symptoms of endocarditis, such as weakness, fatigue, weight loss, anorexia, night sweats, fever, dyspnea, splinter hemorrhages under the nails, and petechiae of the skin, buccal, pharyngeal, or conjunctival mucosa, and to notify the doctor immediately if these symptoms occur
- to get proper rest and conserve energy while performing activities of daily living (ADLs).

Gastroesophageal reflux

Teach the patient:

- about tests, such as esophagoscopy and biopsy and barium swallow with fluoroscopy
- about treatments for mild cases, such as diet therapy and positional therapy
- about treatments for intermittent reflux, such as drugs to control acid secretion in the stomach, and taking antacids 1 to 3 hours after meals and at bedtime or hourly
- about treatments for patients with refractory symptoms or serious complications, such as surgery to create an artificial closure at the gastroesophageal junction (vagotomy or pyloroplasty)
- to eat small, frequent meals and sit upright afterward for 2 to 3 hours
- to avoid highly seasoned foods, acidic juices, bedtime snacks, high-fat foods, foods high in carbohydrates, cigarettes, and alcohol to help prevent occurrences
- to avoid situations or activities that increase intra-abdominal pressure, such as bending, coughing, vigorous exercise, obesity, constipation, and wearing tight clothes.

Glaucoma

Teach the patient:

- about tests, such as tonometry, slit lamp examination, gonioscopy, ophthalmoscopy, perimetry or visual field tests, and fundus photography
- about treatments, such as ophthalmic beta blockers, ophthalmic epinephrine, pilocarpine, and argon laser trabeculoplasty or trabeculectomy (if unresponsive to drug therapy)
- about treatments in angle-closure glaucoma, such as acetazolamide, pilocarpine, I.V. mannitol, oral glycerin, laser or surgical iridectomy (if other treatments unsuccessful), and narcotic analgesics
- that lost vision can't be restored but continued treatment can prevent further loss
- to modify home environment for safety by keeping pathways clear and memorizing room layouts
- to seek prompt medical attention if sudden vision changes or eye pain occurs.

Gout

Teach the patient:

- about tests, such as needle aspiration of synovial fluids or of tophaceous material, serum uric acid levels, urine uric acid levels, and X-ray studies
- about treatments for acute attacks, such as bed rest, immobilization and protection of the inflamed and painful joints, application of cold, analgesics, nonsteroidal anti-inflammatory drugs, I.M. corticotropin, colchicine, and intra-articular corticosteroids
- about treatments for chronic attacks, such as allopurinol, probenecid, and sulfinpyrazone
- to drink plenty of fluids (up to 2 qt [2 L] per day) to prevent renal calculi
- about needle aspiration and explain that it will be very painful
- to have serum uric acid levels evaluated periodically
- to avoid eating purine-rich foods, such as liver, anchovies, sardines, kidneys, sweetbreads, and lentils, because they increase urate levels
- to lose weight to decrease uric acid levels and stress on painful joints (for obese patients)
- to avoid aspirin and other salicylates if taking probenecid or sulfinpyrazone because their combined effect causes urate retention.

Influenza

Teach the patient:

- about tests, such as isolation of the virus through inoculation of chicken embryos with nasal secretions from infected patients, nose and throat cultures, serum antibodies, and WBC count
- about treatments, such as bed rest, forced fluids, acetaminophen, antihistamines, antitussives, antivirals, and expectorants
- about treatments for bacterial pneumonia, such as I.V. fluid and electrolyte replacement, oxygen administration, mechanical ventilation in severe respiratory failure, and antibiotics
- to use mouthwash or warm saline gargles to ease sore throat

Influenza *(continued)*

- to increase fluid intake to prevent dehydration
- to use a vaporizer to provide cool, moist air, and to clean the reservoir and change the water every 8 hours
- to take warm baths or use a heating pad to relieve myalgia
- to follow proper hand-washing technique to prevent the virus from spreading, and dispose of soiled tissues
- and caregivers that children with influenza shouldn't be given aspirin because of the risk of Reye's syndrome
- that high-risk patients should receive influenza immunization
- to recognize possible adverse reactions from the vaccine, such as discomfort at the vaccination site, fever, malaise and, rarely, Guillain-Barré syndrome
- not to take the vaccine if allergic to eggs, feathers, or chickens.

Lyme disease

Teach the patient:

- about tests, such as antibody titers to identify *Borrelia burgdorferi* or enzyme-linked immunosorbent assay, blood studies, and lumbar puncture if central nervous system (CNS) is involved
- about treatments, such as antibiotics
- to avoid tick-infested areas; if unable to avoid these areas, tell patient to cover skin with clothing, use insect repellents, and inspect exposed skin for attached ticks at least every 4 hours
- to remove any ticks found on the body by using tweezers as forceps to pull the tick out, using firm traction; tell the patient to carefully grasp the tick, taking care not to crush the insect or fail to remove the entire embedded body, and thoroughly wash hands after tick removal.

Meningitis

Teach the patient:

- about tests, such as lumbar puncture, chest X-ray, WBC count, and CT scan to rule out other disease processes
- about treatments, such as I.V. antibiotics for two weeks followed by oral antibiotics, mannitol, anticonvulsants, sedatives, and analgesics
- about supportive measures, such as bed rest, hypothermia, and fluid therapy
- about contagion risks to patient and family and to notify anyone who comes in contact with the patient
- to follow proper medical treatment to help prevent meningitis (for the patient with chronic sinusitis or other chronic infections).

Mitral insufficiency

Teach the patient:

- about tests, such as cardiac catheterization, chest X-ray, echocardiography, and ECG
- about treatments (for the patient with heart failure), such as digoxin, diuretics, sodium-restricted diet, oxygen in acute cases, anticoagulants, prophylactic antibiotics, valve replacement, and valvuloplasty
- to plan for periodic rests in daily routine to prevent undue fatigue.

Mitral stenosis

Teach the patient:

- about tests, such as cardiac catheterization, chest X-ray, echocardiography, and ECG
- about treatments (for the patient with heart failure), such as digoxin, diuretics, sodium-restricted diet, oxygen in acute cases, low-dose beta blockers to slow ventricular rate, surgical commissurotomy or surgical valve replacement, and percutaneous balloon valvuloplasty
- to plan for periodic rests in daily routine to prevent undue fatigue.

Mononucleosis

Teach the patient:

- about tests, such as WBC count, antibodies to effective blood volume and cellular antigens shown on indirect immunofluorescence, and liver function tests
- about treatments, such as bed rest, salicylates, steroids for severe throat inflammation, splenectomy if splenic rupture, and antibiotics if streptococcal pharyngotonsillitis
- that convalescence may take several weeks, usually until the WBC count returns to normal
- to observe bed rest during the acute illness and avoid excessive activity that could lead to splenic rupture
- to continue less demanding school assignments (if the patient is a student) and see friends but avoid long, difficult projects until after recovery
- to drink milkshakes and fruit juices and eat cool, bland foods to minimize throat discomfort
- to use warm saline gargles, analgesics, and antipyretics as needed.

(continued)

Pericarditis
Teach the patient:
- about tests, such as blood studies, purified protein derivative skin test, echocardiography, and ECG
- about treatments, such as antibiotics and surgical drainage
- to resume daily activities slowly and schedule rest periods into daily routine for a while.

Peritonitis
Teach the patient:
- about tests, such as WBC count, abdominal X-ray, chest X-ray, paracentesis, and CT scan
- about treatments, such as antibiotics, having nothing to eat or drink, I.V. fluids and parenteral electrolytes, analgesics, NG tube to decompress bowel, rectal tube to facilitate passage of flatus, surgery to control the source of the peritonitis, and peritoneal lavage via laparoscopy
- to complete the full course of antibiotic therapy
- to recognize signs and symptoms of worsening infection, such as recurring fevers.

Pernicious anemia
Teach the patient:
- about tests, such as Schilling test and blood, bone marrow, and gastric analysis
- about treatments, such as I.M. vitamin B_{12} replacement and iron replacement therapy
- about treatments (if severe anemia and cardiopulmonary distress), such as blood transfusions, digitalis glycosides, diuretics, and low-sodium diet
- to guard against infections and report signs of infection promptly, especially pulmonary and urinary tract infection
- to avoid exposing extremities to extreme cold or heat (if the patient has a sensory deficit)
- to avoid clothing with small buttons and ADLs that require fine motor skills (if the patient has neurologic involvement)
- that caregivers should observe for confusion or irritability and report these findings to the doctor
- that vitamin B_{12} replacement isn't a permanent cure; the injections must be continued for life.

Pulmonary edema
Teach the patient:
- about tests, such as ABG analysis, chest X-ray, pulse oximetry, and ECG
- about treatments, such as oxygen administration, mechanical ventilation, bronchodilators, diuretics, positive inotropic agents, pressor agents, arterial vasodilators, and morphine
- to report early signs of fluid overload, such as increased shortness of breath, orthopnea, and a 3- to 5-lb (1.5- to 2-kg) weight gain in 1 week's time
- to follow a low-sodium diet and list high-sodium foods and drugs
- to conserve physical energy.

Pulmonary hypertension
Teach the patient:
- about tests, such as ABG analysis, ECG, pulmonary artery catheterization, and cardiac catheterization
- about tests to determine underlying cause, such as pulmonary angiography, pulmonary function tests, radionuclide imaging, open lung biopsy, echocardiography, and perfusion lung scan
- about treatments, such as oxygen therapy, bronchodilators, and beta-adrenergic agents
- about treatments for patients with right-sided heart failure, such as fluid restriction, digitalis glycosides, diuretics, vasodilators, calcium channel blockers, and heart-lung transplantation
- to report increased shortness of breath, swelling, weight gain, and increasing fatigue to the doctor
- to quit smoking and utilize programs to help stop smoking
- to follow diet restrictions and maintain a low-sodium diet
- to eat foods high in potassium (for the patient receiving a potassium-wasting diuretic)
- to take frequent rest periods between activities to avoid overexertion.

Pulmonic insufficiency
Teach the patient:
- about tests, such as cardiac catheterization, chest X-ray, echocardiography, and ECG
- about treatments, such as low-sodium diet, diuretics, and valve replacement in severe cases
- to elevate legs whenever sitting.

Pulmonic stenosis
Teach the patient:
- about tests, such as chest X-ray, echocardiography, and ECG

Pulmonic stenosis *(continued)*
- about treatments, such as low-sodium diet, diuretics, and cardiac catheter balloon valvuloplasty
- to elevate legs whenever sitting
- to get adequate rest and to space activities to prevent fatigue.

Retinal detachment
Teach the patient:
- about tests, such as direct and indirect ophthalmoscopy and ocular ultrasonography
- about treatments, such as restriction of eye movement until surgical repair can be made, cryotherapy for a hole in the peripheral retina, laser therapy for a hole in the posterior retina, and scleral buckling to reattach the retina
- that laser therapy may be done as same-day surgery and that vision will be blurred for several days afterward
- to rest and avoid driving, bending, heavy lifting, and any other activity that increases intraocular pressure for several days after surgery, and avoid bumping the eyes
- how to administer eyedrops properly if having scleral bulking surgery and, after surgery, to lie in the position recommended by the doctor
- to wear sunglasses if photosensitivity occurs.

Rheumatic heart disease
Teach the patient:
- about tests, such as blood studies, and throat cultures
- about tests used to determine cardiac involvement, such as chest X-ray, echocardiography, and cardiac catheterization
- about treatments, such as diuretics, valve commissurotomy, valve replacement, and balloon valvuloplasty
- to watch for and report early signs of left-sided heart failure, such as dyspnea and a hacking, nonproductive cough
- to follow prophylactic antibiotic therapy before dental procedures.

Salmonellosis
Teach the patient:
- about tests, such as cultures (of blood, stool, urine, pus, and vomitus), bone marrow aspiration for culture, and Widal's test
- about treatments, such as antimicrobials, and surgical drainage of localized abscesses
- about symptomatic treatments, such as bed rest, fluid and electrolyte replacement, and antidiarrheals
- to prevent infection by washing hands after using the bathroom and before and after handling food; cooking all foods thoroughly and refrigerating all foods promptly; thoroughly cleaning cutting board or food preparation area with soapy water and drying it thoroughly after use; using a clean surface each time when preparing more than one food
- that patient's family and close contacts should obtain a medical examination and pursue treatment if cultures are positive.

Shingles
Teach the patient:
- about tests, such as vesicular fluid and infected tissue analysis, staining antibodies from vesicular fluid and identification under fluorescent light, and lumbar puncture and cerebrospinal fluid analysis (with CNS involvement)
- about treatments, such as antipruritics, analgesics, application of demulcent and skin protectant, systemic antibiotics, idoxuridine ointment or other antiviral agents (if trigeminal and corneal structures are affected), systemic corticosteroids for intractable pain of postherpetic neuralgia, tranquilizers, tricyclic antidepressants, acyclovir for immunocompromised patient
- about treatments for pain that's unrelieved by conventional treatment, such as peripheral nerve stimulation, patient-controlled analgesia, and small-dose radiotherapy
- to use a soft toothbrush, eat soft foods, and use a saline or bicarbonate-based mouthwash and oral anesthetics to decrease discomfort from oral lesions
- to get adequate rest during the acute phase
- to practice meticulous hygiene to prevent spreading the infection to other body parts.

Spinal injuries
Teach the patient:
- about tests, such as X-rays, myelography, CT scan, and magnetic resonance imaging
- about treatments for cervical injury, such as skeletal traction, plaster cast, hard cervical collar, and halo device
- about treatments for stable lumbar and dorsal fractures, such as bed rest on a firm surface, analgesics, and muscle relaxants
- about treatments used when fracture of lumbar or dorsal spine stabilizes, such as exercises to strengthen the back

(continued)

Spinal injuries *(continued)*
muscles and a back brace or corset to provide support while walking
- about treatments for unstable dorsal or lumbar fractures, such as plaster cast, laminectomy and spinal fusion with severe fracture, and neurosurgery (if fracture results in compression of the spinal column)
- about traction methods and that the halo traction device or skull tongs don't penetrate the brain
- that the patient with a halo device should follow proper pin care technique.

Syndrome of inappropriate antidiuretic hormone (SIADH) secretion
Teach the patient:
- about tests, such as serum osmolality, serum sodium levels, and urine sodium levels
- about treatments, such as restricted water intake, high-sodium and high-protein diet, urea supplements, demeclocycline or lithium to help block the renal response to antidiuretic hormone, loop diuretics, and administration of 200 to 300 ml of 3% to 5% sodium chloride solution (in severe water intoxication)
- to restrict fluids and use methods to decrease discomfort from thirst
- to self-monitor fluid retention, including measurement of intake and output and daily weights.

Thrombophlebitis
Teach the patient:
- about tests, such as diagnosis of superficial vein thrombophlebitis (based on physical findings), Doppler ultrasonography, plethysmography, and phlebography
- about treatments for deep vein thrombosis, such as bed rest with elevation of the affected arm or leg, application of warm moist compresses, analgesics, anticoagulants, streptokinase or urokinase for acute and extensive cases, ambulation wearing antiembolism stocking after acute episode subsides
- about treatments for deep vein thrombophlebitis causing complete venous occlusion, such as venous ligation, vein plication, vein clipping, embolectomy, and umbrella filter
- about treatments for severe superficial vein thrombophlebitis, such as anti-inflammatory drugs, antiembolism stockings, warm compresses, and elevation of affected extremity
- to properly administer S.C. heparin injections if discharged on this regimen
- to avoid prolonged sitting or standing to help prevent a recurrence.

Tricuspid insufficiency
Teach the patient:
- about tests, such as cardiac catheterization, chest X-ray, echocardiography, and ECG
- about treatments, such as low-sodium diet, diuretics, tricuspid annuloplasty, and tricuspid valve replacement
- to follow the prescribed diet
- to recognize signs and symptoms to report, such as palpitations and dizziness
- to elevate lower extremities when sitting.

Volvulus
Teach the patient:
- about tests, such as biopsy of the affected vessel, arteriography, abdominal X-ray, barium enema, and WBC count
- about treatments, such as reduction by careful insertion of a flexible sigmoidoscope to deflate the bowel, surgical detorsion, bowel resection and anastomosis if the bowel is necrotic, total parenteral nutrition, and I.V. antibiotics
- to complete the full course of antibiotic therapies
- to recognize signs and symptoms to report, such as abdominal pain and vomiting
- to recognize signs and symptoms of infections, such as peritonitis
- to monitor the surgical incision site for signs and symptoms of infection.

Index

A

Abdominal aneurysm, 332
Abdominal breathing, 50i
Abdominal ultrasonography, 3t
Ablation therapy, 10-11
Acquired immunodeficiency syndrome, 151-154, 156-159
  activity and lifestyle and, 154, 156, 157
  diagnosing, 152-154
  diet and, 156-157
  human immunodeficiency virus infection and, 151-152
  infection protection and, 153
  medication for, 157-159
  opportunistic infections associated with, 152
  signs and symptoms of, 152
  transmission of, 151-152, 156
Acute inflammatory demyelinating polyneuropathy. *See* Guillain-Barré syndrome.
Acute renal failure, 219-222, 226-228
  activity and lifestyle and, 221-222
  classifying, 219-220
  complications of, 220, 221
  diagnosing, 220-221
  diet and, 222, 226, 227
  medication for, 227
  procedures for, 227-228
Acute respiratory failure, 332
Acute tubular necrosis, 332
Adrenal medullary autologous transplant, 110
Adult respiratory distress syndrome, 332
AIDS. *See* Acquired immunodeficiency syndrome.
Alzheimer's disease, 79-82, 86-87
  activity and lifestyle and, 80, 82
  diagnosing, 80
  diet and, 81-82, 87
  medication for, 82, 86-87
  signs and symptoms of, 80
Ambulatory monitoring, 3t
Anaphylactic reaction, 332
Angina, managing, 21
Angiography, 3t
Antegrade pyelography, 223t
Anticoagulation therapy, 13, 65-67
Antimalarials, 181-182
Aortic insufficiency, 333
Aortic stenosis, 333
Appendicitis, 333
Appetite, how to improve, 49, 57-58
Arrhythmias, 1-11
  activity and lifestyle and, 2, 6, 7
  causes of, 2
  complications of, 2
  diagnosing, 2
  diet and, 7, 8
  medication for, 7-8
  procedures used to manage, 8-10
  surgery for, 10-11
Arterial blood gas analysis, 44t
Arterial occlusive disease, 11-17
  activity and lifestyle and, 12-13, 14, 15
  complications of, 11
  diagnosing, 12
  diet and, 13
  medication for, 13-15
  procedures for, 15-16
  surgery for, 16-17
Arteriography, 3t
Arteriosclerosis, 11. *See also* Arterial occlusive disease.
Arthrocentesis, 195t
Arthrodesis, 168, 210
Arthrography, 194t
Arthroplasty, 168
Arthroscopy, 194t
Asthma, 40, 41, 42. *See also* Chronic obstructive pulmonary disease.
Atherosclerosis, 11, 18, 34. *See also* Arterial occlusive disease, Coronary artery disease, *and* Myocardial infarction.
Automatic implantable cardioverter defibrillator, implantation of, 10

B

Balloon angioplasty, 15, 36
Barium enema study, 118t
Barium swallow, 118t
Basal gastric secretion test, 118t
Benign prostatic hyperplasia, 281-282, 286-288
  activity and lifestyle and, 286, 287
  complications of, 282
  diagnosing, 282
  medication for, 286-287
  signs and symptoms of, 281
  surgery for, 287-288

i refers to an illustration; t refers to a table.

Biliary colic. *See* Gallstones.
Bleeding time, 155t
Blood and immune system disorders, 151-186
  diagnostic tests for, 155t
Blood pooling, preventing, 65
Blood pressure, 28, 29
Bone biopsy, 194t
Bone marrow aspiration and biopsy, 155t
Bone resection, 168
Bone scan, 195t
Bone scintigraphy, 195t
Breast biopsy, 283t
Breast ultrasonography, 283t
Breathing exercises, 50i, 62
Bronchodilators, oral, 52, 53
Bronchoscopy, 44t
Bypass graft surgery, 16-17

C

CAD. *See* Coronary artery disease.
Cancer, 307-330
  diagnosing, 318, 319-320t, 320-321
  helping patient adjust to diagnosis of, 308-310, 315-316
  helping patient cope with recurrence of, 316-318
  teaching about, 307, 311-315
  treatments for, 321-330
Cane, how to use, 91i
Cardiac blood pool imaging, 3t
Cardiac catheterization, 3-4t
Cardiac computed tomography scan, 4t
Cardiovascular disorders, 1-37
  diagnostic tests for, 3-6t
Carotid endarterectomy, 17, 91-92
Carpal tunnel syndrome, 187-192
  activity and lifestyle and, 189, 191i
  diagnosing, 188, 190
  diet and, 190, 192
  medication for, 189-190
  risk factors for, 188
  surgery for, 191-192
  symptoms of, 188, 189
Cataract, 333
Cerebral angiography, 83t
Cerebral arteriography, 83t
Cerebral blood flow studies, 83t
Cerebrospinal fluid analysis, 83-84t
Cerebrovascular accident, 87-92
  activity and lifestyle and, 88-90, 91i
  diagnosing, 88
  diet and, 90
  medication for, 90, 92
  surgery for, 91-92
Chest physiotherapy, 54, 63, 77
Chest radiography, 44t
Chest X-ray, 44t
Cholangiography, 119t
Cholecystectomy, 128-129
Cholecystotomy, 128
Choledochostomy, 128
Cholelithiasis. *See* Gallstones.
Chronic bronchitis, 40. *See also* Chronic obstructive pulmonary disease.
Chronic low back pain, 192-193, 197-200
  activity and lifestyle and, 193, 197, 198, 199
  causes of, 192
  diagnosing, 193
  diet and, 197
  medication for, 198-199
  risk factors for, 193
  surgery for, 199-200
Chronic obstructive pulmonary disease, 39-54. *See also specific type.*
  activity and lifestyle and, 43, 49, 50i
  diagnosing, 43
  diet and, 49
  medication for, 51-53
  medications to avoid in, 54
  procedures for, 54, 55
  risks of, 42-43
  self-care for, 51
  types of, 39-40
Chronic pancreatitis, 142-144
  activity and lifestyle and, 143
  diagnosing, 142-143
  diet and, 143-144
  medication for, 144
  signs and symptoms of, 142
  surgery for, 144
Chronic renal failure, 228-231
  activity and lifestyle and, 229
  diagnosing, 228
  diet and, 229
  managing signs and symptoms of, 230
  medication for, 229
  procedures for, 229-230
Chylothorax, 56. *See also* Pleural disorders.
Cirrhosis, 115-117, 122-123
  activity and lifestyle and, 116, 117
  causes of, 115
  complications of, 116
  diagnosing, 116
  diet and, 116-117
  medication for, 117
  surgery for, 117, 122-123
Closed reduction of fracture, 203
Clotting factor replacement products, 162

i refers to an illustration; t refers to a table.

Coagulation tests, response to therapy and, 64-65
Colonoscopy, 119t
Colostomy, 136-137
Colposcopy, 283t
Compartment syndrome, 201, 202
Computed tomography scan, 45t, 84t, 119-120t, 195t. *See also specific type.*
Congestive heart failure. *See* Heart failure.
Continent ileostomy, 138
COPD. *See* Chronic obstructive pulmonary disease.
Coronary artery bypass graft, 21-23, 37
Coronary artery disease, 17-23
  activity and lifestyle in, 19, 20, 21
  complications of, 18
  diagnosing, 18-19
  diet and, 19-21
  medication for, 21
  procedures for, 21
  risk factors for, 18
  surgery for, 21-23
Corticosteroid therapy, 53, 135, 181
Credé's method, 238
Crohn's disease, 132, 132t, 136. *See also* Inflammatory bowel disease.
Culdocentesis, 303-304
Cutaneous ureterostomy, 240
CVA. *See* Cerebrovascular accident.
Cystitis. *See* Urinary tract infection.
Cystometry, 223t
Cystoscopy, 223t
Cystourethroscopy, 224t, 284t

D

Decortication, 59-60
Degenerative joint disease. *See* Osteoarthritis.
Diabetes mellitus, 249-251, 254-263
  activity and lifestyle and, 251, 254
  complications of, 250, 251
  diagnosing, 250
  diet and, 255, 256
  forms of, 249-250
  medication for, 255-258
  self-care for, 259-263
Diabetic ketoacidosis, 251
Digital subtraction angiography, 84-85t
Dilatation and curettage, 284t
Diskography, 195t
Dissolution therapy, oral, for gallstones, 125
Diuretic therapy, considerations for, 27
Diverticular disease, 333
Doppler ultrasonography, 5t
Dumping syndrome, 149
Dysfunctional uterine bleeding, 288-292
  activity and lifestyle and, 290, 291
  complications of, 289
  diagnosing, 289-290
  medication for, 290-291
  surgery for, 291-292

E

ECG. *See* Electrocardiography.
Echocardiography, 5t
Electrocardiography, 5t, 45t
Electrocardioversion, 9-10
Electroencephalography, 85t
Electromyography, 85t
Electrophysiologic studies, 5t, 190
Emphysema, 40. *See also* Chronic obstructive pulmonary disease.
Empyema, 56. *See also* Pleural disorders.
Endocarditis, 333-334
Endocrine disorders, 249-279
  diagnostic tests for, 252-253t
Endometriosis, 292-298
  activity and lifestyle and, 294, 295
  causes of, 292
  complications of, 293
  diagnosing, 293-294
  medication for, 294-296
  risk factors for, 293
  signs and symptoms of, 292
  surgery for, 296-298
Endoscopic retrograde cholangiopancreatography, 120t, 126
Endoscopic sphincterotomy, 126
Enzyme-linked immunosorbent assay, 153
Epilepsy. *See* Seizures.
Esophagogastroduodenoscopy, 1225
Esophagography, 118t
Estrogen replacement therapy, 215
Evoked potential studies, 85t
Evoked responses, 85t
Excretory urography, 284t
Exercise ECG, 6t, 45t
Extracorporeal shock-wave lithotripsy, 127-128

F

Fasting plasma glucose test, 252t
Fat embolism, 201
Fibrinolytic therapy, 67
Fibrocystic breast changes, 298-302
  activity and lifestyle and, 300
  diagnosing, 299-300
  diet and, 301
  medication for, 301-302

i refers to an illustration; t refers to a table.

Fibrocystic breast changes *(continued)*
- signs and symptoms of, 298-299
- surgery for, 302

Fluid intake and output, measuring, 226
Fractures, 200-204
- activity and lifestyle and, 202, 203
- complications of, 201
- diagnosing, 201
- diet and, 202
- medication for, 202-203
- preventing, 203
- procedures for, 203
- signs and symptoms of, 201
- surgery for, 203-204

G

Gallstones, 123-129
- diagnosing, 118-122t, 124
- diet and, 124
- medication for, 124-126
- procedures for, 126-128
- surgery for, 128-129

Gastric acid stimulation test, 120t
Gastroesophageal reflux, 334
Gastrointestinal disorders, 115-149
- diagnostic tests for, 118-122t

Glaucoma, 334
Glomerulonephritis, 232-236
- activity and lifestyle and, 234
- complications of, 233, 234
- diagnosing, 233-234
- diet and, 234-235, 236
- medication for, 235
- procedures for, 235-236
- types of, 232-233

Glycosylated hemoglobin test, 252t
Gout, 334
Graded exercise test. *See* Exercise ECG.
Graves' disease, 264. *See also* Hyperthyroidism.
Guillain-Barré syndrome, 92-96
- activity and lifestyle and, 94-95
- complications of, 93
- diagnosing, 93-94
- diet and, 95
- medication for, 95-96
- procedures for, 96
- symptoms of, 93

H

Hardening of the arteries. *See* Arteriosclerosis.
Heart failure, 23-28
- activity and lifestyle and, 25-26
- causes of, 24
- diagnosing, 3-6t, 25
- diet for, 26-27
- early signs of, 26
- medication for, 27-28
- risk factors for, 24

Hemodialysis, 227
Hemophilia, 159-164
- activity and lifestyle and, 160-162
- complications of, 159-160, 163, 164t
- diagnosing, 160
- managing bleeding in, 164t
- medication for, 162
- procedures for, 162-163
- types of, 160

Hepatitis, 129-131
- activity and lifestyle and, 130-131
- causes of, 129
- complications of, 129
- diagnosing, 130
- diet and, 131
- medication for, 131
- preventing spread of, 130
- signs and symptoms of, 129

Histamine-2 receptor antagonists, 147
HIV. *See* Human immunodeficiency virus.
Holiday heart syndrome, 8
Holter monitoring, 3t
Home oxygen therapy, 54, 55
Human immunodeficiency virus, 151-152. *See also* Acquired immunodeficiency syndrome.
- antibody tests for, 152-153
- progression of, to acquired immunodeficiency syndrome, 152
- transmission of, 151-152

Hydration therapy, 62
Hyperkalemia as renal failure complication, 221
Hypertension, 28-33
- activity and lifestyle and, 29-30, 31
- diagnosing, 29
- diet and, 30-32, 33
- medication for, 32
- types of, 29

Hyperthyroidism, 263-269
- activity and lifestyle and, 265, 266
- complications of, 264-265
- diagnosing, 265
- diet and, 265
- forms of, 264
- medication for, 265-266
- radioactive iodine therapy and, 266-267
- signs and symptoms of, 264
- surgery for, 267-269

Hypervolemia as renal failure complication, 221

i refers to an illustration; t refers to a table.

Hypoglycemia, 273-279
 activity and lifestyle and, 276, 277
 complications of, 274-275
 diagnosing, 276
 diet and, 276, 278
 forms of, 275-276
 medication for, 278-279
 signs and symptoms of, 279
 surgery for, 279
Hypothyroidism, 269-273
 activity and lifestyle and, 271
 complications of, 270
 diagnosing, 270-271
 diet and, 271-272
 effects of, 270
 forms of, 269
 medication for, 272-273
Hypovolemia as renal failure complication, 221
Hysterectomy, 291-292
Hysterosalpingography, 285t

I

Ileal conduit, 240
Ileostomy, 137-138
Immunosuppressant therapy, 110, 135-136, 182
Indwelling catheter care, 239
Inflammatory bowel disease, 131-138
 activity and lifestyle and, 133, 134
 comparing forms of, 132t
 complications of, 132-133
 diagnosing, 133
 diet and, 133-135
 medication for, 135-136
 surgery for, 136-138
Influenza, 334-335
Inhalation therapy, 51-52
Inhaler, how to use, 52
Insulin therapy, 255-256, 257, 258
Intra-aortic balloon pump, 37
Irritable bowel syndrome, 139-142
 activity and lifestyle and, 140
 causes of, 139
 diagnosing, 139-140
 diet and, 140-141
 medication for, 141-142
Irritable colon. *See* Irritable bowel syndrome.
Isometric exercises, 209i
I.V. glucose tolerance test, 252t

J

Joint aspiration, 195t
Joint debridement, goals of, 210
Joint replacement, 210

K

Kaposi's sarcoma, 152, 158, 159
Kidney stones. *See* Renal calculi.
Kidney-ureter-bladder radiography, 224t

L

Laminectomy, 200
Laparoscopy, 285t
Laparotomy, 296
Laser-assisted angioplasty, 15-16
Latex allergy, 169-172
 activity and lifestyle and, 170-171, 172
 diagnosing, 155t, 169-170
 forms of, 170
 medication for, 171-172
Liver-spleen test, 121t
Low-salt diet, 26, 30-31
Lung perfusion scan, 45t
Lyme disease, 335

M

Magnetic resonance imaging, 4t, 46t, 86t
Mammography, 285t
Mediastinoscopy, 46t
Meningitis, 335
MI. *See* Myocardial infarction.
Mitral insufficiency, 335
Mitral stenosis, 335
Mononucleosis, 335
Mucous colitis. *See* Irritable bowel syndrome.
Multiple sclerosis, 96-101
 activity and lifestyle and, 97-98, 99
 complications of, 97
 diagnosing, 97
 diet and, 98
 medication for, 100
 procedures for, 100
 surgery for, 100-101
Musculoskeletal disorders, 187-217
 diagnostic tests for, 194-196t
Myasthenia gravis, 101-104
 activity and lifestyle and, 102
 diagnosing, 101-102
 diet and, 102-103
 medication for, 103-104
 procedures for, 104
 surgery for, 104
Myelography, 196t
Myocardial infarction, 33-37
 activity and lifestyle and, 34-35, 36, 37
 causes of, 34
 diagnosing, 34
 diet and, 35

i refers to an illustration; t refers to a table.

Myocardial infarction *(continued)*
medication for, 35-36
procedures for, 36-37
risks of, 34
surgery for, 37
Myxedema, 270

N

Narcotic analgesics, 58, 59
Nephrotic syndrome, 233, 234
Nephrotomography, 224t
Neurogenic bladder, 236-240
activity and lifestyle and, 237, 238
causes of, 236
complications of, 237
diagnosing, 237
diet and, 237-238
medication for, 238-239
procedures for, 239
surgery for, 239-240
types of, 236, 237
Neurologic disorders, 79-113
diagnostic tests for, 83-86t
Nonsteroidal anti-inflammatory drugs, 206

O

Open reduction of fracture, 203-204
Oral antidiabetic drugs, 257, 258
Oral cholecystography, 121t
Oral glucose tolerance test, 252t
Osteoarthritis, 204-210
activity and lifestyle and, 205-209, 206-207i, 208i
diagnosing, 205
diet and, 209
effects of, 205
forms of, 204-205
medication for, 209
surgery for, 209-210
Osteoporosis, 210-215
activity and lifestyle and, 212, 213, 214
classifying, 211-212
diagnosing, 212
diet and, 213
medication for, 213-215
risk factors for, 211
Osteotomy, 168, 210
Oxygen therapy at home, 54, 55

PQ

Pacemaker
permanent, implantation of, 10
temporary, 8-9
Parkinson's disease, 104-110
activity and lifestyle and, 106-108, 109
diagnosing, 105-106
diet and, 108-109
medication for, 109-110
signs and symptoms of, 105
surgery for, 110
Pelvic inflammatory disease, 302-306
activity and lifestyle and, 304, 305
causes of, 303
complications of, 303
diagnosing, 303-304
medication for, 304-305
risk factors for, 302, 303
signs and symptoms of, 303, 304
surgery for, 305-306
Pelvic ultrasonography, 286t
Peptic ulcer disease, 144-149
activity and lifestyle and, 146
causes of, 145
complications of, 145
definition of, 145
diagnosing, 145
diet and, 146
medication for, 146-148
surgery for, 148-149
Percutaneous liver biopsy, 121t
Percutaneous transluminal coronary angioplasty, 15
Pericarditis, 336
Peritoneal dialysis, 227
Peritonitis, 336
Pernicious anemia, 336
Photodensitometry, 196t
Photon absorptiometry, 196t
Plasmapheresis, 96, 235-236
Platelet infusion, 184-185
Pleural biopsy, 46t
Pleural disorders, 54, 56-60
activity and lifestyle and, 56-57
diagnosing, 44-48t, 56
diet and, 57-58
medication for, 58-59
procedures used to control, 59
surgery for, 59-60
types of, 54, 56
Pleural effusion, 54, 56. *See also* Pleural disorders.
Pleural fluid aspiration, 48t
Pleurisy, 56, 57. *See also* Pleural disorders.
Pneumocystis carinii pneumonia, 152, 158, 159
Pneumonia, 60-63
activity and lifestyle and, 61, 62, 63
classifying, 60
complications of, 60-61
diagnosing, 61

i refers to an illustration; t refers to a table.

Pneumonia *(continued)*
medication for, 61-62
procedures to treat, 62-63
risk factors for, 60, 61
signs and symptoms of, 60
Portosystemic shunting, 117, 122-123
Positron emission tomography, 86t
Proctosigmoidoscopy, 119t
Prostatectomy, 287-288
Pseudodysfunctional uterine bleeding, causes of, 288. *See also* Dysfunctional uterine bleeding.
PTCA. *See* Balloon angioplasty.
Pulmonary angiography, 47t
Pulmonary arteriography, 47t
Pulmonary artery catheterization, indications for, 37
Pulmonary edema, 26, 336. *See also* Heart failure.
Pulmonary embolism, 63-68
activity and lifestyle and, 65, 66
causes of, 64
complications of, 66
diagnosing, 64-65
medication for, 65-67
surgery for, 67-68
Pulmonary function tests, 47t
Pulmonary hypertension, 336
Pulmonic insufficiency, 336
Pulmonic stenosis, 336-337
Pursed-lip breathing, 50i
Pyelonephritis. *See* Urinary tract infection.

R

Radioactive iodine therapy, 266-267
Radioactive iodine uptake test, 252t
Radionuclide thyroid imaging, 253t
Random plasma glucose test, 253t
Range-of-motion exercises, 207-208i
Renal and urologic disorders, 219-247
diagnostic tests for, 223-225t
Renal biopsy, 225t
Renal calculi, 241-244
activity and lifestyle and, 242
complications of, 242
diagnosing, 242
diet and, 243-244
medication for, 244
procedures for, 243
risk factors for, 241
Renal computed tomography, 224t
Renal ultrasonography, 225t
Reproductive disorders, 281-306
diagnostic tests for, 283-286t
Respiratory disorders, 39-77
diagnostic tests for, 44-48t
Retinal detachment, 337
Retrograde cystography, 225t
Rheumatic heart disease, 337
Rheumatoid arthritis, 164-169
activity and lifestyle and, 165-167
cause of, 165
complications of, 165
diagnosing, 165
diet and, 167, 168
medication for, 167-168
surgery for, 168-169

S

Salmonellosis, 337
Seizures, 110-113
activity and lifestyle and, 112, 113
diagnosing, 111
diet and, 112
medication for, 112-113
signs and symptoms of, 111
surgery for, 113
types of, 111
Shingles, 337
Sickle cell anemia, 172-177
activity and lifestyle and, 173-174, 175
cause of, 172
complications of, 173
diagnosing, 173
diet and, 174
medication for, 174, 176-177
precipitating factors for, 172-173, 174
surgery for, 177
Skin testing, 155t
Spastic colon. *See* Irritable bowel syndrome.
Spinal injuries, 337-338
Sprains, 215-217
activity and lifestyle and, 216
diagnosing, 216
medication for, 216-217
procedures for, 217
surgery for, 217
Sputum analysis, 48t, 71
Sputum sample, collecting, 71
Status epilepticus, 112. *See also* Seizures.
Stereotaxic thalamotomy, 100, 110
Stool culture, collecting specimen for, 140
Strains, 215-217
activity and lifestyle and, 216
diagnosing, 216
medication for, 216-217
Stress test. *See* Exercise ECG.
Stroke. *See* Cerebrovascular accident.
Sympathectomy, 17

i refers to an illustration; t refers to a table.

Syndrome of inappropriate antidiuretic hormone secretion, 338
Synovectomy, 168
Synovial fluid analysis, 155t
Systemic lupus erythematosus, 177-182
  activity and lifestyle and, 179, 180
  complications of, 179
  diagnosing, 178-179
  diet and, 179
  medication for, 181-182
  signs and symptoms of, 177-178

T

Technetium scan, 6t
Thallium scan (resting), 6t
Thoracentesis, 48t, 59
Thoracic computed tomography, 45t
Thrombocytopenia, 182-186
  activity and lifestyle and, 183, 184, 185
  causes of, 182
  complications of, 182-183
  diagnosing, 182
  medication for, 183-184
  procedures for, 184-185
  surgery for, 185-186
Thrombolytic therapy, 67, 92
Thrombophlebitis, 338
Thyroid hormone replacement therapy, 272-273
Thyroid scan, 253t
Thyroid storm, 264-265
Thyroidectomy, 267-269
Transiliac bone biopsy, 196t
Transurethral resection, 287
Treadmill test. *See* Exercise ECG.
Tricuspid insufficiency, 338
T tube care, 129
Tuberculin skin test, 71
Tuberculosis, 68-77
  activity and lifestyle and, 72
  classifying, 70t
  complications of, 69-70
  diagnosing, 70-71
  diet and, 72-73
  medication for, 73-74, 75-76t, 77
  preventing spread of, 73
  procedures for, 77
  signs and symptoms of, 68-69

U

Ulcerative colitis, 132, 132t, 135-136. *See also* Inflammatory bowel disease.
Ultrasonography, 122t, 253t. *See also specific type.*
Upper GI endoscopy, 122t
Uremia as renal failure complication, 221
Ureteropyelography, 225t
Urethritis. *See* Urinary tract infection.
Urethrography, 225t
Urinary tract infection, 244-247
  activity and lifestyle and, 246, 247
  complications of, 245
  diagnosing, 245-246
  diet and, 246
  medication for, 246-247
  signs and symptoms of, 244-245
  surgery for, 247

V

Vagotomy, 148
Valsalva's maneuver, 8, 238
Vasodilator therapy, 13-14
Vaso-occlusive crisis, 173. *See also* Sickle cell anemia.
Ventilation scan, 48t
Viral hepatitis, 129. *See also* Hepatitis.
Volvulus, 338

WXYZ

Walker, how to use, 90

i refers to an illustration; t refers to a table.